Arthritis For Dummies

D1137929

Getting the Facts When Considering Surgery

Surgery is either the end of all your troubles or the beginning of a whole new set of problems. Before agreeing to go under the knife, ask your orthopaedic surgeon the following questions:

- Do my symptoms and test results go hand-in-hand; is my diagnosis really confirmed?
- Does the type of arthritis I have respond well to surgery?
- Is surgery a permanent fix for my symptoms, or will it need redoing eventually?
- What results can I expect from this surgery?
- What risks are involved?
- What is involved in the post-surgery rehabilitation?
- Am I physically able to withstand the surgery?
- What does the future hold if I don't have surgery?

Making the Most of the NHS

New changes rolling out across the country mean many people now have more choice when it comes to making hospital or clinic appointments and booking dates for surgery. While these innovations are rolling out, it's possible that not all have reached your area, but it's worth asking.

- Remember, you are entitled to ask your GP for a referral to a specialist for a second opinion.
- Ask about available choices in deciding when and where to receive specialist treatment such as hip replacement.
- Ask whether you can book hospital appointments yourself, from home or work, after you've thought through all your options.
- Ask whether you can choose between NHS trust hospitals, diagnosis and treatment centres, specialists operating from GP surgeries, or even a private hospital (with the NHS footing your bills).
- If you need surgery, those having to wait longer than six months can often choose a different hospital in a different region if this means they'll get quicker treatment.
- Ask about your eligibility to go abroad for NHS treatment.

Identifying False Claims for Alternative Therapies

Most alternative practitioners are honest and sincere, but a few will tell you tales to take your money. Watching for the following warning signs will help safeguard your health and your wallet:

- The "miracle cure" that eliminates every form of arthritis and will allow you to throw away your crutches, stop taking your medicine, and/or ignore your physician's advice.
- The "secret formula" that is not revealed.
- The remedy that's based on only one small study.
- Shady practices, such as demands for full payment up front or a promise that you won't tell your physician what you're doing.

For Dummies: Bestselling Book Series for Beginners

Arthritis For Dummies®

Cheat Sheet

Easing Arthritis Symptoms with Supplements

Research has shown that the following supplements can help in easing arthritis-related symptoms, especially pain and inflammation:

- **Bromelain:** May reduce the swelling and pain of arthritis as effectively as an NSAID. Recommended dose is 80 to 320 milligrams per day, divided into two or three doses.
- **Gamma linolenic acid (GLA):** Helps decrease inflammation and pain, especially in patients with rheumatoid arthritis. Recommended dose is 1 to 2 grams of GLA daily.
- **Ginger:** Shown to reduce OA knee pain, thanks to its analgesic, anti-inflammatory abilities. Recommended dose is 225 milligrams of highly purified ginger extract twice daily.
- **Glucosamine sulphate & chondroitin sulphate:** Increases production of cartilage and the molecules that keep it moist and decreases cartilage breakdown, thereby easing the pain of osteoarthritis and even slowing its progression. Recommended dose is 500 milligrams of glucosamine and 400 milligrams of chondroitin, each taken three times daily.
- **Grapeseed extract:** Eases arthritis pain and joint damage by fighting inflammation and preventing or repairing free radical damage to cells. Recommended dosage is 75 to 300 milligrams daily for three weeks and 40 to 80 milligrams daily for maintenance.
- **Niacin:** Helps improve joint mobility in OA, decrease skin lesions in lupus, and reduces the frequency and duration of Raynaud's attacks. Recommended dosage is 15 milligrams daily in the form of niacinamide. (Only take larger doses under the supervision of your doctor.)
- **Omega-3 fatty acids:** Helps relieve the pain and inflammation seen in rheumatoid arthritis, prevents Raynaud's spasms, and eases some symptoms of lupus. Some suggest taking omega-3's containing 3 grams of DHA or EPA daily.
- **Selenium:** Helps fight free radical damage to the joints and surrounding tissues. Recommended dose is 100 to 200 micrograms daily.
- **Vitamin E:** Fights pain by slowing the action of the prostaglandins. Also helps control free radical damage to joint tissues. Recommended dose is 400 to 800 international units daily.
- **Vitamin C:** Works together with vitamin E to scavenge free radicals. Researchers have reported that vitamin C may help halt the progression of osteoarthritis, as well as decreasing OA pain. An often-suggested dose is 500 to 1,000 milligrams of vitamin C per day. A non-acid form known as ester-C is especially helpful for those prone to indigestion, as it is non-acidic.

Talking to Your Doctor about Alternative Therapies

At least 40 percent of people use alternative therapies, but an estimated three-quarters don't tell their doctors what they're doing. Talking to physicians about alternative approaches is often difficult. Here are some tips to help you discuss complementary therapies with your physician:

- Begin with the assumption that your physician is supportive.
- Ask what she knows about the therapy in which you're interested.
- If your physician doesn't know about the therapy you like, offer him information — you can get material from many organizations on the Web.
- If your doctor doesn't approve of the therapy you're interested in, ask for a detailed explanation.
- If there's no time to discuss your alternative therapy during this visit, ask for another appointment.
- If your doctor does approve of the therapy, ask if the approach is available on the NHS. If you have private health insurance, see if they will cover the costs of your chosen complementary treatment.
- If your physician gives you trouble, ask why.
- If your physician refuses to discuss alternatives with you and/or refuses to work with you if you're using a non-conventional approach, think about changing your doctor.

For Dummies: Bestselling Book Series for Beginners

Arthritis
FOR
DUMMIES®

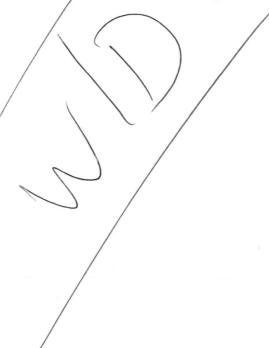

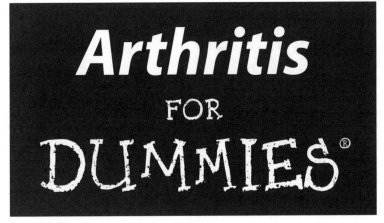

Arthritis
FOR
DUMMIES®

by Barry Fox, PhD
Nadine Taylor, MS, RD
Jinoos Yazdany, MD
Sarah Brewer, MD

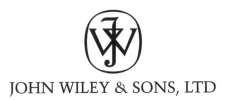

JOHN WILEY & SONS, LTD

Arthritis For Dummies®

Published by
John Wiley & Sons, Ltd
The Atrium
Southern Gate
Chichester
West Sussex
PO19 8SQ
England

E-mail (for orders and customer service enquires): cs-books@wiley.co.uk

Visit our Home Page on www.wiley.com

For general information on our other products and services, please contact our Customer Care Department within the U.S. at 800-762-2974, outside the U.S. at 317-572-3993, or fax 317-572-4002.

For technical support, please visit www.wiley.com/techsupport.

Wiley also publishes its books in a variety of electronic formats. Some content that appears in print may not be available in electronic books.

British Library Cataloguing in Publication Data: A catalogue record for this book is available from the British Library

ISBN-13: 978-0-470-02582-6

ISBN-10: 0-470-02582-4

Printed and bound in Great Britain by Bell & Bain Ltd., Glasgow

10 9 8 7 6 5 4 3 2 1

WILEY

About the Authors

Barry Fox and Nadine Taylor are a husband-and-wife writing team living in Los Angeles, California.

Dr Sarah Brewer qualified as a doctor in 1983 from Cambridge University. She was a full-time GP for five years and now works in nutritional medicine and sexual health. Sarah is currently completing an MSc in Nutritional Medicine at the University of Surrey, Guildford.

Although her first love is medicine, her major passion is writing. Sarah writes widely on all aspects of health and has written over 40 popular self-help books. She is a regular contributor to a number of newspapers and women's magazines, and appears regularly on TV and radio. She was voted Health Journalist of the Year 2002.

Barry Fox, PhD, is the author, coauthor, or ghostwriter of numerous books, including the *New York Times* number one best-seller, *The Arthritis Cure* (St. Martin's, 1997). He also wrote its sequel, *Maximizing The Arthritis Cure* (St. Martin's, 1998), as well as *The Side Effects Solution* (Broadway Books, 2005), *What Your Doctor May Not Tell You About Hypertension* (Warner Books, 2003), *What Your Doctor May Not Tell You About Migraines* (Warner Books, 2001), *Syndrome X* (Simon & Schuster, 2000), *The 20/30 Fat and Fiber Diet Plan* (HarperCollins, 1999), and *Cancer Talk* (Broadway Books, 1999). His books and over 160 articles covering various aspects of health, business, biography, law, and other topics have been translated into 20 languages.

Nadine Taylor, MS, RD, is the author of *Natural Menopause Remedies* (Signet, 2004), *25 Natural Ways To Relieve PMS* (Contemporary Books, 2002), and *Green Tea* (Kensington Press, 1998), as well as co-author of *Runaway Eating* (to be published by Rodale in 2005), *What Your Doctor May Not Tell You About Hypertension* (Warner Books, 2003), and *If You Think You Have An Eating Disorder* (Dell, 1998). After a brief stint as head dietitian at the Eating Disorders Unit at Glendale Adventist Medical Center, Ms. Taylor lectured on women's health issues to groups of health professionals throughout the country. She has also written numerous articles on health and nutrition for the popular press.

Jinoos Yazdany, MD, MPH, is a board certified internist and a Rheumatology Fellow at the University of California, San Francisco. She completed her undergraduate education at Stanford University, where she received the Deans' Award for Academic Achievement and graduated with Honors and Distinction. She completed medical school at the University of California, Los Angeles, where she received a Humanism in Medicine award from the Health Care Foundation of New Jersey and graduated Alpha Omega Alpha. Dr. Yazdany also studied public health at Harvard University. Her research involves examining health disparities in the care of patients with chronic diseases. This is her first book.

Dedication

Dedicated to Nina Ostrom Taylor, world's greatest mom and mom-in-law.

Authors' Acknowledgements

Nadine and Barry thank Arnold Fox, MD, for providing us with a great deal of information on arthritis; Jinoos Yazdany, MD, for her invaluable contributions to the text; Anthony Padula, MD, for his careful review of the manuscript; and of course, Natasha Graf, Traci Cumbay, and the editorial staff at Wiley.

Jinoos thanks the many patients who have shared with her their lives and wisdom regarding living with arthritis.

Sarah thanks Barry Fox, Nadine Taylor, and Jinoos Yazdany, authors of the original US version of *Arthritis For Dummies*. The quality of their original script made my job easy, as I had so very little to do when adapting their excellent book for the UK market.

Publisher's Acknowledgements

We're proud of this book; please send us your comments through our Dummies online registration form located at www.dummies.com/register/.

Some of the people who helped bring this book to market include the following:

Acquisitions, Editorial, and Media Development

Executive Editor: Jason Dunne

Executive Project Editor:
Amie Jackowski Tibble

Commissioning Editor: Alison Yates

Project Editor: Simon Bell

Copy Editor: Kate O'Leary

Technical Reviewer:
Dr Charles Mackworth-Young. MA, MD, FRCP

Cover Photos: Getty Images/Robert Harding

Cartoons: Ed McLachlan

Composition Services

Project Coordinator: Maridee Ennis

Layout and Graphics: Carl Byers, Andrea Dahl, Lynsey Osborn, Heather Ryan

Proofreaders: Laura Albert, Dwight Ramsey

Indexer: TECHBOOKS Production Services

Publishing and Editorial for Consumer Dummies

  Diane Graves Steele, Vice President and Publisher, Consumer Dummies

  Joyce Pepple, Acquisitions Director, Consumer Dummies

  Kristin A. Cocks, Product Development Director, Consumer Dummies

  Michael Spring, Vice President and Publisher, Travel

  Kelly Regan, Editorial Director, Travel

Publishing for Technology Dummies

  Andy Cummings, Vice President and Publisher, Dummies Technology/General User

Composition Services

  Gerry Fahey, Vice President of Production Services

  Debbie Stailey, Director of Composition Services

Contents at a Glance

Table of Contents

Introduction

*W*hether it appears as a bit of creaky stiffness in the hip or knee or as a major case of inflammation that settles in several joints, arthritis is an unwelcome visitor that knocks on just about everyone's door sooner or later. Although no out-and-out cure for arthritis exists, there are many techniques for *managing* this disease – that is, controlling its symptoms so you can get on with your life! Arthritis does *not* mean you must spend your days relegated to a rocking chair or shuffling from your bed to an armchair and back again. Most of the time, you can take charge of your disease instead of letting it take charge of you. By following the simple techniques outlined in this book, you can do much to control your pain, exercise away your stiffness, keep yourself on the move, and slow down or prevent progression of your disease. All you need to manage your disease is a little know-how – and you can find that in these chapters.

About This Book

The goal of this book is to provide you with the best and most up-to-date information on arthritis treatments in an easy-to-read format that you can simply thumb through. The best-of-the-best of many different healing systems are included – ranging from standard Western medicine (including medications and surgery), to Eastern hands-on healing methods (including acupuncture, acupressure, and reiki), to alternative therapies (including homeopathy, herbs, methylsulphonylmethane (MSM), glucosamine, and even far-out approaches such as bee venom therapy). You can read this book straight through from cover to cover if you like, but it's not necessary. Reading the first chapter as an introduction is worth your while, then you can home in on the description of your particular kind of arthritis, found in Chapters 2, 3, 4, or 5. After that, feel free to flip through the book and read whatever catches your fancy.

Because arthritis impacts your life in so many different ways, different chapters address the many complex issues you may face, including the technical aspects of arthritis (tests, medicines, and operations), the practical aspects (diet, exercise, and day-to-day living), and the emotional aspects (depression and anger). You can also find tips on how to assemble your health-care treatment team, how to talk to your doctor, and what to do about chronic pain.

Foolish Assumptions

This book makes certain educated guesses about you. Rightly or wrongly, this book assumes that:

- ✔ You either have arthritis yourself or you're close to someone who has it.
- ✔ You're interested in finding out more about arthritis and its treatments.
- ✔ You want to do something to ease arthritis pain and other symptoms.
- ✔ You want to play an active part in managing the disease, rather than just going along with whatever your doctor tells you.
- ✔ You're interested in finding out about some alternative ways to treat arthritis.
- ✔ You want to find out how to handle the emotional issues that go hand-in-hand with the disease.

How This Book Is Organised

The organisation of *Arthritis For Dummies* is meant to correspond with the way that you may experience arthritis in your daily life. When you first realise that you have arthritis, you probably want to know what it is, what the common symptoms are, and what you can expect as the disease progresses. The next step is to visit your doctor for tests. Then, medicines are prescribed, pain-management strategies discussed, and surgery (if applicable) is contemplated as a last resort.

After you make it through all that, you go back to living your life. Suddenly, the everyday things you used to take for granted become important parts of your arthritis management, such as diet, exercise, and the way you use your joints. Stress and depression are new and confounding problems, and getting through the day is often a tougher prospect, both physically and mentally, than it was before.

Eventually, you may start wondering about alternative healing methods and have an urge to explore them. And, you may become curious about certain superfoods that can help ease arthritis symptoms and what cutting-edge medical treatments are on the horizon. This book answers all your questions.

Part 1: Getting a Grip on Types of Arthritis

These five chapters give an overview of arthritis in its many forms – the symptoms, disease processes, causes, and likeliest victims. Chapter 1 discusses arthritis in general, Chapter 2 tackles osteoarthritis (the type of arthritis that most people get), Chapter 3 explains rheumatoid arthritis (another fairly common kind of arthritis), Chapter 4 discusses the other forms the disease may take, and Chapter 5 is dedicated to other conditions that are linked to arthritis. This part also explains what doctors do for each type of arthritis and what you can do for yourself.

Part 11: Tests and Treatments: What to Expect

Chapters 6 to 9 walk you through the maze of medical treatments, beginning with a trip to the doctor's office. This part explains how doctors diagnose the many forms of arthritis and discusses the high-tech and low-tech tests they may use. Equally important, this part shows you how to work with your doctor to make your treatment decisions. Chapter 8 outlines the medicines you may take, and Chapter 9 explains the operations that are applicable. Finally, Chapter 10 thoroughly explains the strategies you can use for managing pain.

Part 111: Is Complementary Medicine for You?

Alternative medicine is now incredibly popular, and scientific studies are beginning to show that many of these methods have merit. This part discusses the most popular complementary therapies for arthritis including massage, herbs, homeopathy, acupuncture, reflexology, and others. Part III also provides tips on finding a reputable alternative practitioner and identifying false claims.

Part 1V: The Arthritis Lifestyle Strategy

Many of the keys to arthritis management lie in the little things you do every day, such as what you eat, the kind and amount of exercise you get, and how you use your joints. This part tells you how to fight arthritis pain through diet and supplements; how to keep your joints in shape through exercise; how to protect your joints by walking, sitting, and moving correctly; and how to deal effectively with depression and anger. Part IV also provides loads of tips on how to make day-to-day living with arthritis easier.

Part V: The Part of Tens

This part divides some of the key information on managing your arthritis into lists, each containing ten 'information bites'. These information bites include ten tips for travelling with arthritis, ten drug-free ways to manage the pain and stiffness of arthritis, ten health professionals that can help you fight arthritis, and ten new treatments for arthritis that you may not have heard about yet.

Part VI: Appendixes

Appendix A contains a glossary of arthritis terms to help keep you straight as you wend your way through the information in this book. Appendix B lists lots of interesting organisations that may help you find the treatment you seek. This appendix gives detailed information on the foundations associated with most kinds of arthritis or arthritis-related conditions, as well as major medical and complementary associations so you can request practitioner referrals or more information. Information on support groups is also included in Appendix B. Appendix C discusses strategies for losing weight the safe and healthy way, because getting rid of extra pounds is one of the best things you can do for your weight-bearing joints.

Icons Used in This Book

The icons tell you what you must know, what you need to be aware of, and what you may find interesting but can live without.

The Medical Speak icon marks a more in-depth medical passage or gives you further information about confusing medical terms.

When you see this icon, it means that the information is essential, so pay attention to it.

This icon marks important information that can save you time and energy.

The Warning icon cautions you against potential problems.

Where to Go from Here

Someone once said, 'Knowledge is power.' You have the power to take charge of your arthritis; all you have to do is educate yourself and apply what you discover. This book is a good place to start, but you have to commit and recommit yourself to maintaining your health on a daily basis. Remember, the little things you do every day are what count. As you embark on your journey, may the universe grant you luck, strength, and many active, pain-free years!

Part I
Getting a Grip on Types of Arthritis

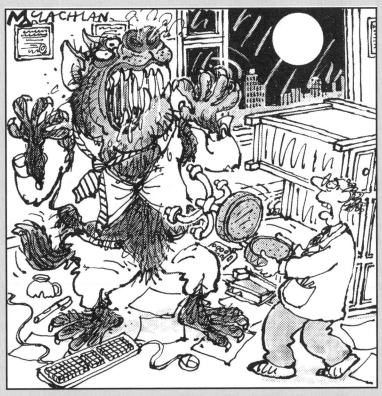

"If it only happens every full moon,
then it's not systemic lupus erythematosus,
Mr Etherington."

In this part . . .

Arthritis can really put a damper on your life . . . if you let it. But the good news is that most forms of arthritis and the pain they cause can be managed (if not completely done away with) through medical techniques and lifestyle changes.

Part I gives you an overview of arthritis in its many forms: the symptoms, diseases, processes, causes, and most likely victims. You also learn what doctors can do for each type of arthritis and what you can do for yourself. We give special attention to the most common forms of this disease: osteoarthritis and rheumatoid arthritis.

Chapter 1

Looking at Arthritis Basics

*O*uch! There it goes again! That grinding pain in your hip, those aching knees that make walking from the kitchen to the bedroom a chore, the stiff and swollen fingers that won't allow you to twist the lid off a jam jar or even sew on a button. Arthritis seems to get to everybody sooner or later – slowing you down, forcing you to give up some of your favourite activities, and just generally being a pain in the neck (sometimes literally!). In more advanced cases, the disease can seriously compromise your quality of life as you may have to surrender your independence, mobility, and sense of usefulness, as well as cope with the relentless pain.

The good news is that you can manage your arthritis, if not cure it, with a combination of medical care, simple lifestyle changes, and good, old common sense. Sitting at home in an armchair, gritting your teeth from pain, or hobbling around the garden with a walking stick aren't obligatory. Although you may not run a marathon or do back-flips like you did at the age of 13, if you follow the programme outlined in this book, you can usually manage to do things you really want to do – such as take a brisk walk in the park, carry a sleeping child upstairs to bed, or swing a golf club with the best of them. Arthritis may affect a lot of people, but thanks to intensive research over the past several years, medical professionals now know a lot more about how to handle it.

Understanding How Arthritis Affects Your Joints

So what exactly is arthritis, this disease that brings you so much misery and pain? Unfortunately, that question has no easy answer because arthritis involves a group of diseases – each with its own causes, set of symptoms, and treatments. However, these diseases do have the following symptoms in common:

- ✔ They affect some part of the joint.
- ✔ They cause pain and (possibly) loss of movement.
- ✔ They often bring about some kind of inflammation (heat).

As for the causes of these different kinds of arthritis, they run the gamut from inheriting an unlucky gene to physical trauma to getting bitten by the wrong mosquito.

The word *arthritis*, which literally means joint inflammation, is derived from the Greek words *arthros* (joint) and *itis* (inflammation), and the condition's major symptom is joint pain. Although the same group of ailments is sometimes called rheumatism, they're usually referred to as arthritis, so that's the term in use throughout this book. The word *arthralgia*, a term that's used much less frequently, refers to joint pain alone.

According to Arthritis Care, arthritis affects some 9 million people in the UK (almost one out of every six people) – that's a big chunk of the population.

Saying hello to your joints

Before you can understand what's wrong with your joints, you need to understand what a joint is and how it works. Any place in the body where two bones meet is called a *joint.* Sometimes those bones actually fuse; your skull is an example of an area with fused bones. But in the joints that can develop arthritis, the bones don't actually touch. As shown in Figure 1-1, a small space exists between the two bone ends. The space between the ends of the bones keeps them from grinding against each other and wearing each other down.

Other structures surrounding your joints, such as muscles, tendons, and *bursae* – small sacs that cushion your tendons – support your joints and provide the power that makes your bones move. The joint capsule wraps itself around the joint, and its special lining, the *synovial membrane* or *synovium*, makes a slick, slippery liquid called the *synovial fluid.* This liquid fills that little space between the bone ends. Finally, the bone ends are capped by *cartilage* – a slick, tough, rubbery material that is eight times more slippery than ice and a better shock absorber than the tyres and springs on your car! Together, these parts make up the joint, one of the most fascinating bits of machinery found in your body.

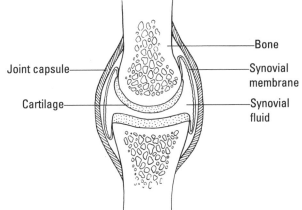

Bone

Synovial membrane

Joint capsule

Synovial fluid

Cartilage

Figure 1-1:
Anatomy of
a healthy
synovial
joint.

Bones are living tissue – hard, porous structures with a blood supply and nerves – that constantly rebuild themselves. Bones protect your vital organs and provide the supporting framework for your body. Without bones, you would consist of nothing more than blobs of tissue – like a tent without any supporting poles!

But bones are more than broomsticks that prop you up and, fortunately, they don't leave you rigid and awkward. The 200-plus bones found in your body are connected together by some 150 joints, giving you a remarkable flexibility and range of motion. You only have to watch a gymnast, ballet dancer, or figure skater execute a handspring, arabesque, or triple axle to see how well designed the joint connections are. But you don't have to have athletic or contortionist tendencies to enjoy the benefits of joint flexibility. Just think about some of the things you do regularly – such as twisting around while you sit in the front seat of your car to grab something off the back-seat floor. Now imagine how limited you would feel if you had fewer joints, or if they didn't move the way they do!

Cushioning cartilage: The human shock absorber

Cartilage is extremely important for the healthy functioning of a joint, especially if that joint bears weight, like your knee. Imagine that you're looking into the inner workings of your left knee as you walk down the street. When you shift your weight from your left leg to your right, the pressure on your left knee is released. The cartilage in your left knee then 'drinks in' synovial fluid, in much the same way that a sponge soaks up liquid when immersed in water. When you take another step and transfer the weight back onto your left leg, much of the fluid squeezes out of the cartilage. This squeezing of joint fluid into and out of the cartilage helps it respond to the off-and-on pressure of walking without shattering under the strain.

Can you imagine the results if you didn't have this watery cushion within your joints? With the rough, porous surfaces of the bone ends pitted against each other, bones would grind each other down in no time.

Typing joints

To accommodate the bends, twists, and turns that you perform without even thinking, the skeletal system is made up of different shapes and sizes of bones, which connect to form different kinds of joints. The joints are categorised according to how much motion they allow:

- **Synarthrodial joints** allow no movement at all. These joints are found in the skull, where the bones meet to form tough, fibrous joints called *sutures*. Because synarthrodial joints don't move, arthritis doesn't affect them.

- **Amphiarthrodial joints,** such as those in the pelvis, allow limited movement. Generally, these joints aren't attacked by arthritic conditions as often as others. (A slipped disc is not arthritis.)

- **Synovial joints** contain synovial fluid and allow a wide range of movement. Most joints fall into this class. Synovial joints come in all kinds of interesting variations including those that glide, hinge, pivot, look like saddles, or have a ball-and-socket type structure. (For more on these joints, take a look at the next section, 'Looking at the types of synovial joints'.) Because of the synovial joints, you can bend over and pick a flower, kick up your heels while line dancing, reach for a glass on a high shelf, and turn around to see what's going on behind you. Unfortunately, these joints are also the ones most likely to be hit with arthritis, precisely because they do move!

Looking at the types of synovial joints

Because of their tendency to become arthritic, this book focuses mostly on synovial joints. Synovial joints come in a wide variety of shapes and sizes to accommodate a wide variety of movements.

Strange but true joint points

Here are a few things you may not know about bones and joints:

- By the time a foetus is four months old, its joints and limbs are in working order and ready to move.

- A newborn baby has 350 bones, many of which fuse to form the 206 bones of the adult body.

- Cartilage is 65–85 per cent water. (The amount of water in your cartilage generally decreases as you get older.)

- When you run, the pressure on your knees can increase to ten times your body weight.

- Not a single man-made substance is more resilient, a better shock absorber, or lower in friction than cartilage.

Gliding joints

A *gliding joint* contains two bones with somewhat flat surfaces that can slide over each other. The vertebrae in your spine are connected by gliding joints, allowing you to bend forward to touch your toes and backward to do a back-bend (well, maybe!). See Figure 1-2 for an example of a gliding joint.

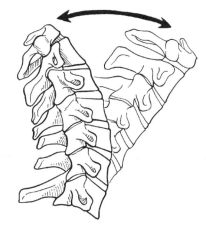

Figure 1-2: A gliding joint helps keep your vertebrae aligned when you bend and stretch.

Hinge joints

You have *hinge joints* in your elbows, knees, and fingers. These joints open and close like a door. But just like a door, hinge joints only go one way – you can't bend your knee up toward your face, only back toward your rear. See Figure 1-3 for an example of a hinge joint.

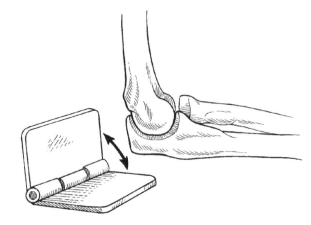

Figure 1-3:
A hinge joint
bends only
one way.

Saddle joints

This type of joint looks like a horse's back with a saddle resting on it. One bone is rounded outwards (convex) and fits neatly into the other bone, which is rounded inwards (concave). Figure 1-4 shows an example of a saddle joint at the elbow, and you have other examples in your wrist and at the base of your thumb. A saddle joint moves up and down and side to side, but it doesn't rotate. So, although you can move your thumb down and around to describe a circle, for example, you can't rotate it around on itself like you can pivot your head on your neck.

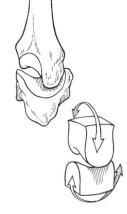

Figure 1-4:
A saddle
joint moves
up and
down and
side to side.

Ball-and-socket joints

This is truly a freewheeling joint – it's ready for anything! Up, down, back, forth, or around in circles. The bone attached to a ball-and-socket joint can move in just about any direction. The end of one bone is round, like a ball, and the other bone has a little cave that the ball fits into. Your shoulders and hips have ball-and-socket joints. Swimming the backstroke is a perfect example of the range of motion made possible by these joints. See Figure 1-5 for an example of a ball-and-socket joint.

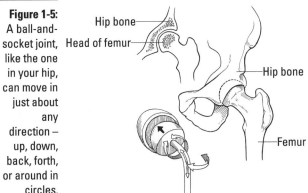

Figure 1-5: A ball-and-socket joint, like the one in your hip, can move in just about any direction – up, down, back, forth, or around in circles.

Hip bone
Head of femur
Hip bone
Femur

Distinguishing Between Arthritis and Arthritis-related Conditions

Some organisations define arthritis as a group of more than 100 related diseases, ranging from bursitis to osteoarthritis. But this book uses the following classifications, which conform to those widely accepted by the medical community:

- ✔ 'True' arthritis
- ✔ Arthritis as a 'major player'
- ✔ Arthritis as a 'minor player'
- ✔ Arthritis as a 'companion condition'

The following subsections go over the various types of arthritis and arthritis-related diseases and their classifications. Each disease is also discussed in greater detail in Chapters 2, 3, 4, and 5.

Defining 'true' arthritis

True arthritis isn't a medical term; it's just a convenient way of referring to the group of ailments in which arthritis is the primary disease process and is a major part of the syndrome. Osteoarthritis and rheumatoid arthritis are the best-known members of this group, which can cause problems ranging from mild joint pain to a permanently bowed spine.

The following is a list of conditions in which arthritis is the major part of the syndrome and the primary disease process:

- **Ankylosing spondylitis:** A chronic inflammation of the spine, this disease can cause the vertebrae to grow together, making the spine rigid. Its appearance on an X-ray is often referred to as *bamboo spine*. Although the cause is unknown, heredity is a factor.

- **Gonococcal arthritis:** The most widespread of the infectious forms of arthritis, originates from the *gonococci* bacterium (which also causes the venereal disease gonorrhoea). Symptoms include pain flitting from one joint to another, with small blisters appearing on the skin over all or parts of the body.

- **Gout:** Known as the 'king of diseases' and the 'disease of kings', this 'regal' form of arthritis is caused by the build-up of uric acid. The uric acid forms sharp crystals that are deposited in a joint causing inflammation and leading to severe pain. These needle-like crystals are most commonly found in the knees, wrists, and the 'bunion' joint of the big toe. Genetic factors, diet, and certain drugs can cause gout.

- **Infectious arthritis:** Bacteria, viruses, or fungi that enter the body can settle in the joints, causing fever, inflammation, and loss of joint function.

- **Juvenile arthritis:** This is a catch-all term for the different kinds of arthritis that strike children under the age of 16. The most common type is *juvenile rheumatoid arthritis* (JRA). Typical symptoms of JRA include pain or swelling in the shoulders, elbows, knees, ankles, or toes; chills; a reappearing fever; and sometimes a body rash. The cause remains unknown.

- **Osteoarthritis (OA):** In this, the most common type of arthritis, the cartilage breaks down, exposing bone ends and allowing them to rub together. The resulting pain, stiffness, loss of movement, and sometimes swelling can have a profound effect on quality of life. Osteoarthritis is most often found in weight-bearing joints, such as the hips, knees, ankles, and spine, but it can also affect the fingers. Osteoarthritis often results from trauma, metabolic conditions, obesity and may also have a hereditary basis.

✔ **Pseudogout:** Like gout, pseudogout is caused by crystals being deposited in the joint. But, instead of uric acid crystals as in 'real' gout, these crystals are made from calcium. The results can include pain, swelling, and sometimes the destruction of cartilage.

Note: These calcium crystals are not related to the dietary intake of calcium.

✔ **Psoriatic arthropathy:** This form of arthritis occurs in people who have a skin condition called *psoriasis*, which causes scaly, red, rough patches on the neck, elbows, and knees, as well as pitting of the nails. Often settling in the joints of the fingers and toes, psoriatic arthritis can cause the digits to swell up like little sausages.

✔ **Reiter's syndrome:** Sufferers are usually young men, who commonly experience inflammation of the urogenital tract, conjunctivitis, plus swollen, stiff joints (usually the knees or ankles). The disease is an immune reaction to Chlamydia, but can follow a bout of Salmonella food poisoning. There is no cure, but painkillers and rest can help to relieve symptoms.

✔ **Rheumatoid arthritis (RA):** In this, the second-most common form of arthritis, the immune system turns against the body, causing inflammation and swelling that begins in the joint lining and spreads to the cartilage and the bone. It often affects the same joint on both sides of the body (for example, both wrists), when it is described as 'symmetrical'.

Classifying arthritis as a 'major player'

In the following conditions, arthritis is present and is usually a major part of the syndrome, but is *not* the main, underlying, or primary disease process:

✔ **Lyme disease:** Caused by a certain type of bacteria transmitted to humans via tick bites, Lyme disease causes a fever, distinctive red skin lesion in the shape of a bull's eye, problems with the nerves and/or heart, and arthritis. Antibiotics are the main treatment for this disease.

✔ **Reactive arthritis:** An inflammation of the joints, reactive arthritis strikes along with, or shortly after, the onset of a sexually transmitted or intestinal infection. The three problems generally associated with reactive arthritis are arthritis, *conjunctivitis* (inflammation of the eye lining), and *urethritis* (inflammation of the urethra, which is the urinary tube).

✔ **Scleroderma:** The word *scleroderma* means hard skin and results when the body responds to inflammation of tiny blood vessels (capillaries) with the overproduction of collagen. This condition leads to stiffening of tissues in the skin, blood vessels, internal organs, and joints. The joint stiffness in scleroderma is actually due to hardening of the overlying skin. An autoimmune disease, scleroderma usually attacks adults rather than children.

✔ **Systemic lupus erythematosus (SLE):** Yet another disease caused when your immune system goes wrong. In *lupus* (or SLE), the body attacks its own tissues, causing inflammation, joint pain, stiffness, permanent damage to the joints, and exhaustion. Although lupus most often affects women of child-bearing age, it *does* strike some men and can occur at nearly any age, including childhood and post-menopause. There is another, more limited form of the disease, *discoid lupus,* which generally confines itself to the skin and usually doesn't venture into your body to attack other organs.

Describing arthritis as a 'minor player'

In these conditions, arthritis may appear, but is a minor part of the syndrome:

✔ **Bursitis and tendonitis:** Caused by overusing or injuring a joint, *bursitis* is an inflammation of the fibrous sac that cushions your tendons. *Tendonitis* is an irritation of the *tendons*, which attach your muscles to your bones. The sheaths surrounding certain tendons can also get inflamed, producing a condition known as *tenosynovitis.*

✔ **Paget's disease:** With Paget's disease, the breakdown and rebuilding of your bones is speeded-up. The resulting bone is larger but also softer and weaker, making it more likely to fracture. These weakened and deformed bones cause arthritis to develop in their respective joints, which typically include those of the hip, skull, spine, knee, and ankle. The cause is unknown.

✔ **Polymyalgia rheumatica:** Often known simply as *PMR,* this condition can strike seemingly overnight, causing severe pain and stiffness in the lower back, hips, shoulders, and neck that can make it difficult even to get out of bed. The pain is similar to that of RA, but there's no evidence of any active arthritis. PMR can occur by itself or together with a life-threatening inflammation of the blood vessels called *giant cell arteritis (GCA).* Symptoms of GCA can occur before, after, or at the same time as PMR, and include headaches, scalp tenderness, hearing problems, jaw pain, difficulty swallowing, and coughing. Anyone experiencing these symptoms should be evaluated by a medical professional immediately as, if left untreated, GCA can lead to serious problems such as sudden blindness.

✔ **Raynaud's disease:** A disease, in its primary form, that affects the small blood vessels in the fingers and toes, causing discolouration, pain, tingling, burning, and sometimes numbness, which are brought on by cold or stress. The secondary form, *Raynaud's phenomenon,* is less common and more serious, and usually accompanies scleroderma or lupus.

✔ **Sjögren's syndrome:** Another autoimmune disease, Sjögren's syndrome brings about inflammation of the tear and saliva glands, causing dryness of your eyes and mouth, hazy vision, cracks at the corners of your mouth, and problems with chewing and swallowing. Inflammation of the brain, nerves, thyroid, lungs, liver, kidneys, and, of course, the joints can also occur.

Experiencing arthritis as a 'companion condition'

These conditions are linked to arthritis; that is, arthritis may be present, but it constitutes another separate disease process:

✔ **Carpal tunnel syndrome:** This syndrome results when pressure on a nerve in your wrist makes your fingers tingle and feel numb. This syndrome is usually caused by overuse of the wrist. Permanent muscle and nerve damage can occur if carpal tunnel isn't treated.

✔ **Fibromyalgia:** Also known as *fibromyalgia syndrome (FMS),* this condition involves pain in your muscles and tendons that occurs without a specific injury or cause. Fibromyalgia can make you 'hurt all over', particularly in certain tender points in the neck, upper back, elbows, and knees. Those with fibromyalgia often develop sleep abnormalities, fatigue, stiffness, and depression. The cause is unknown. Physical or mental stress, fatigue, or infections may trigger this condition.

✔ **Myositis:** This disease causes inflammation of your muscles, which can take one of two forms: *polymyositis* – an inflammation of the muscles that causes weakening and breakdown, as well as pain, and *dermatomyositis* – polymyositis plus rashes that can lead to skin scarring and changes in pigmentation.

Deciding Whether It's Really Arthritis: Signs and Symptoms

With all the different kinds of arthritis, how do you know whether or not you have one of them? Remember two things: Arthritis can strike anyone at any time, and you may find it difficult to tell whether the pain you're experiencing is serious enough to warrant medical attention. Almost everyone has an ache or pain at some time or other, after overextending themselves physically, but you need to know what is minor and temporary, and what may be serious and long term. Knowing what symptoms to watch for can make a difference in your treatment and physical comfort. Typical warning signs of arthritis include:

- ✔ **Joint pain:** This includes not only steady, ever-present pain, but also off-again-on-again pain or pain that occurs only when you move or only when you sit still. In fact, if your joints hurt in *any* way for more than two weeks, you should see your doctor.

- ✔ **Stiffness or difficulty in moving a joint:** If you have trouble getting out of bed, unscrewing a jar lid, climbing the stairs, or doing anything else that involves moving your joints, consider it a red flag. Although difficulty moving a joint is most often the result of a muscular condition, it is sometimes a sign of arthritis.

- ✔ **Swelling:** If the skin around a joint is red, puffed up, hot, throbbing, or painful to the touch, you're experiencing joint inflammation. Don't wait. See your doctor.

The warning signs may come in triplicate (pain plus stiffness plus swelling), two together, or one all alone. Or, as Chapters 3 and 4 point out, you may experience other early signs, such as malaise or muscle pain. But if you experience *any* of these or other symptoms in or around a joint for longer than two weeks, see your doctor.

You may be tempted to read this book's descriptions of various diseases, pick out the one with symptoms most closely matching yours, and make your own diagnosis. Some people may make the right diagnosis. But a lot of people make the wrong one because the symptoms of many forms of arthritis overlap with those of other forms of the disease – they can even be confused with entirely different ailments. Making the wrong diagnosis can lead to the wrong treatment, which can be dangerous. Do not self-diagnose. No matter how obvious your situation seems, go to a medical doctor, have a complete examination, and get a professional diagnosis.

Considering the Causes of Arthritis

Just as many different kinds of arthritis exist, many different causes also exist – and some of them are still unknown. However, scientists have found that certain factors can contribute to the development of joint problems:

- ✔ **Heredity:** Your parents gave you your beautiful eyes, strong jawline, exceptional maths ability, and, possibly, a tendency to develop rheumatoid arthritis. Scientists have discovered that the genetic marker HLA-DR4 is linked to rheumatoid arthritis, so if you happen to have this gene, you're more likely to develop the disease. Ankylosing spondylitis is

---

Arthritis by the numbers

Arthritis affects a surprisingly large number of us, as you can see by the following numbers:

✔ Nine million people in the UK currently have arthritis, or related conditions – almost one in six people.

✔ Arthritis is the reason behind one in five visits to general practitioners, with more than two million people consulting their GP for osteoarthritis over the past year.

✔ Osteoarthritis leads the pack in prevalence, affecting around 8.5 million people, most of whom develop the disease after the age of 45 years.

✔ Over 4 million people in the UK show signs of moderate-to-severe osteoarthritis in X-rays of their hands; over 500,000 have signs of moderate-to-severe osteoarthritis in X-rays of their knees; and over 200,000 have signs of moderate-to-severe osteoarthritis in X-rays of their hips.

✔ Almost 390,000 people have rheumatoid arthritis (RA) in the UK, with at least 12,000 new cases diagnosed each year.

✔ Ankylosing spondylitis caused 250,000 people to visit their GP with gout over the last year.

✔ Around 12,000 children in the UK under the age of 16 – 1 in every 1,000 – has juvenile arthritis.

✔ Surprisingly, 9 out of 10 people with arthritis and joint pain in the UK are not receiving specialist help from a rheumatologist or orthopaedic consultant.

✔ In any one year, over 3,000 deaths in the UK are directly attributable to arthritis and related conditions.

---

linked to the genetic marker HLA-B27, and although having this gene doesn't mean that you absolutely *will* get this form of arthritis, you *can* – if the conditions are right.

✔ **Age:** It's a fact of life that the older you get, the more likely you are to develop arthritis, especially osteoarthritis. Like the tyres on your car, cartilage can wear down over time, becoming thin, cracked, or even wearing through. Bones may also break down with age, bringing on joint pain and dysfunction. However, osteoarthritis is not just a wear-and-tear disease. Research suggests it involves an active process in which the cartilage lining a joint becomes weakened, followed by an over-zealous healing response.

✔ **Overuse of a joint:** What do ballet dancers, cricket bowlers, and tennis players have in common? A great chance that they may develop arthritis due to the tremendous repetitive strain they put on their joints. The dancers, who go from flat foot to *pointe* hundreds of times during a prac-tise session, often end up with painful arthritic ankles. In cricket, fast bowlers, who propel balls at speeds of up to 100 mph, regularly develop arthritis of the shoulder and/or elbow. But you don't need to be a tennis pro to develop *tennis elbow*, a form of tendonitis that has sidelined many a player.

- **Injury:** Sustaining injury to a joint (from a household mishap, a car accident, playing sports, or doing anything else) increases the odds that you may develop arthritis in that joint in the future. Rugby players are well-known victims of arthritis of the knee, which is certainly not surprising: They often fall smack on their knees or other joints when they're tackled – then have a ton of 'rugby flesh' crash down on top of them.

- **Infection:** Some forms of arthritis are the result of bacteria, viruses, or fungi that can either cause the disease or trigger it in susceptible people. Lyme disease comes from bacteria transmitted by the bite of a tick. Infectious arthritis can arise following surgery, trauma, a needle being inserted into the joint, bone infection, or an infection that's travelled from another area of the body.

- **Tumour necrosis factor (TNF):** TNF is a substance the body produces that causes inflammation and may play a part in initiating or maintaining rheumatoid arthritis. Although scientists are unsure exactly what triggers rheumatoid arthritis, they have found that drugs that counteract the effects of TNF, called *TNF antagonists*, are often helpful in managing the symptoms of this disease.

Understanding Who Gets Arthritis

Statistically speaking, the typical arthritis victim (if there is such a thing) is a middle-class, Caucasian woman between the ages of 65 and 74, who has a high school education, is overweight, and who has osteoarthritis. But arthritis isn't all that picky and doesn't worry too much about statistics: It strikes young and old, male and female, rich and poor, and doesn't seem to care where you live. Like nits, arthritis, in one form or another, can affect just about anybody from any walk of life.

However, arthritis does seem to hit women particularly hard. Nearly two-thirds of those who get the disease are women, and the facts about females and arthritis make interesting reading:

- In surveys, 34 per cent of the female population say they currently have arthritis or joint pains compared with 23 per cent of males.

- Women are almost 5 times more likely to have rheumatoid arthritis than men, and girls are 2.5 times more likely to develop RA than boys.

- For every male with moderate-to-severe X-ray evidence of osteoarthritis of the hands, 2 women are affected, and 4 times as many women as men have X-ray evidence of OA of the knees. The incidence of OA of the hips is similar in both sexes but, overall, women usually develop the disease at a younger age.

- In a typical year, over 5 million women consult their GP about arthritis-related problems compared with around 3.7 million men.

- Women are over 5 times more likely to develop ankylosing spondylitis than men.

- Ninety per cent of those who have either lupus or fibromyalgia are women.

- Women are more likely to develop back pain, which is often a symptom of arthritis, than men.

Ethnicity also appears to be important in the arthritis stakes. For example, a study in the West Midlands found that, for systemic lupus erythematosus (SLE), 11 times more women than men were affected among the White population, but among people of African Caribbean origin, women were 22 times more likely to be affected than their menfolk; for those of Asian descent, women were a staggering 35 times more likely to develop the condition than men of the same ethnicity. The reason for these gender and cultural oddities is unknown.

Assessing Your Treatment Options

The good news is that, in many cases, arthritis can be managed. Finding the right treatment(s) for your particular version of the disease may take some time and effort, but answers, like the truth, are out there.

Medications and surgery are only a part of the answer. Following an arthritis-fighting diet, exercising, using joint protection techniques, controlling stress, anger, and depression, and organising your day-to-day activities can offer relief from pain and a new lease of life. And the world of herbs, homeopathy, hands-on healing, and other alternative medicine treatments may offer you additional ammunition in the fight against arthritis pain and other symptoms.

Looking into medications

When you're in pain, your joints are hot or swollen, and you can hardly walk from one end of the house to the other, you want relief *now*. In many cases, the fastest way to relieve arthritis symptoms is to take medication. Arthritis medications fall into five main classes, which are described here in order of the complexity of their action:

- **Simple analgesics:** These fight pain but do not interfere with the inflammation process. The best-known and most commonly-used simple analgesic is paracetamol.

- ✔ **Non-steroidal anti-inflammatory drugs (NSAIDs):** The NSAIDs help to relieve pain and reduce inflammation by interfering with an enzyme called *COX (cyclo-oxygenase)*. Milder versions (aspirin, ibuprofen) of NSAIDs are available over the counter, but the more powerful ones (naproxen, diclofenac sodium, flurbiprofen) require a prescription.

- ✔ **Corticosteroids:** These drugs are man-made versions of naturally occurring hormones in the body that help to quell inflammation. Although corticosteroids have powerful anti-inflammatory actions, they can also have powerful side effects, including elevated blood pressure, stomach ulcers, thinning of the bones and skin, and increased risk of infection.

- ✔ **Disease-modifying antirheumatic drugs (DMARDs):** Although these drugs are used to treat rheumatic arthritis, they won't quite make you worth your weight in gold – they include gold injections – along with antimalarials and other drugs, such as sulfasalazine and methotrexate, which modify certain rheumatic disease processes in your body.

  DMARDs are usually used in inflammatory forms of arthritis (such as RA, psoriatic arthritis, and ankylosing spondylitis) that haven't responded to other medicines. These drugs change the way the immune system works, slowing or stopping its attack on the body. This change helps to damp down symptoms that are linked with over-zealous activity of certain immune cells, which release inflammatory substances such as TNF (mentioned in the previous section on 'Considering the Causes of Arthritis').

- ✔ **Biologic response modifiers (BRMs):** The newest drugs to help fight stubborn cases of inflammation, they work by inhibiting certain components of the immune system called *cytokines*. The cytokines play a part in the inflammation that accompanies rheumatoid arthritis, and drugs such as adalimumab and infliximab inhibit their inflammatory action.

Chapter 8 gives you the complete low-down on arthritis medications.

Considering surgery

If pain is interfering with your ability to lead a happy and productive life, you have to take the maximum amount of pain relievers just to get through the day, and you've tried all other pain-relieving methods with no luck, you may want to consider surgery. Although joint surgery is complex and never undertaken lightly, some people enjoy excellent results, to the point of feeling that they have a new lease of life.

Surgical techniques can involve flushing a joint with water, resurfacing rough bone ends or cartilage, removing inflamed membranes, growing new bone, or putting in a whole new joint. Turn to Chapter 9 to find out more about surgical treatments.

Making lifestyle changes

Chances are excellent that you can significantly ease your arthritis-related pain, stiffness, swelling, and decreased range of motion just by changing certain things you do every day. The following list goes over some options you may want to consider:

- ✔ **Eat an arthritis-fighting diet.** This means consuming plenty of fish, fresh fruit, fresh vegetables, and whole-grains, with a minimum of processed meats and salad oils (corn, safflower, or sunflower). However, the Mediterranean diet fits the bill, as olive oil and fish oils are good for joints, while also warding off both heart disease and certain types of cancer. See Chapter 15 for the low-down on the elements of a good arthritis-fighting diet.

- ✔ **Consider taking joint-saving supplements.** Many supplements can help to ease the symptoms of different kinds of arthritis. Among them are antioxidants (betacarotene, vitamins C and E, grapeseed extract, green tea, and selenium), boron, vitamin B6, niacin, vitamin D, zinc, flaxseed oil, glucosamine sulphate, chondroitin, bromelain, and others. These supplements are discussed at length in Chapter 15.

- ✔ **Exercise daily (whenever possible).** Countless studies have shown that exercise can help lubricate and nourish your joints by forcing joint fluid into and out of your cartilage. Under-exercised joints don't get much of this in-and-out action, so cartilage can thin and become dry. Brisk walking may be one of the best exercises for those with arthritis, because it doesn't put undue stress on your joints and is easy and fun to do. For a rundown of exercises that help ease arthritis symptoms, see Chapter 16.

- ✔ **Watch your joint alignment.** Ensuring that you stand, sit, walk, run, and lift correctly can help protect your joints from injury and excess wear and tear. The best joint-saving techniques are discussed in detail in Chapter 17, along with tips on how to make them a part of your life.

- ✔ **Control stress, aggression, and depression.** The way you think and feel about your arthritis pain can actually make it worse. So can stress, anger, hostility, aggression, and depression. Luckily, you can reduce your pain just by reducing your stress levels and tapping into your natural potential for relaxation. Chapter 18 covers positive thinking, biofeedback, controlling your breathing, laughter, prayer, and spirituality – all effective ways of improving your mood, easing your pain, and making you feel better over all.

- ✔ **Organise your life for maximum efficiency.** Studies show that people who actively manage their arthritis and find new ways to cope with physical problems feel less pain and fatigue. Chapter 19 gives you helpful tips for managing arthritis on a day-to-day basis. Included are ideas for conserving your energy, getting a good night's sleep, using assistive devices, making household jobs easy, and holding on to your sex life. An occupational therapist can offer valuable assistance.

Stargazing: Famous people with arthritis

Does the idea of having arthritis make you feel like you may as well just give up? Well, many people have felt the same, but persevered anyway. Take a look at what some people have done with their lives while coping with arthritis:

- **Lucille Ball** was diagnosed with rheumatoid arthritis at the age of 17, but she went on to live a long and healthy life, enjoying a top-notch career in films and television.

- The famous French artist **Pierre-Auguste Renoir** developed RA in his late fifties, but painted nearly 6,000 pictures during his lifetime, many of them great masterpieces.

- Actress **Mary McDonough**, best known for her role as Erin on the TV show *The Waltons*, has lupus, yet is a wife and mother and continues a successful career as an actress and spokesperson for the Lupus Foundation of America.

- **Dr Christian Barnard** developed rheumatoid arthritis as a youngster but went on to perform the world's first human heart transplant in 1967.

- **Billie Jean King** has osteoarthritis of the knees, probably the result of a car accident when she was 18 years old. Yet she won the Wimbledon singles title for the sixth time when she was in her early thirties.

- **Rosalind Russell,** star of the silver screen, had severe RA and did much to garner support for the advancement of research into this disease.

- **Ainsley Harriott,** TV chef who had surgery to resurface his hip in 2004.

Looking at alternative approaches

Because there isn't any one magic bullet that cures arthritis, a great many people are turning to more holistic approaches – either as an alternative to traditional medicine or as that extra something that just may do the trick. In Chapters 11 through 14, the most popular complementary treatments for arthritis are discussed, – from herbs to homeopathy, from acupuncture to reflexology, from aromatherapy to hydrotherapy. The text describes each therapy, explains what it can do for you, and gives important tips on how to find a reputable practitioner.

Chapter 2

Osteoarthritis, the Most Common Form

*W*hether you call it *osteoarthritis (OA)*, degenerative arthritis, or degenerative joint disease, this annoying condition is the painful result of cartilage breakdown. When the tough, rubbery substance that cushions the ends of your bones no longer does its job properly, the bone ends can't slide easily across each other when your joints move. Pain and stiffness then strike. Suddenly, your knee aches, your hip burns, a finger joint swells and throbs, or your shoulder stiffens up. You can't bend and flex the painful joint like you used to; its range of movement is limited. Most of all, the joint just plain hurts!

But what happened to mess up your cartilage in the first place? To understand what went wrong, this chapter looks at how things work in healthy cartilage.

Considering Cartilage

Healthy cartilage is absolutely essential for joints to function properly and painlessly. Slick as polished marble and tough as galvanised rubber, cartilage covers and protects the ends of your bones from wearing each other away where they meet inside a joint. Cartilage also provides a smooth, slick surface so bone ends can glide easily across each other and is an excellent shock absorber, cushioning your bones and soaking up the impact created by movement and physical stresses.

Without intact cartilage, bones grind away at each other and bear the brunt of the impact of movement. Eventually, the joint itself can be damaged or even destroyed.

Four elements help cartilage do its all-important job:

- **Water:** Sixty-five to eighty per cent of cartilage is water – a crucial substance that lubricates your joints, cushions your bones, and absorbs shock.

- **Collagen:** Elasticity and a superb capability to absorb shock make collagen an integral part of healthy cartilage. A connective tissue that helps hold bones, muscles, and other bodily structures together, collagen is the mesh-like framework that provides a home for the proteoglycans.

- **Proteoglycans:** These large, oblong molecules are covered with centipede-like 'legs' that weave themselves securely into the collagen mesh and soak up water like a sponge. Then, when pressured, proteoglycans release water. Thanks in part to the proteoglycans, cartilage can mould itself to the shape of the joint and respond to the ever-changing amount of pressure within the joint.

- **Chondrocytes:** These cells follow the principle 'out with the old and in with the new' as they break down and get rid of old proteoglycan and collagen molecules, forming new ones to take their place.

Water, collagen, proteoglycans, and chondrocytes all work together to keep your joints moving like well-oiled machinery. When the pressure is released from a joint – say your knee when you lift your leg to take a step – water rushes into the cartilage, nourishing, bathing, and plumping it up. The water-loving proteoglycans, woven securely into the collagen web, soak up water and hold on to it until pressure is applied to the joint (that is, you take another step). Then the water and wastes rush out of the cartilage. But as soon as the pressure is off, the proteoglycans thirstily soak up the water again. The resilient collagen stretches and shrinks to accommodate joint pressure and water content, so your cartilage can bounce back after being flattened out – rather like your own inbuilt bouncy castle.

But if your cartilage loses its ability to attract and hold water, it becomes thin, dry, cracked, and unable to provide a slippery surface (see Figure 2-1). No longer plump and resilient, the cartilage makes a poor shock absorber and cushion for the bones, particularly affecting the weight-bearing joints.

You can visualise the action of the cartilage by thinking of two tins of soup facing each other end-to-end with an almost-filled water balloon in between them. As you press the tins together, the water balloon changes shape to accommodate the pressure, but it never lets the tins actually touch. When you release the pressure, the water balloon (like your cartilage) resumes its old shape.

Identifying the Signs and Symptoms of Osteoarthritis

Figure 2-1 shows the sites that are most commonly affected by osteoarthritis – the neck, lower back, knees, hips, ends of the fingers, and the base of the thumbs.

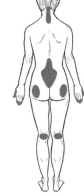

Figure 2-1: Places where OA makes its presence felt.

How do you know if the joint pain you're experiencing is due to osteoarthritis? Most of those with the disease have at least one of the following symptoms:

- ✔ **Joint pain:** Most people experience joint pain as a deep-seated ache radiating from the inner core of the joint. The feeling is distinctly different from a muscular ache and may come and go according to changes in the weather ('I can feel it in my bones when it's going to rain'). The pain typically increases as you use the joint and eases off with joint rest. As the disease worsens, though, the pain can become fairly steady. If joint pain occurs during the night, poor sleep and next-day fatigue may be two unpleasant side effects.

  Some people really can feel it in their joints when it's going to rain because as the barometric pressure falls, the lining of an arthritic joint can become inflamed, causing pain and the release of excess fluid (swelling).

- ✔ **Stiffness and loss of movement:** Stiff joints, limited range of motion and, in the later stages, joints that freeze into a bent position are all signs of osteoarthritis.

✔ **Tenderness, warmth, and swelling around the joint:** Although swelling is not usually a big problem with osteoarthritis, some joints do swell in response to cartilage damage and irritation, especially if they've been overused. The finger joints and the knees are most often affected.

✔ **'Cracking' joints:** If you hear popping or crunching sounds when you move a joint, you may have osteoarthritis. These cracking sounds (doctors call them *crepitus*) can be created by roughened cartilage. (The crunching sound you hear when you move a joint isn't the same thing as 'cracking' your joints by applying pressure to them, which causes a harmless release of nitrogen bubbles and isn't associated with OA.)

✔ **Bony growths on the fingers:** Bony lumps, either at the ends of the fingers (called *Heberden's nodes*) or on the middle joint of the fingers (called *Bouchard's nodes*) are signs of osteoarthritis. These bony growths may be hereditary.

Don't assume that you have osteoarthritis just because you have one or more of these symptoms. Get a thorough examination and diagnosis from your doctor.

Discovering What Causes Cartilage Breakdown

Sometimes, doctors really don't know why the cartilage disintegrates. In these cases, they designate the problem as *primary osteoarthritis*, or osteoarthritis of unknown cause. In other cases, it's clear that osteoarthritis is triggered by another problem, in which case it's called *secondary osteoarthritis*.

Considering causes of primary osteoarthritis

The ultimate cause of primary osteoarthritis remains a mystery. Although scientists aren't sure why, the collagen mesh of the cartilage becomes scrambled; it weakens and can't hold its structure. The proteoglycans, once so cosily intertwined in the collagen mesh, suddenly find themselves evicted from their secure homes. As they float off into the joint fluid, the protoglycans take their water-retaining abilities with them. The cartilage is left high and dry; it thins and may even crack. At the same time, the newly-freed proteoglycans draw excess fluid into the joint, causing swelling. (Unfortunately, this fluid can't get back into the cartilage, where it's desperately needed – like dying of thirst in the middle of the ocean.)

Although no one is absolutely certain what causes primary osteoarthritis, here are a few theories:

- ✔ **The chondrocytes become too efficient at breaking down the collagen and proteoglycan molecules.** In healthy cartilage, the amount of breaking down enzymes is equal to the amount of building up enzymes. An over-abundance of destructive enzymes leads to weakened collagen and a lack of proteoglycans.

- ✔ **The chondrocytes go wild and start making too many proteoglycan and collagen molecules.** The opposite of the previous condition, these chondrocytes are too good at making new cartilage components. The excess proteoglycan and collagen molecules, in turn, pull extra fluid into the joint, flooding it and washing away most of the chondrocytes. The cartilage, then, is left bereft of cartilage-producing molecules.

Sorting out the sources of secondary osteoarthritis

Although the origins of primary osteoarthritis remain murky, experts are quite sure what causes secondary osteoarthritis: Various types of trauma to the joints. Trauma includes sudden, high-velocity trauma (the kind you'd experience in a car accident), as well as little insults to your joints that occur time and time again, like repeated poor posture or running on a concrete surface every day for years. The causes of secondary osteoarthritis can be further broken down as follows:

- ✔ **Joint injury:** Weekend warriors beware! Once a joint is injured, whether through a sports mishap, car accident, slipping at home, or anything else, it is much more likely to develop osteoarthritis.

- ✔ **Repetitive motion injury:** Joints that are stressed over and over again in the same way (for example, a ballerina's ankles, a football player's knees, or a data processor's wrists) are more likely to experience a cartilage breakdown than joints subjected to normal use.

- ✔ **Damage to the bone end:** Usually due to trauma or continual stress, a bone may chip or sustain small fractures. In the body's zeal to repair the damage, it may cause an overgrowth of bone in the injured area. The result of this overgrowth is a bone end that's bumpy, not smooth, and joint problems can ensue.

✔ **Bone disease:** A bone disease, such as Paget's disease, weakens the bone structure, making it more likely to fracture and develop bony overgrowth.

✔ **Carrying too much body weight:** The heavier you are, the more stress you place on your knees, hips, and ankles. Osteoarthritis of the knee is clearly linked to excess body weight. That fact is not surprising, considering that every time you take a step the stress on your knee is roughly equivalent to three times your body weight. This figure increases to ten times your body weight when you run!

Regarding the repair problem

Unfortunately, once your cartilage is damaged, your body can make the problem worse if it repairs itself in certain ways. Like injured bone, injured cartilage can overdo the repair process, piling too much new cartilage into a crack or tear. The result of this repair is a lumpy, bumpy surface that doesn't glide smoothly against the cartilage on the opposing bone end. Sometimes the cartilage doesn't repair itself at all though, and remains in its damaged state – cracked, pitted, frayed, and even worn-through. Pieces of loose cartilage and/or bone may break off and float freely through the joint fluid. Then, the bone ends, which are no longer well cushioned, start to rub against each other and can develop bony spurs (osteophytes) that further interfere with smooth joint movement. Figure 2-2 shows this problem. The joint space narrows, and the entire shape of the joint can change. All this mayhem from a little damaged cartilage!

Figure 2-2:
Osteoarthritic joints have narrowed joint space, and thin, rough, broken-down, or completely missing cartilage.

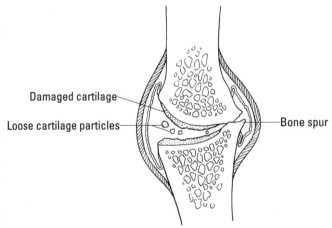

Damaged cartilage

Loose cartilage particles

Bone spur

You may hear your doctor use some of these technical terms: *Eburnation* (increased and abnormal bone density), *subchondral bone* (the bone right below the cartilage), or *subchondral cyst* (an abnormal pocket of fluid in the bone beneath the cartilage).

Recognising Risk Factors for Osteoarthritis

Although osteoarthritis affects nearly 9 million people in the UK at any one time, not everyone will eventually develop it. Some people actually sail into their golden years with joints unaffected by pain, stiffness, or other symptoms, while others are hobbling around by the time they're 35. So how come one person gets osteoarthritis while another gets away scot-free? And how can you tell if you happen to have a particular susceptibility to arthritis?

Your chances of developing osteoarthritis are increased if:

- ✔ **You're past the age of 45:** Cartilage and other joint structures, like most body tissues, tend to degrade and become weaker over time. After decades of use, they start to wear out. Luckily, research has shown that osteoarthritis isn't inevitable as you age – the odds just go up.

- ✔ **You've had a joint injury:** If you've been in a car accident, played rough-and-tumble sports, or injured any of your joints in any way, you're more likely to develop osteoarthritis in those areas.

- ✔ **Your joints have been repeatedly stressed:** Ballet dancers, assembly-line workers, bowlers in cricket, keyboard operators, and anyone else who overuses and stresses a joint or joints can develop cartilage breakdown in those areas.

- ✔ **You're a woman:** Women are three times more likely than men to develop osteoarthritis. This greater susceptibility may be due to smaller joint structures or some link to oestrogen, although possible reasons are still under investigation.

- ✔ **Your parents had it:** A genetic component to osteoarthritis exists and, in fact, one study concludes that genes are responsible for 50 per cent of cases of osteoarthritis of the hip. Osteoarthritis in the hands is also at least partially due to genetics. An inherited tendency toward defective cartilage or poorly structured joints can certainly put you on the road to osteoarthritis, although you won't necessarily develop it.

- ✔ **You're overweight:** Excess weight puts a great deal of strain on your weight-bearing joints, especially your hips, knees, and ankles. For every ten pounds of excess weight you carry, you increase the force exerted on these joints anywhere from three to ten times, depending on the type of activity you pursue. Researchers have already found a definite link between excess weight and osteoarthritis of the knee joints.

If you can believe it, using chopsticks increases your risk of developing OA of the hand! Researchers studying 2,507 60-year-old residents of Beijing, China found significantly more OA in the first, second, and third fingers of the hand that used chopsticks than the non-chopstick-using hand. Repeated mechanical stress to these joints, via chopstick use, is the undoubted culprit.

Determining Whether It Really Is Osteoarthritis

Nearly 50 per cent of people with osteoarthritis don't know what kind of arthritis they have; therefore, they can't make good decisions about their treatment.

Say your knee hurts. The first time you visit your doctor complaining of pain, he or she puts you through the standard round of questions, examinations, and tests. The doctor reviews your medical history and makes a detailed list of the injuries you have sustained, especially to your knees. He or she may palpate your knee to see if it's painful to the touch, carefully bend your knee and straighten it several times (it may hurt a little and seem stiff), and listen for cracking or popping in the joint. If your arthritis is inflammatory in nature, your doctor may request some blood tests to rule out other forms of the disease, such as rheumatoid arthritis. At this point, all your doctor has to go on is any history of knee injury, some pain and stiffness upon movement, and a little cracking in the joint. Your symptoms may sound like osteoarthritis, but the diagnosis is not yet a sure thing.

The next step is to order an X-ray of your knee to see if one or more of the following signs are present:

- Cartilage degradation
- Cartilage overgrowth
- Narrowing of the joint space
- Bone spur – bony outgrowth that resembles the goading instrument on a rider's heel (although it won't make YOU go faster, just the opposite)
- Bits of cartilage or bone floating in the joint fluid
- Joint deformity

Treating Osteoarthritis

After a diagnosis of osteoarthritis is confirmed, you and your doctor can begin devising a treatment programme – confident that you're heading in the right direction. Although your symptoms may not disappear completely, you still have a good chance that, with proper treatment, your pain is diminished significantly and further deterioration of your joint is kept to a minimum.

A good treatment plan for osteoarthritis includes the elements in the following sections to help you manage pain and discomfort on a daily basis.

Muting the pain with medication

Both prescription and over-the-counter remedies are commonly used to relieve osteoarthritis pain. These drugs usually fall into one of two categories:

- ✔ **Paracetamol:** This relieves pain and fever, but doesn't reduce swelling.

- ✔ **Non-steroidal anti-inflammatory drugs or NSAIDs:** These relieve pain and fever and *do* reduce swelling (for example, aspirin and ibuprofen).

If your joints are swollen, the doctor may prescribe an NSAID. If swelling isn't a problem, he or she may suggest paracetamol.

To avoid drug interactions, overdoses, or side effects, check with your doctor before taking any over-the-counter medications. (See Chapter 8 for more information on medicines.)

Lubricating your joints with exercise

If you're in pain, you probably want to *stop* moving, and it's certainly advisable to rest your joints when you're feeling achy. But too much sitting around is actually the *worst* thing for you in the long run. Exercise is a great way to 'oil and feed' your cartilage. Under-exercised joints don't get the lubricating and nourishing benefits of the in-and-out action of the joint fluid, so cartilage can become thin and dry, losing its resilience and ability to cushion your bones.

Include three types of exercises in your overall physical fitness programme:

- ✔ **Flexibility exercises:** Do stretching, bending and twisting exercises every day to increase your range-of-motion and reduce stiffness. Flexibility exercises help keep your joints loose and flexible.

- ✔ **Strengthening exercises:** Do weight-lifting or isometric exercises every other day to build up your muscles and to help keep your joint-supporting structures stable. These types of exercises help increase your muscle strength.

- ✔ **Endurance exercises:** Do aerobic exercises at least three times a week for 20 to 30 minutes each session as these increase overall fitness, strengthen your cardiovascular system, and help to keep your weight under control. Brisk walking (especially uphill), jogging, cycling, dancing, skipping, and so on, all help to increase your fitness and capacity for exercise.

Before starting a new exercise programme, check with your doctor to find out what kinds of exercise and levels of activity are appropriate for you. Doing the wrong exercises – or doing the right exercises in the wrong way – can cause you further injury. (See Chapter 16 for more information on exercise.)

Protecting your joints through good alignment

Applying the techniques of body alignment, proper standing, sitting, walking and running, and correct lifting can go a long way toward sparing your joints from excessive wear and tear and protecting them from future injury. Wrapping affected joints with elastic supports may be helpful or using assistive devices, such as a walking stick or crutches. Other joint-protective techniques include alternating your activities with rest periods, varying your tasks to avoid too much repetitive stress on any one area, and pacing yourself. Don't try to do too much at once. (See Chapter 17 for more information on joint protection.)

Heating and cooling the pain away

Some people prefer heat, others prefer cold, so use whatever works for you. Hot baths, heating pads, electric blankets, and hot tubs can relax painful muscles, while ice packs can numb the affected area. To avoid damaging tissues, just make sure you don't use either method for longer than 20 minutes at a time. (See Chapter 10 for more information on physical therapy for pain relief.)

Always give your skin time to return to its usual temperature before reapplying hot or cold packs.

Taking a load off with weight control

If you're overweight, your hips, knees, and ankles are probably suffering. Not only are these joints subjected to a force equal to three times your body weight each time you take a step, they can be pummelled by ten times your body weight if you jog or run! So that extra 10 pounds (4½ kilograms) around your middle may translate to an extra 100 pounds (45 kilograms) slamming away on certain joints at certain times. And, that strain on your joints is only *one* reason why keeping your weight at an acceptable level is so important. (See Appendix C for more information on diet and weight control.)

Fifty per cent of people who develop knee osteoarthritis have battled with excess weight for between three and ten years.

Knowing how to help yourself

Strategies for pain management, foods and supplements that can help to heal, positive thinking, prayer, spirituality, massage, relaxation techniques, and complementary healing methods can add to your arsenal in the fight against pain and disability. Don't ignore the enormous potential of these resources to improve the quality of your life. (Look at Chapters 10 through 19 for more information on these topics.)

Considering surgery

When you have a painful joint that isn't getting better, and the pain is seriously compromising the quality of your life, you may need to consider surgery. These days, routine operations like arthroscopic surgery, cartilage transplants, and joint replacement surgery can make a huge difference for those who live in pain. (See Chapter 9 for more information on surgery.)

Chapter 3

Fighting a War Within: Rheumatoid Arthritis

*R*heumatoid arthritis (RA) is a case of the human body's good intentions gone awry. Your body is equipped with a very effective immune system that fights off bacteria and other foreign bodies. Specialised cells attack these invaders, surround them, paralyse them, and destroy them. A strong, intact immune system is absolutely essential for your survival – without it, you can quickly succumb to infections and disease. But if your immune system should suddenly go haywire and start attacking your body's own tissues, it could become your worst enemy. When you have RA, your immune system attacks the tissues that cushion and line your joints, eventually causing entire joints to deteriorate.

Turning on Itself: The Body Becomes Its Own Worst Enemy

For reasons that aren't completely understood, in rheumatoid arthritis the white blood cells of your immune system suspects that your joint lining *(synovial membrane)* is a foreign object and sets about attacking it, causing pain, loss of movement, and joint destruction. Your immune system's attack on your joint lining follows these steps:

1. The assaulted membrane becomes inflamed and painful, your entire joint capsule swells, and the synovial cells start to grow and divide in an abnormal way.

2. Almost as if they're launching a counter-attack, these abnormal cells invade your surrounding tissues – mostly the bone and cartilage of the affected joint.

3. Your joint space begins to narrow, and the joint's supporting structures become weak. At the same time, the cells that trigger inflammation release enzymes that start eating away at the bone and cartilage, causing joint erosion and scarring.

4. Reeling under this many-sided attack, the joint itself deteriorates, eventually becoming misshapen and misaligned.

Figure 3-1 compares a healthy joint to one with RA. Notice that in the healthy joint in Figure 3-1a.), the synovial membrane is thin and free from inflammation; the cartilage is smooth, thick, and even; the joint space is well defined; and the joint capsule assumes a normal shape. In Figure 3-1b., which shows a joint affected by RA, the synovial membrane is inflamed and swollen, with inflammatory cells invading both bone and cartilage. The cartilage is thin, the joint space narrowed, and the joint capsule swollen.

Rheumatoid arthritis insidiously makes its way through your body and (in more severe cases) can eventually spread to all of your joints. But joints are not RA's only target. RA is a *systemic disease*, which means that it can attack many body systems and is capable of triggering numerous problems in various other parts of your body. RA can cause inflammation of the membranes surrounding your eyes, heart, lungs, and other internal organs, generally wreaking havoc on your body as a whole.

If your tear and salivary glands partially 'dry up', Sjögren's syndrome can develop in association with RA. See Chapter 5 for more on this 'drying disease'.

Some people have RA for just a short time – a few months or a couple of years – and then it disappears forever. Other people develop painful periods (flare-ups) that come and go, although they can feel quite well in between episodes. However, those people with severe forms of RA are in pain a good deal of the time, experience symptoms for many years, and experience serious joint damage.

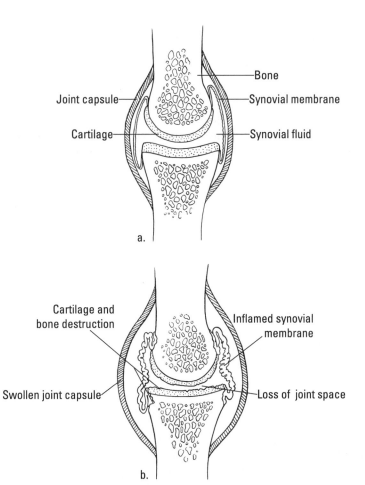

Bone

Synovial membrane

Synovial fluid

Joint capsule

Cartilage

a.

Cartilage and
bone destruction

Inflamed synovial
membrane

Swollen joint capsule

Loss of joint space

b.

Figure 3-1:
The a. part
shows a
healthy
joint; the
b. part
shows
a joint
affected
by RA.

Although rheumatoid arthritis can have some very serious consequences, this disease is manageable in a medical sense. Many people with RA live long, successful lives. But remember: Early treatment can make a big difference in RA, so don't wait to see a doctor.

Recognising the signs and symptoms of RA

If you have rheumatoid arthritis, the first thing you may notice is a dull ache, stiffness, and swelling in two matching joints – for example, both elbows, both knees, or both index fingers. The most typical sites for RA are the fingers and wrists, but it can also settle in the hands, elbows, shoulders, neck, hips, knees, ankles, and feet. Figure 3-2 shows these areas.

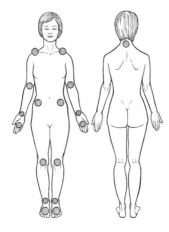

Figure 3-2:
The areas where rheumatoid arthritis is most likely to strike.

RA typically begins with minor symptoms and slowly makes its presence known. But RA can also strike dramatically, causing several joints to become inflamed all at once. Although the symptoms of RA vary, most people with the condition experience one or more of the following:

- Pain, warmth, redness, swelling, or tightness in a joint

- Swelling of three or more joints for six or more weeks

- Joints affected in a symmetrical pattern (for example, both knees, both shoulders, and so on)

- Joint pain or stiffness lasting longer than an hour upon arising or after prolonged inactivity

- Pea-shaped bumps under the skin (called *rheumatoid nodules*), especially on pressure points like the elbows or the feet. In people who are bedridden, nodules may also occur at the base of the scalp or on the back of the hips

✔ Evidence of joint erosion on X-ray

✔ Loss of mobility

✔ General soreness, aching, and stiffness

✔ A general 'sick' feeling *(malaise)*

✔ Fatigue and weakness, especially in the early afternoon

✔ Periodic low-grade fever and/or sweats

✔ Difficulty sleeping

✔ Anaemia

✔ Blood tests showing the presence of rheumatoid factor (an abnormal substance found in the blood of about 80 per cent of people with RA)

Although pain and inflammation are early signs of RA, they're not always the first to herald the arrival of the disease. *Still's disease* is a type of RA in which the first indicators are fever, rash, chills, and other general symptoms affecting the entire body, not just the joints. Among children with juvenile rheumatoid arthritis, some 10 per cent have Still's disease.

As RA progresses, the joints enlarge and can become deformed. The joints may even freeze in a semi-contracted position, making complete extension impossible. The fingers can start to curl up, pointing away from the thumb, as tendons slip out of place.

In general, the older you are when rheumatoid arthritis first strikes, the milder your symptoms.

Scanning associated conditions and their symptoms

RA may also attack other parts of the body, causing the following conditions:

✔ **Episcleritis:** If RA attacks the tissues covering the white part of the eye (a condition called *episcleritis*), it can cause eye pain, sensitivity to light, and excessive tear production.

✔ **Pericarditis:** If RA settles in the membrane surrounding the heart (a condition called *pericarditis*), it can cause abnormal heart function.

✔ **Pleurisy:** If RA attacks the lungs, it can cause *pleurisy* (inflammation of the membranes around the lungs), prompting difficulty in breathing, chest pain, and lung scarring.

✔ **Vasculitis:** If RA affects the blood vessels (*vasculitis*), the circulation to other parts of the body can reduce, causing nerve damage and even tissue death.

Comparing rheumatoid arthritis and osteoarthritis

Rheumatoid arthritis and osteoarthritis have two things in common: namely, joint pain and damage to certain joint structures, such as the cartilage and the bone. Other than these two elements, the two conditions are about as different as night and day. Table 3-1 outlines the differences between RA and OA.

Table 3-1	Rheumatoid Arthritis Compared to Osteoarthritis
Rheumatoid Arthritis	**Osteoarthritis**
Joint inflammation and swelling are prominent symptoms.	Joint inflammation and swelling are less common.
Usually begins between the ages of 25 to 50, but can also strike children.	Usually begins after the age of 40. Rarely strikes children.
Settles in a majority of joints, especially fingers, wrists, shoulders, knees, and elbows.	Affects the weight-bearing joints primarily (for example, knees, hips, ankles, and spine).
Affects joints symmetrically (for example, both wrists).	Affects isolated joints or one joint at a time.
Morning stiffness lasts more than one hour.	Brief periods of morning stiffness.
Often causes systemic symptoms, such as fatigue, fever, weight loss, and general malaise.	Does not cause systemic symptoms.

Understanding the causes of RA

The truth is that nobody really knows what causes RA, although some believe it is linked to a defect in the immune system. Many people with RA have a particular genetic marker – HLA-DR4 – so it's reasonable to suspect that this gene is involved. Yet, not everyone with this gene ends up with RA, and not everyone with RA has this gene. And scientists are certain that more than just one gene is involved: Perhaps HLA-DR4 is only one of several genes that can tip the scales in favour of developing RA. Most likely, genetic markers play a part in the development of the disease but aren't the determining factor.

Some researchers believe that RA is triggered by a virus, or perhaps an unrecognised type of bacterium, that 'wakes up' a dormant genetic defect and sets it in motion. As yet, no such infectious agent is identifiable, and RA is definitely not considered contagious.

Hormones or hormone deficiencies may also play a part in developing RA, although their possible role is unclear. Women are more likely than men to develop RA, suggesting a possible link to oestrogen. But, at present, as you can see, doctors have more questions than answers about RA.

Describing the most likely victim of RA

Rheumatoid arthritis can strike just about anyone – children, the elderly, the middle-aged, and people of almost all racial or ethnic groups. But RA has a particular affinity for women, especially those between the ages of 20 and 50. Women account for around 285,000 of the 390,000 UK adults who have RA, making them almost three times more likely than men to get the disease, although scientists have yet to determine why.

Overcoming RA: Lucy's story

Lucille Ball, the famous comedienne and zany star of the *I Love Lucy* television series, was just 17 years old and working as a model when she suddenly developed a fiery pain in both her legs. 'It was so bad, I had to sit down,' she wrote in her autobiography, *Love, Lucy*. She had recently recovered from a bout of pneumonia and a high fever; now this!

Hurrying to her doctor, Lucy received the terrifying news: She had rheumatoid arthritis, a crippling disease that becomes progressively worse over time. In fact, it was conceivable that Lucy would spend her life in a wheelchair. Lucy's doctor sent her to an orthopaedic clinic where she waited for three hours, nearly fainting from the pain, before the doctor informed her that there was no cure. The doctor did ask if Lucy wanted to try an experimental treatment, though – injections of 'horse serum'. Lucy agreed and received these injections over the next several weeks until she finally ran out of money. Unfortunately, the pain continued.

Discouraged but not about to give up, Lucy went back home to her parents, who massaged her legs, gave her money to continue the horse serum injections, and encouraged her to take better care of her health. Finally, months later, the pain began to ease, and Lucy was able to stand up on weak and shaky legs. Her left leg had shortened a bit during the course of the disease, so Lucy added a 20-pound weight to her corrective shoe to stretch the leg out.

Lucy's hard work and perseverance paid off. Lucy was able to return to New York; she made several films and eventually starred in her own television series, one that required vigorous physical comedy, stamina, and energy. Lucy also starred in Broadway plays, performing eight shows a week while managing to sail through energetic song and dance numbers with a seemingly effortless grace and ease. Lucy remained active and healthy until her death in 1989, and in spite of her doctor's ominous prediction, never spent a single day in a wheelchair.

Diagnosing Rheumatoid Arthritis

Unfortunately, no one test can tell your doctor that you definitely have RA. Instead, your doctor looks for a tell-tale pattern in the information taken from many sources, such as your medical history, physical examination, laboratory tests, X-rays, a fluid sample taken from affected joints and, if rheumatoid nodules are present, a biopsy of those nodules.

Searching for clues: The medical history and physical examination

During your initial examination, your doctor asks you about the onset of your symptoms, whether you experience any morning stiffness, the kind and amount of pain you feel, the presence of swelling, whether or not joints are affected on both sides of your body, and so on.

Looking into your medical history is a way to see if your symptoms fit the general pattern of RA or suggest another disease instead. During your physical examination, your doctor also checks for tenderness, range of motion, and the presence of rheumatoid nodules.

Taking tests

Several tests are typically used to help diagnose rheumatoid arthritis; all involve taking a sample of your blood and sending it to the laboratory for examination:

- **Rheumatoid factor (RF) test** checks for the presence of a particular antibody that appears in the blood of the majority of people who have RA. But a positive RF test doesn't necessarily mean that you have rheumatoid arthritis. The RF antibody can occur with other rheumatic diseases as well as many other medical conditions.

- **Erythrocyte sedimentation rate (ESR)** checks for the presence of inflammation in your body.

- **Plasma viscosity (PV)** can also measure the level of inflammation in your body.

- **C-reactive protein (CR)** is another test that is increasingly used to assess inflammation in the body.

- **Red blood cell count (RBC)** checks for anaemia, a common symptom associated with systemic types of arthritis.

(See Chapter 7 for a complete description of these tests.)

In addition to the preceding tests, your doctor may also perform the following:

- **Joint fluid sample:** The doctor inserts a needle into your affected joint(s) to remove some fluid, which is examined under a microscope for evidence of infection or inflammation.

- **Joint X-ray:** An X-ray of your joints is taken to detect early bone and cartilage loss or to serve as a baseline for future X-rays.

- **Biopsy of rheumatoid nodules:** If you have rheumatoid nodules, the doctor may want to cut a piece of tissue from one of them and examine it under a microscope to confirm the diagnosis.

  Here's how the test is done: After carefully cleansing the skin and injecting a local anaesthetic, the doctor makes a tiny cut near the nodule. If the nodule is easily accessible, the doctor may decide to reach in with a scalpel and shave off a piece of tissue. Or, he or she may push a thin, hollow needle into the nodule and gently suck out a few cells using a syringe.

Treating Rheumatoid Arthritis

Although RA is often a chronic (long-term) disease, most people respond well to treatment and lead active, productive lives. A few years back, someone with RA could look forward to a dreary life spent bedridden or in a wheelchair. But today, those with rheumatoid arthritis have a much better prognosis: Only about one person in ten with RA progresses to the point of disability (although one-third leave work prematurely). In a full 70 per cent of cases, symptoms are relieved or controlled by treatment for long periods of time. And one out of ten people completely recovers from RA, usually within the first year, never to be bothered by it again.

Treatment usually begins with the least aggressive, most conservative measure, which is rest, and gradually moves on to more aggressive methods – medication and surgery – if necessary.

Mental outlook appears to affect RA symptoms. Stress tends to make flare-ups worse, whereas a positive outlook can help keep complications at bay.

Relying on rest

Resting your affected joints during a flare-up is a must, because using them tends to increase inflammation. You can build regular rest periods into your daily schedule, and when necessary, indulge in total bed rest without feeling guilty. Immobilising a severely affected joint with a splint may help, but aim to move the joint from time to time to keep it from locking up. You can wear a splint during the most active times of the day, and take it off when you are least active – for example, 12 hours on and 12 hours off.

Delving into your diet

What you do and don't eat can make a difference to the arthritis-disease process and how much pain you feel. Because many forms of arthritis and arthritis-related conditions involve inflammation, eating foods that reduce the inflammation response (such as fish, fish oils, flaxseed oil, black walnuts, and green soya beans) can make a positive difference. By eating plenty of fruit, vegetables, and whole-grains, which supply ample amounts of antioxidants like vitamins C and E and selenium, you can fight the cellular damage that contributes to arthritis. And taking the dietary supplements glucosamine sulphate and chondroitin sulphate can not only reduce pain but, in some cases, even stop the arthritis process in its tracks. (See Chapter 15 to find out more about how what you eat affects how you feel.)

Easing into exercise and physical therapy

An overall exercise programme helps strengthen joint-supporting structures, increase endurance, and helps maintain or improve flexibility. Exercising inflamed joints even a little helps prevent them from freezing up.

A physiotherapist can provide exercises that gently take your joints through their full range of movement. Exercising in water, especially during flare-ups, is usually easier than exercising on land, because it's low impact and the cool water may help to ease inflammation. (Chapter 16 has more on helpful exercises.)

Protecting your joints

Not only do you make your mum happy when you stand up straight, but you reduce the pressure on your joints. Maintaining proper posture while walking, standing, and sitting can go a long way toward easing joint stress. And understanding how to lift or move heavy objects correctly is also a must. (Chapter 17 covers moving well.)

Applying hot or cold compresses

Applying hot or cold packs to inflamed joints eases the pain and helps reduce inflammation. Use heat to ease sore muscles and increase circulation, and try cold to dull the pain and reduce inflammation. (See Chapter 10 for more on pain management.)

Taking medication

Many drugs are used to combat RA symptoms. The following subsections give you details on the main types commonly prescribed.

All drugs can potentially cause side effects. If you experience a problem that concerns you, always tell your doctor.

Non-steroidal anti-inflammatory drugs (NSAIDs)

NSAIDs (pronounced *n-seds*) reduce swelling, relieve pain, and are the most commonly prescribed drugs for RA. Aspirin and ibuprofen are two well-known NSAIDs, but these drugs are typically prescribed in much larger doses than recommended when you buy them over the counter. A dose of 600 milligrams of ibuprofen taken three times a day is a standard treatment for pain for most people newly diagnosed with RA. (Do not take this dosage of ibuprofen or any other medication unless your doctor prescribes it.)

Interestingly, although differences in the anti-inflammatory activity of different NSAIDs are small, there is a lot of variation in the way individual people respond to them. Overall, around 60 per cent of people experience pain relief with *any* NSAID. Of the remaining people, those who do not experience relief with one NSAID may well respond to another – it's all down to your genes and the enzymes you inherited to handle each drug.

As with all drugs, certain side effects can occur when taking NSAIDs, including upset stomach, nausea, diarrhoea, and stomach bleeding. Take this type of medication with food to prevent these physical reactions.

Analgesics

Analgesic pain fighters don't relieve inflammation, which makes them less irritating to the stomach than NSAIDs. Paracetamol, the best-known and most commonly used analgesic, is often recommended as a first-line treatment for RA pain.

Paracetamol is available over-the-counter and on prescription, sometimes in combination with other analgesics, such as codeine and dihydrocodeine. Sometimes a combination of an analgesic and an NSAID is prescribed for intense pain.

Disease-modifying antirheumatic drugs (DMARDs)

If NSAIDs aren't effective, or if your disease seems to be progressing quickly, your doctor may prescribe a *DMARD*, which can potentially alter the course of your disease by reducing inflammation and joint damage, while preserving joint function. This category of drugs includes gold; methotrexate; the anti-malarial drug, chloroquine; sulfasalazine; and leflunomide; to name but a few.

DMARDs are also known as *remittive drugs* and *slow-acting drugs* – slow acting because you may not see the results for weeks or months.

These drugs influence the immune system – whose errant behaviour leads to RA – to slow the formation of bone deformities, affect cell growth, or otherwise slow the progress of RA. These drugs can even send the disease into remission, at least temporarily. Depending upon which drug is used, you may take it until symptoms improve, until unacceptable side effects appear, or until it's clear that the medicine isn't helping you.

Potential side effects of DMARDs include increased infections, gastrointestinal distress (diarrhoea, loss of appetite, vomiting, and so on), liver problems, rashes, and blood cell disorders. If you notice any possible side effects, always tell your doctor.

Corticosteroids

Corticosteroids (or steroids), such as prednisone, are powerful weapons against inflammation. These drugs work by suppressing the immune system, which triggers the errant inflammation seen in RA. Corticosteroids work well because they're 'souped-up' versions of cortisone, the body's natural immune suppressor, and the latest data suggests that they may also have disease-modifying properties. Two studies published in 2002 indicate that steroids reduce bone damage in early RA.

Unfortunately, these strong drugs can trigger severe side effects, including high blood pressure, osteoporosis, an increase in blood glucose, cataracts, and bruising and thinning of the skin. When used in high doses for a month or longer, corticosteroids may cause fluid retention in the face ('moon face'), abdomen, legs, and so on. Because of this side effect, corticosteroids are typically reserved for severe cases, and then used for only short periods of time.

Because they work more quickly than most other therapies, these drugs can serve as a bridge until other medications take effect.

If you suddenly stop taking corticosteroids, you may develop pain, swelling, critical illness, or even death from adrenal crisis. Always taper off your use of these drugs exactly as your doctor advises.

Biologic response modifiers (BRMs)

BRMs are the latest weapons in the war against RA, and have exotic other-worldly names like adalimumab, anakinra, etanercept, and infliximab. These exciting, new therapies – also known as *cytokine inhibitors* – block inflammation by inhibiting certain components of the immune system to alter the course of your disease.

These drugs are quite expensive because they are either injected or infused, but researchers are currently working on less expensive versions to take by mouth.

Each BRM partially disables a 'part' of your immune system; therefore, making you more susceptible to certain infections. For example, those BRMs that block a substance called *tumour necrosis factor* (the anti-TNF BRMs) can increase your risk of tuberculosis and similar infections. Ask your doctor about these risks before taking BRMs.

Saving your joints via surgery

When all else fails and RA becomes severe or disabling, surgery remains an option. Surgeons have different approaches to relieving symptoms, some of which include:

- ✔ Surgically removing diseased joint linings.
- ✔ Replacing a joint to correct deformity and ease pain.
- ✔ Fusing or removing joints in the foot to relieve pain when walking.
- ✔ Fusing vertebrae in the neck to prevent spinal cord compression.
- ✔ Fusing the thumb joint to aid grasping.

Other sophisticated surgical techniques are also on the horizon, which may help to ensure that a healthier and less painful future is available for people with RA.

Modifying risk factors for heart disease

Many studies show that the risk of developing coronary heart disease is much higher in people with RA; in fact, it's the number-one cause of death. Coronary heart disease is most likely the result of chronic inflammation caused by RA speeding up the progression of hardening and furring up of the arteries *(atherosclerosis)*. Most rheumatologists recommend that people with RA exercise, watch their weight, eat a nutritious diet, keep their cholesterol and blood pressure under control, and stop smoking as part of their routine care. Check out *Heart Disease For Dummies* (Wiley) to find out more.

Predicting the outcome

Predicting how a person with RA will fare is difficult as every individual is so different. But certain factors can suggest whether your disease is likely to follow an easier or more difficult path. For example, RA is often less severe if one or more of the following factors applies to you:

- ✔ **You're female.** Women are more likely to get RA, but the disease often takes a greater toll on men.
- ✔ **You have a university degree or better.** Educated people tend to seek help earlier, are more likely to follow doctor's orders to the letter, often have less physically strenuous jobs, and have better access to health care.
- ✔ **You're middle-aged or older when RA strikes.**
- ✔ **Your cartilage and bone ends are not worn away, and you don't yet have joint deformities.**
- ✔ **You don't have rheumatoid nodules.**
- ✔ **Your level of rheumatoid factor is low.** However, remember that some people who have little or no rheumatoid factor can still develop severe symptoms.
- ✔ **You're pregnant.** Some women enjoy nine months or longer with fewer arthritis symptoms.

Perhaps as many as 10 per cent of people with RA enjoy what doctors call *spontaneous remission,* or the disappearance of their disease for no apparent reason – it's almost as if your body miraculously heals itself!

Looking to the future

Today, rheumatoid arthritis rarely manifests as the crippling, deforming disease of just a few years ago. Researchers in genetics and immunology are constantly uncovering new and fascinating parts of this puzzle, and have recently introduced some 15 new drugs to treat RA. Surgeons have also made great strides in surgical techniques, offering renewed hope to those with deformed, painful joints. Through a rapidly expanding arsenal of knowledge, medications, certain lifestyle changes, and new surgical techniques, the medical profession can soon tame, if not conquer, the beast known as rheumatoid arthritis.

Chapter 4

Investigating Other Forms of Arthritis

*T*he various forms of arthritis all have one thing in common: They produce pain, swelling, and other problems in or near one or more joints. Symptoms may appear suddenly and obviously or sneak up so gradually that you can't remember when they began; they may strike with the force of a jackhammer or feel more like a chilly breeze. Sometimes the diagnosis is obvious; other times it eludes doctors for a year or longer. The varied treatments may seem quick and effective, produce delayed reactions or in some cases, hardly work at all.

Osteoarthritis and rheumatoid arthritis, the subjects of Chapters 2 and 3, are the best-known forms of arthritis. This chapter examines some of the lesser-known and less-prevalent, but still troublesome, 'true' forms of the disease, namely gout, pseudogout, juvenile rheumatoid arthritis, infectious arthritis, gonococcal arthritis, Reiter's syndrome, psoriatic arthropathy, and ankylosing spondylitis.

Gaining Insight into Gout: It's Not Just for Royalty

Gout is traditionally viewed as a disease reserved for corpulent kings and beefy barons, but it can affect anyone, even those who are slim and never drink alcohol.

Summarising the symptoms

Some 250,000 people experience gout in the UK, each year, with four times as many men affected as women. Officially known as *acute gouty arthritis*, the problem usually begins with a sudden, overwhelming assault on a joint. You may go to bed feeling fine, with no inkling of trouble ahead, only to wake up in the middle of the night with excruciating pain in the bunion joint of your big toe. The joint feels stiff and warm to the touch and swelling lends a shiny, tight, reddish or purplish look to the skin, which is severely stretched over the area. Sometimes, the joint is so inflamed and painful that even the touch of a bed sheet causes agonising pain. You may also have a fever, chills, a rapid heart rate, and a general blah feeling.

Gout is linked to excess *uric acid* in the blood. (Doctors call this *hyperuricaemia*.) When the blood has more uric acid than it can handle, the body may convert the excess into sharp, pointed crystals and store them in one or more joints. See Figure 4-1 for an example of what the crystal deposits look like in a joint.

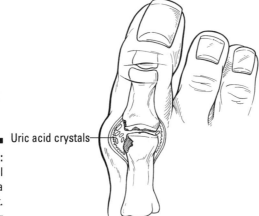

Uric acid crystals

Figure 4-1:
Crystal
deposits in a
gouty joint.

The big toe is often the first site that gout strikes. The elbows, wrists, fingers, knees, ankles, heels, and instep are often also attacked during the first or subsequent bouts, while the shoulders, spine, and hips are rarely touched. No matter where gout strikes first, the odds are three out of four that the big toe is affected at some point.

Your first attack of gout is often also your last, as gout frequently disappears forever after several days, even without treatment, and without lingering after-effects. However, sometimes gout heralds the beginning of a series of attacks on one or more joints, leading to progressive and irreversible joint injury. Fortunately, medical treatment can help ward off recurring attacks while preventing or minimising permanent joint damage.

To guard against gout, the best strategies are to choose your parents carefully, and to request femininity. Women's uric acid levels are lower than men's until after the menopause when women's uric acid levels start to rise (although up to 20 years may pass before they're equal to levels found in males).

Several situations can lead to an excessive amount of uric acid, including:

- ✔ Genetics – 6 to 18 per cent of those with gout have a family history of the disease.

- ✔ Eating lots of offal and other meats, gravies, peas, anchovies, dried peas, and beans. These foods contain large amounts of building blocks called *purines*, which stimulate the body's production of uric acid.

- ✔ Blood cancer or other diseases that cause rapid multiplication and destruction of body cells, leading to higher levels of purines and uric acid.

- ✔ Certain diseases that hamper the kidneys' capability to filter out uric acid.

- ✔ Drinking too much alcohol (which can upset kidney function).

- ✔ Taking drugs that increase uric acid production.

Gout is also associated with high blood pressure, high levels of blood fats, excess weight, and obesity.

Though the disease comes about when excess uric acid is deposited in the joints as crystals, elevated blood levels of uric acid on their own don't necessarily lead to gout. Many people with excess uric acid suffer nary a twinge, while others, with terrible pain, have fairly standard amounts in their circulation. Strangely, you can also have fully-formed uric acid crystals in a joint or two, yet feel no pain.

Diagnosing and treating gout

Sometimes the symptoms of gout speak loudly, making the diagnosis fairly easy; other times, the symptoms are vague, making the diagnosis extremely difficult.

Microscopic examination of fluid taken from the stricken joint is an important diagnostic step. If needle-like uric acid crystals are visible, gout is the probable diagnosis. As part of the inflammation process, white blood cells are often also present in the joint fluid. To diagnose gout, your doctor can order a blood test to check your uric acid levels as well as look for *tophi* (lumps of uric acid crystals stored under your skin). Your doctor may also X-ray the afflicted joint.

Gout has no sure-fire cure, although medications and lifestyle changes can help. Treatment often begins with high doses of *non-steroidal anti-inflammatory drugs* (NSAIDs) for pain and inflammation, and a drug called colchicine to help prevent further attacks. (See Chapter 8 for in-depth coverage of medications.) This regimen is usually only a short-term measure (12 weeks or so), as side effects may occur with long-term usage.

If you have recurrent or disabling attacks of gout, tophi in your blood, your X-rays show evidence of joint destruction, or you have recurrent kidney stones, your doctor may prescribe a urate-lowering drug, such as allopurinol or probenecid, to keep your uric acid levels under control. Corticosteroids are sometimes injected into an affected joint to reduce inflammation.

In addition to offering medicines, your doctor can tap your joint by inserting a needle to draw out any excess fluid. This procedure often helps relieve pressure pain and sometimes is all the treatment that's needed.

Helping yourself heal

The following measures help heal gout and prevent its recurrence:

- Losing weight if you are overweight
- Eliminating alcohol intake, especially beer, which contains *purines*
- Eliminating foods containing purines (for example, organ meats, fatty meats, meat gravies, wild game, sardines, anchovies, herring, mackerel, and scallops) and limiting meat, fish, poultry, dried peas, and beans to one serving per day
- Working with your doctor to keep your blood pressure under control, if it's a problem
- Consulting with your doctor to make sure you're not taking any medicines or supplements that encourage gout or interfere with your treatment
- Exercising regularly

Studying Pseudogout: The Royal Pretender

Although gout is an ancient disease that ruined many a medieval VIP's day, *pseudogout* is a new affliction. Although psuedogout has probably been around as long as regular gout, doctors didn't realise it was a separate problem until recently.

Summarising the symptoms

The symptoms and signs of pseudogout are similar to those of gout but without needle-like uric acid crystals in the joint. Instead, pseudogout is characterised by rhomboid-shaped crystals made up of *calcium pyrophosphate dihydrate* (a complete mouthful, which you can promptly forget – just think calcium crystals). And, although gout typically affects the big toe joint, pseudogout more often targets the knee.

The disease itself may be acute or chronic. Acute attacks strike suddenly, settle in, and last for several days or even weeks. (Fortunately, they are usually not as painful as acute attacks of true gout.) Chronic attacks last longer, typically target more than one joint at the same time and can eventually cause severe joint damage.

The causes of pseudogout are unknown. Surgery, a hormonal imbalance, or a metabolic upset may trigger the problem. Sometimes pseudogout strikes together with other problems, such as low blood magnesium or too much iron in body tissues. Pseudogout affects men and women at about the same rate and prefers older people, especially those over the age of 60 years.

Diagnosing and treating pseudogout

Because pseudogout can masquerade as gout, rheumatoid arthritis, or other ailments, diagnosis is usually made by inspecting fluid taken from the affected joint, although crystals are also visible on X-rays. If you have pseudogout, your joint's fluid contains calcium pyrophosphate dihydrate crystals.

Unfortunately, a complete cure for pseudogout does not exist, and there's no method for removing the offending crystals from the joints. Therefore, treatment mainly involves taking NSAIDs to reduce pain and inflammation.

Sometimes, simply tapping the joint and drawing out excess fluid is enough to relieve pressure pain. Although treatment brings relief during an attack, it can't prevent joint damage.

Understanding Juvenile Rheumatoid Arthritis

Arthritis is bad for everyone, but somehow it seems worse when it strikes children. Youngsters can develop most of the forms that affect adults, and juvenile arthritis affects around 12,000 children in the UK. Many of these have *juvenile rheumatoid arthritis* (JRA), which is similar to adult rheumatoid arthritis (refer to Chapter 3), except that many children outgrow the problem (adults, unfortunately, don't).

An autoimmune disease, JRA causes the body to turn on itself and destroy its own tissue. No one knows just why the immune system goes wrong, but researchers suspect it's a two-part process: The child has a genetic tendency toward JRA to begin with; then something in the environment (such as a virus) sets it off, allowing the disease to develop.

Summarising the symptoms

Three kinds of juvenile rheumatoid arthritis exist with different patterns of symptoms:

- **Pauciarticular JRA:** The most common form of JRA, *pauciarticular JRA* involves no more than four joints. About 50 per cent of children with JRA have pauciarticular JRA, which usually strikes in the knees and other large joints, attacks mostly girls aged 8 and younger, and may only strike one of a pair of joints (one knee rather than both, one elbow instead of two, and so on).

  In 20 to 30 per cent of cases, pauciarticular JRA triggers eye inflammation that, if untreated, can become serious. This particular kind of eye inflammation, called *uveitis*, can occur even in the absence of any eye symptoms, so children with this form of JRA are routinely referred to an ophthalmologist for screening. Fortunately, many children outgrow this disease (although the eye problems can continue into adulthood).

- **Polyarticular JRA:** This form of JRA attacks five or more joints. Striking some 40 per cent of children with JRA, the *polyarticular* form usually settles in the fingers and other small joints, although large joints are not immune. The disease is typically symmetrical, which means that it attacks fingers on both hands, and so on. Fever and rheumatoid nodules can also occur. Girls are more likely than boys to develop polyarticular JRA.

✔ **Systemic JRA:** The *systemic* form of JRA travels throughout body systems, causing trouble wherever it settles. The least common form of juvenile rheumatoid arthritis, systemic JRA can result in a variety of symptoms, including fever, pale red spots on various parts of the body, anaemia, swollen lymph nodes, as well as inflammation of the linings of the lungs and heart.

Regardless of the form JRA takes, it causes joint stiffness, pain, and swelling that is usually worse upon waking from a full night's sleep or even a nap. Symptoms usually come and go. Sometimes a child is lucky – the symptoms arise just a few times and then disappear forever – but a large percentage of children continue to have arthritis into adulthood. Luckily, most of these adults have only mild problems.

Diagnosing and treating JRA

Someone under the age of 17 must experience joint inflammation and stiffness for at least six weeks in order to receive a diagnosis of JRA. JRA is similar to adult rheumatoid arthritis, except for a few key differences:

✔ Many children with JRA outgrow the problem, while most adults with RA do not.

✔ JRA may affect bone development and growth in children, causing slow, rapid, or uneven growth in affected joints.

✔ Less than 50 per cent of those with JRA test positive for rheumatoid arthritis factor, compared with 70 to 80 per cent of adults.

Doctors diagnose and treat JRA in much the same way as the adult version; the treatments are discussed in Chapter 3. In addition to the strict medical treatment, children with JRA need special emotional and social support.

Figuring Out Infectious Arthritis

Infectious arthritis is caused by viruses, bacteria, or fungi that enter the body and settle into one or more joints. Depending upon which germs have invaded, which joint(s) they inhabit, the strength of your immune system, and the speed and accuracy of any treatment, a bout of infectious arthritis is either brief and relatively painless, or serious and unpleasantly painful.

Infectious arthritis is an infection of the joint tissues and/or fluid. Several different germs, ranging from staphylococci to HIV to tuberculosis, can infect a joint. But remember, these are not specifically arthritis germs; they're regular germs that cause staph infections, mumps, hepatitis B, and other diseases. Infectious arthritis only occurs when these germs settle in the joints.

Summarising the symptoms

The nature and extent of the symptoms of infectious arthritis depend on which germ has taken-up residence in your joint(s). In the joint itself, you may experience pain to the touch or with movement, as well as swelling and stiffness. The skin around the joint may be red and puffy. If the infection spreads beyond the joint, a fever or other symptoms may accompany it (although fever can occur for other reasons). Some forms of infectious arthritis can hit strong and fast, so it's important to see your doctor immediately if you have any symptoms. If left untreated, infections can seriously damage your joints within just a few days or weeks.

Diagnosing and treating infectious arthritis

If your doctor suspects infectious arthritis, he or she quickly calls for various tests to firm up the diagnosis. Blood, urine, and joint fluid samples are analysed for infectious organisms but even before the lab results come back, your doctor usually starts giving you antibiotics, commencing with those that kill the usual suspects. Other medicines may follow after your doctor is sure what infection's got you in its grip.

Antibiotics are effective against bacterial infections, and antifungal medicines fight fungus infections, but viruses are another story. Unfortunately, no effective antiviral medications exist. But don't despair if you have a virus; many viruses cause short-lived problems, which clear up on their own.

As well as medicines, your doctor may drain pus from your joint, splint the joint, if necessary, and arrange for physiotherapy. Certain infections can require surgery to wash out the joint.

Getting a Grip On Gonococcal Arthritis

Caused by the *gonococci* bacterium – the same culprit responsible for gonor-rhoea – *gonococcal arthritis* is the most widespread of the infectious forms of arthritis. Summarising the symptoms

Gonococcal arthritis typically strikes hard and fast, with pain flitting from one joint to another. Small blisters can appear on the skin over some or many parts of your body, and your tendons may swell and ache.

Diagnosing and treating gonococcal arthritis

Both men and women can develop gonococcal arthritis. Men are much more likely to know something is wrong because of penile discharge and painful urination; thus, they are more likely to receive treatment for gonorrhoea before it progresses to gonococcal arthritis. Women, who don't have such obvious symptoms, are less likely to receive early treatment for gonorrhoea and more likely to develop arthritis. Women may also develop pain in the abdomen and fever.

The typical patient with this disease is a young, sexually active person with signs and symptoms of venereal disease, so the doctor can often home-in on the diagnosis of gonococcal arthritis during the medical history and physical examination. The doctor then checks for skin blisters and sends samples of various body fluids to the laboratory before making a definitive diagnosis.

Treatment of gonorrhoea with antibiotics is usually successful, although in recent years certain strains have become resistant to both penicillin and tetracycline. Today, the disease is treated by a large number of new and potent antibiotics and, in most cases, vanishes without permanently damag-ing the joints

Running Down Reiter's Syndrome

Reiter's syndrome is the commonest cause of arthritis in young men as it's an immune reaction to *Chlamydia* – one of the commonest sexually transmitted infections. The syndrome can also follow food poisoning with bacteria, such as Salmonella and Campylobacter. Eight out of ten people affected with Reiter's syndrome have the HLA-B27 gene.

Summarising the symptoms

If you develop inflammation of the urogenital tract (especially the *urethra* – the tube that passes urine out of your body), *conjunctivitis* (inflammation of the clear eye lining, and sometimes *uveitis* or inflammation of the iris), plus inflammation of one or more joints, then you're probably affected with Reiter's syndrome. The arthritis usually affects one or two joints – commonly a knee or ankle – which become hot, swollen, stiff, and painful. Fever, painless ulceration of the end of the penis (males only!), mouth ulcers, skin rashes, hard nodules on the soles of the feet, and occasionally heart valve problems or *pericarditis* (inflammation of the heart membrane) can also develop.

Diagnosing and treating Reiter's syndrome

Reiter's syndrome affects 3 per cent of men with a sexually transmitted infection; it's much less common in women, in whom symptoms are usually mild. Diagnosis of the syndrome is based on history and symptoms because no single test can confirm its presence, but investigations are helpful in ruling out other forms of arthritis.

Although no cure for Reiter's syndrome exists, rest, painkillers, and anti-inflammatory drugs usually relieve your symptoms. Antibiotics eradicate Chlamydia, if present, and resolve embarrassing discharge. Sometimes, immunosuppressive drugs, such as sulfasalazine or methotrexate, are needed.

Most first attacks resolve within 2 to 6 months, but recovery can take as long as a year. Unfortunately, the arthritis flares up again in a third of cases, especially after further episodes of sexually transmitted infections. Don't forget those condoms!

Surveying Psoriatic Arthropathy

This form of arthritis adds insult to the injury of psoriasis, because it strikes those already suffering from this scaly skin condition. Fortunately, only about 5 per cent of psoriasis sufferers develop *psoriatic arthropathy*.

Arthropathy means 'disease of the joints', while *arthritis* means 'inflammation of the joints'.

Summarising the symptoms

In psoriatic arthritis, the joints of your fingers and toes get inflamed, swollen, and, in more severe cases, deformed. Your spine, hips, and other joints can suffer, too.

Diagnosing and treating psoriatic arthritis

As specific tests for psoriatic arthritis don't exist, doctors base the diagnosis on your symptoms and, to some extent, your family medical history because it's often hereditary.

Treatment is important, because psoriatic arthritis can cause severe joint damage, but unfortunately, no cure for psoriatic arthritis exists. NSAIDS help to reduce joint inflammation but if these don't work, more aggressive drugs such as methotrexate or sulfasalazine are needed. Certain *biologic response modifiers* (BRMs), such as etanercept and infliximab, have also proven tremendously effective in fighting psoriatic arthritis. Chapter 8 tells you more about medications.

Considering Ankylosing Spondylitis

Ankylosing spondylitis (AS) attacks the cartilage, ligaments, and tendons of your spine, so your back becomes stiff, inflamed, and sore. As the disease progresses, your ligaments and tendons may harden, forming bony bridges between your vertebrae and locking them into place. In more severe cases, AS can turn the spine into an unbending rod, but the disease usually doesn't advance that far. Figure 4-2 shows the difference between a normal spine and one with AS.

In the UK, 200,000 people consult their GP every year because of AS. Five times more men than women are affected with AS, and the young and middle-aged are its favourite targets. As with several other forms of arthritis, AS is most common in those inheriting the HLA-B27 gene, which increases susceptibility; something else (perhaps an infection) must trigger the disease itself, however.

Summarising the symptoms

AS generally comes on gradually, with pain or stiffness settling in the lower back or other joints, such as the shoulders, hips, or knees. The pain or stiffness is often worse at night or upon rising, and then gets better as you start moving around. AS can remain a constant companion, or can come and go.

AS can also cause skin and eye problems, loss of appetite, fatigue, and fever. Some people develop shortness of breath, damage to the heart valves, and problems caused by pressure on the nerves.

a. Normal vertebrae

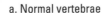

Vertebra

b. Vertebrae with ankylosing spondylitis

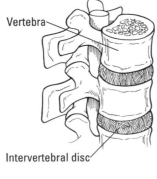
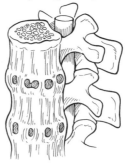

Intervertebral disc

Figure 4-2: Normal vertebrae compared to those with ankylosing spondylitis.

Diagnosing and treating ankylosing spondylitis

No one test can detect ankylosing spondylitis, so doctors usually make the diagnosis on the basis of your symptoms, family history, and a physical examination. Your doctor may ask you to perform various bending exercises to test joint flexibility, and he or she may request X-rays to look for characteristic spinal bone damage. Blood tests can rule out rheumatoid arthritis or other diseases.

Treatment with NSAIDs and muscle relaxants aims to relieve pain and inflammation as well as preventing spasms, which may lead to deformities of your spine and other problems. Although the damage that causes any spinal deformities is permanent, exercises and physiotherapy can help you to remain as strong and flexible as possible, as you work on coping with any deformities that arise. More extreme cases of ankylosing spondylitis may require surgical replacement of a joint.

Though AS has no cure, most people with the disease have mild-to-middling symptoms and do fairly well. One of the most exciting developments in rheumatology over the last few years is the effectiveness of BRMs in treating ankylosing spondylitis; they improve mobility while fighting progression of the disease.

Chapter 5

Exploring Other Conditions Linked to Arthritis

In This Chapter
▶ Discovering the diseases linked to arthritis
▶ Recognising symptoms
▶ Finding out about diagnosis and treatment

*M*illions of people develop symptoms ranging from joint stiffness to skin rashes to difficulty swallowing. Some people's conditions are diagnosed quickly; others are forced to endure myriad tests and bounce from doctor to doctor until they discover what's wrong. Along the way, health-care professionals may mistakenly assume a person's symptoms are due to stress, lack of sleep, or depression, when in reality they're suffering from a condition related to arthritis.

These conditions, which are linked to arthritis, are categorised in one of three ways:

✔ Arthritis is a 'major player' in the disease.

✔ Arthritis is a 'minor player' in the disease.

✔ Arthritis is a 'companion condition' to the disease.

In this chapter, we look at the role of arthritis in each situation.

Experiencing Arthritis as a Major Player

In ailments such as systemic lupus erythematosus and scleroderma, the joint problems that characterise arthritis are a major part of the syndrome. But even though arthritis is present – often in a big way – it isn't the primary disease process.

Systemic lupus erythematosus: The wolf disease

Systemic lupus erythematosus (commonly known as *lupus* or *SLE*) is a body-wide disease that often marks those it affects with a red, wolf-like facial rash. Today, common opinion is that the characteristic SLE rash looks more like a butterfly with its wings spread, but the French doctor who gave the disease its name back in the 1800s thought of a wolf when he saw the rash. The name *lupus*, which means *wolf* in classical Latin, has endured.

Lupus can attack your joints, heart, nervous and vascular systems, skin, lungs, and other parts of the body. Symptoms strike because your body produces large numbers of antibodies – called *autoantibodies* – that attack your own body tissues. No one knows exactly why this assault occurs, but as a result, those with lupus have a higher risk of heart attack, stroke, kidney failure, and osteoporosis than those without the disease.

Ninety per cent of people with lupus are women, and most are in their childbearing years (ages 15 to 45). An estimated 10,000 people in the UK have this disease. A study in the Midlands found that lupus is 2.5 times more common in Asian women and 5.7 times more common in women of African Caribbean origin than in women of European descent. Among men, lupus occurs with equal frequency in Asian and European men, but is 2.7 times more common in men with African Caribbean roots.

Summarising the symptoms of lupus

Symptoms can range from mild to deadly, with problems appearing in your joints, skin, organs, and elsewhere. Typical symptoms of lupus include fever, feeling under the weather, joint pain and inflammation (in other words, arthritis), rash, hair loss, excessive sensitivity to sunlight, anaemia, immune system weakness, problems with the kidneys and other organs, nervous system disorders, and, perhaps not surprisingly, depression.

Lupus settles in for the long haul but tends to hit and run, causing symptoms that flare-up and then retreat. For many people, the good periods can last for weeks, months, or even years.

Diagnosing and treating lupus

Lupus can cause a bewildering variety of symptoms that may mirror those of other diseases, making the diagnosis difficult. Doctors sometimes follow a hunch, tying the fact that the person affected is a young woman to one or more of her symptoms, then ordering tests to confirm or rule out the diagnosis. Blood tests are used to look for antibody abnormalities, abnormal blood chemistries, problems with the immune system, kidney damage, and so on. Biopsies of the kidneys, lungs, or other tissues may be required, as well as X-rays, computerised tomography (CT) scans, magnetic resonance imaging (MRI) scans, electrocardiograms (ECGs), and more.

Treatment of lupus is as varied as the disease. In mild cases, the main thrust may centre on treatments to relieve the symptoms: Non-steroidal anti-inflammatory drugs (NSAIDs) for arthritis symptoms and fever, blood thinners to prevent blood clots, drugs for skin problems, and so on. More severe cases may require prednisone or other corticosteroids to bring down inflammation, immunosuppressants to keep the haywire immune system in check, and antimalarial medications for both skin and joint problems.

Fortunately, you can do several things to cope with lupus. You can't make the symptoms disappear, but you can certainly improve your quality of life by:

- ✔ Cutting back on work or home duties if you tire easily.

- ✔ Looking for ways to reduce stress. (See Chapter 18 for tips on coping with stress.)

- ✔ Protecting yourself from the sun. (This is crucial, because excessive sun exposure leads to both worsening skin disease and disease flare-ups. Complete sun avoidance is advisable but, for even short exposure, use sun blocks *and* protective clothing.)

- ✔ Following your doctor's dietary advice carefully.

Discoid lupus erythematosus: A less dangerous form of lupus

A limited form of the disease, *discoid lupus* generally confines itself to the skin and usually doesn't venture into your body to attack other organs. Approximately 5 per cent of people with discoid lupus progress to the systemic form of lupus; however, a quarter of those with SLE demonstrate discoid disease at some time during the course of their disease.

Summarising the symptoms of discoid lupus

Like systemic lupus, discoid lupus tends to attack women and produces a characteristic skin rash. The rash begins with little, red, disc-like patches, similar in circumference to a drinking straw. Typically appearing on the face, scalp, and ears, the patches may also appear on the upper chest and back, the backs of the arms, and even the shins. Untreated, the rashes may enlarge, growing outwards, with a scar developing in the central area of each disc.

Over time, severe scarring and pitting of the skin, as well as hair loss, can occur.

The rash can come and go, or remain in place, and is often accompanied by joint aches. A drop in your white blood cell count, indicating immune suppression, is also common.

Diagnosing and treating discoid lupus

Discoid lupus is difficult to diagnose because the primary symptom – the rash – can lead doctors to suspect other diagnoses such as psoriasis, actinic keratosis, seborrhoeic dermatitis, SLE (in fact, tests may confirm that it *is* SLE), or other diseases. Because there is no single, conclusive test for discoid lupus, much of the diagnostic investigation is aimed at eliminating other diseases, then diagnosing discoid lupus by default. (A skin rash biopsy is often helpful in determining the diagnosis of discoid lupus.)

Treatment usually consists of sun avoidance and the use of antimalarial drugs to control the disease. If an active rash is present, topical or oral steroids are added to quiet things down. If discoid lupus is detected and treated early, scarring is kept to a minimum.

Scleroderma: Hardening skin

Although it attacks various parts of your body, scleroderma is best known for its effects on the skin. In fact, the name of the disease comes from the Greek words for *hard* and *skin*.

Scleroderma is a collagen vascular disease: Collagen because an excessive deposit of collagen damages body tissue, and vascular because the blood vessels suffer.

No one knows why, but the 1,500 people with scleroderma in the UK produce too much *collagen*, a fibrous, structural material found in your cartilage, skin, and bones.

Unable to dispose of the excess collagen properly, your body starts storing it in harmful ways. Too much collagen in your skin, for example, makes it tight and hard; too much in the internal organs makes it difficult – if not impossible – for them to work properly. To make matters worse, the cells in the lining of your blood vessels begin to grow abnormally. With these vital delivery and waste roads hampered, your body has even more difficulty operating effectively.

Medical professionals don't know exactly why scleroderma develops but immune system errors are a likely candidate. Hormonal upsets are also possible culprits, which may explain why women are much more likely to get this disease than men.

Summarising the symptoms of scleroderma

Symptoms of scleroderma vary from person to person. Scleroderma often begins with joint pain, but sometimes the first problem is difficulty swallowing. The disease may progress rapidly and fatally, or it may confine itself to the skin for years or decades before moving on to attack other parts of your body. Symptoms of scleroderma include:

- **Skin problems:** Thickening, hardening, roughness, and/or dryness of the skin on your fingers, arms, face, and elsewhere. Spider veins (so-called because their thread vein legs radiating out from a central dot resemble a tiny spider) may develop on your face, tongue, chest, and fingers, as well as lumpy calcium deposits under your skin.

- **Joint pain, swelling, and locking:** Pain in your joints can make scleroderma resemble rheumatoid arthritis. As the disease advances, your elbows, wrists, and fingers may lock in a closed position.

- **Difficulty swallowing:** If collagen is deposited in your oesophagus, you may experience trouble with swallowing.

- **Shortness of breath:** Scleroderma can cause scar tissue to accumulate in your lungs and cause changes in blood vessels servicing these vital organs.

- **Digestive difficulties:** If your intestines are strewn with collagen, you may have trouble digesting food and absorbing nutrients.

- **Raynaud's phenomenon:** Many people with scleroderma develop this extreme sensitivity to cold in the fingers and/or toes. (There's a section on Raynaud's phenomenon later on in this chapter.)

Those with scleroderma can also develop a host of other problems, depending upon which organs are over-run with collagen. If your heart is involved, for example, possible symptoms range from an irregular heartbeat to heart failure.

Diagnosing and treating scleroderma

Diagnosing scleroderma is often difficult in the early stages, especially if joint pain and tenderness are your only symptoms. After skin changes or difficulty swallowing show themselves, the identification process is much easier.

After a medical history and physical examination, you usually have special X-rays to check your oesophagus and gastrointestinal system, blood tests to assess lung function, a skin biopsy to search for excess collagen, and other tests to help measure the extent of the problem.

Although there's no cure for scleroderma, various drugs can improve your symptoms, including NSAIDs for pain and inflammation, antihypertensives to lower a raised blood pressure, antacids for heartburn, and so on. Exercise and physiotherapy are important to strengthen muscles and lubricate your affected joints. Severe problems with swallowing may require placement of an artificial feeding tube.

Several self-help measures can help relieve your symptoms and improve your quality of life:

- Protect your skin by keeping it moist with creams and lotions, limiting yourself to short showers or baths, and avoiding strong soaps and household chemicals.

- Use a humidifier if indoor heaters are drying out your skin.

- Diligently perform the flexibility and strengthening exercises that your doctor or physiotherapist recommends. Even if the exercises are difficult to do, they help to maintain your joint function.

- If swallowing is difficult, chew your food well, avoid foods that are hard to swallow, and drink plenty of liquids with your meals.

- If night-time heartburn is a problem, buy an adjustable bed so you can elevate your head. You can get the same effect more easily and cheaply by placing blocks under the legs of the bed frame at the head of your bed. Also, you can try eating dinner earlier than usual or having only a light meal so your stomach is less full at bedtime.

Scleroderma is a daunting condition, and doctors have not yet found a way to stop the overactive collagen production. Still, many people with scleroderma do well for years or even decades, and some enjoy spontaneous remissions, especially when the disease first manifests in the joints and skin rather than in the organs.

Lyme disease: Making you the bull's-eye

This new version of arthritis popped up during the 1970s in the town of Lyme, Connecticut. Local doctors were puzzled when individuals, groups of friends, and even entire families began developing a disease that looked a lot like arthritis, but didn't fall into any of the known categories.

Fortunately, doctors realised that more people developed the disease during the summer than in any other time of the year, that many developed a large, round bull's eye rash, and that the town of Lyme was surrounded by wooded areas harbouring deer and other wild animals. By putting these and other facts together, doctors discovered they were looking at a new disease caused by bacteria called *Borrelia burgdorferi*, which were carried by certain ticks hitching rides on deer in the nearby woods. When these ticks bit people, the bacteria passed into their bodies. And you don't even need to go into the woods to contract Lyme disease – your dog or cat can bring the offending ticks into your home.

Summarising the symptoms of Lyme disease

Lyme disease usually starts with a large red spot on your rear-end, thigh, trunk, or armpit, wherever the tick's had a nibble. The rash may have a blank spot area in the centre, making it look like a bull's eye. The rash may itch and cause pain or feel hot.

About half of those with untreated Lyme disease develop recurrent attacks of arthritis, which manifest as swelling and pain in your knees and other joints, including your shoulders, elbows, wrists, and ankles. These arthritis attacks may last for several months. Unfortunately, up to 20 per cent of those infected may go on to suffer from chronic arthritis.

Other common symptoms of Lyme disease include fever, fatigue, chills, joint pain, muscle aches, headache, and stiff neck; less common symptoms include sore throat, swollen lymph nodes, nausea, vomiting, backache, and other problems. These early symptoms may come and go. Nerve disorders, memory deficits and difficulty concentrating, heart and liver problems, skin disorders, and eye inflammation can also occur.

Diagnosing and treating Lyme disease

The diagnosis of Lyme disease is usually made from a combination of your personal history and the presence of the classic rash. Knowing that you went walking in the woods and that the problems began in the summer, for example, are significant clues.

A blood test looking for the presence of antibodies to *Borrelia burgdorferi* gives a definitive diagnosis. In people showing nervous system disorders, doctors may perform a lumbar puncture to look for antibodies in the spinal fluid. Unfortunately, antibodies don't show up immediately, so it can take a while before a definitive diagnosis is made.

Arresting the spread of Lyme disease is often fairly easy if treatment is started early. Antibiotics, taken orally or given intravenously, can often halt

Staying in the clear(ing): Avoiding Lyme disease

The best way to keep clear of Lyme disease is to make your body a tick-free zone. If you go into the woods or other areas where deer or other wild animals roam:

✔ Use insect repellent.

✔ Use your clothing as a shield over exposed areas of skin.

✔ Wear light-coloured clothes so the dark-coloured ticks stand out if they get on you.

✔ Walk on paths if possible, and stay in the centre of the paths, giving a wide berth to ticks in the grass and bushes.

✔ Admire any animals you come across from a distance.

✔ Afterward, carefully check yourself and your children for ticks. Pay special attention to the hairy areas of your body.

✔ If you live in a tick-infested area or near the woods, make sure your pets have flea and tick collars.

✔ Watch for the tell-tale bull's eye spot on your trunk, rear-end, thighs, or in your armpit. If you find a spot, see your doctor immediately.

✔ If you find a tick and a rash develops, bring the tick to your doctor, because only a certain species of tick carries the bacteria that cause Lyme disease.

the disease's progress and prevent the appearance of arthritis and other later-stage symptoms. More severe cases of Lyme disease can require treatment with intravenous (IV) antibiotics for several weeks. In some people, years may pass before all symptoms finally vanish. Non-steroidal anti-inflammatory drugs (NSAIDs) can help to reduce pain and swelling.

Experiencing Arthritis as a Minor Player

In bursitis, polymyalgia rheumatica, and the other diseases in this category, arthritis is not the major disease process, but symptoms of arthritis (joint pain, inflammation, limitation of movement) are often present in varying degrees. Arthritis thus shows up as a symptom of the disease but doesn't cause the disease itself.

Bursitis: Swelling bursae

Bursae are little fluid-filled sacs strategically placed throughout your body to help reduce the friction of joint movements. Unfortunately, if injured or overused, a bursa becomes inflamed. Infections and certain forms of arthritis, such as gout, can also prompt this inflammation. When one or more bursae become inflamed, you have bursitis.

Summarising the symptoms of bursitis

The normally flat bursae sacs swell with excess fluid, producing pain and often limiting movement. Your shoulders, elbows, and foot joints are common targets for bursitis. See Figure 5-1 for an example of where bursae are located in your shoulder.

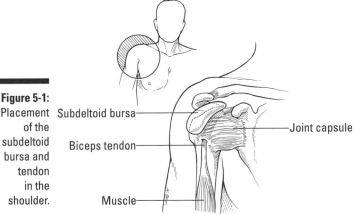

Figure 5-1: Placement of the subdeltoid bursa and tendon in the shoulder.

Subdeltoid bursa

Biceps tendon

Muscle

Joint capsule

The pain and resulting movement limitation caused by bursitis can range from mild to severe. You may have a nagging little pain in one hip or such severe shoulder pain that dressing is difficult.

Diagnosing and treating bursitis

Ultrasound and MRIs are very good at identifying bursitis. Your doctor can also rely on your history and symptoms, as well as carrying out a physical examination of the affected areas to make the diagnosis. Drawing some fluid out of the bursae also helps determine the cause of your inflammation.

In many cases, treatment of bursitis is limited to NSAIDs, rest, and perhaps joint immobilisation. If these strategies don't work, you can have an injection of a corticosteroid directly into the bursa. If a bursa is infected, your doctor may drain it before prescribing antibiotics. Very rarely, in the case of chronic and severe bursitis, oral corticosteroids are required. Exercise can help restore your range of movement and rebuild weakened muscles.

Tendonitis and tenosynovitis: Inflammation of the bone–muscle link

When certain muscles contract or relax, your bones move accordingly. But the bone-and-muscle, contract-and-relax-system depends on your *tendons* – the tough, fibrous extensions at the ends of your muscles that attach themselves to your bones. *Tendonitis* occurs when one or more of these tendons are inflamed. The sheaths surrounding certain tendons can also get inflamed, producing a condition known as *tenosynovitis*.

Summarising the symptoms of tendonitis and tenosynovitis

Most often associated with repetitive motions, over-use, strenuous activity, and advancing years, tendonitis leaves tendons red, raw, and painful to the touch or upon movement.

If the sheath surrounding a tendon dries out and rubs against the tendon, it produces a horrible grating sound or sensation called *crepitus*, which is a part of tenosynovitis. Although usually due to over-use, various diseases, including scleroderma, gout, and gonorrhoea can cause tenosynovitis.

Diagnosing and treating tendonitis and tenosynovitis

Diagnosis of tendonitis and tenosynovitis is based on your symptoms, medical history, and physical examination. Your doctor may prescribe medications such as NSAIDs to counteract pain and inflammation. Corticosteroids or local anaesthetics are sometimes injected right into the sheath surrounding the tendon. Chronic problems may require surgery to remove calcium deposits or release contracted tendons.

The outlook for those with tendonitis and tenosynovitis is good, and the problem often clears up on its own.

A few easy, inexpensive strategies can help to alleviate your pain. You may want to try the following:

- Stop the activity that caused the inflammation.
- Rest.
- Apply hot or cold packs to the area.
- Immobilise the involved joints.

Raynaud's: A chilling problem

Raynaud's involves changes to the small blood vessels in the hands and feet (or less commonly, the nose, lips, or ear lobes) when a person gets cold.

Raynaud's comes in two forms:

- ✔ **Raynaud's disease:** Also known as Primary Raynaud's, this is the more common form. Typically a milder version of the problem, it acts alone when it attacks.

- ✔ **Raynaud's phenomenon:** Also known as Secondary Raynaud's, this is less common. The more serious form of the ailment, it usually accompanies another disease or condition, such as scleroderma or lupus.

Certain types of work increase a person's vulnerability to Raynaud's. Those who operate vibrating tools, who are exposed to vinyl chloride, and who type, play the piano, or otherwise subject their fingers to repetitive stress are more likely to develop Raynaud's.

Summarising the symptoms of Raynaud's

The hallmark of Raynaud's is discoloration in one or more fingers or toes, or the nose, lips, or ear lobes. The colour changes can occur on their own or with tingling, burning, pain, and/or numbness in the affected area. Although many people have cold hands and feet, the characteristic colour changing (fingers or toes turning white or blue, followed by red) indicates Raynaud's.

Spasm of the small arteries that supply blood to these areas causes these symptoms through diminished blood supply. Brought on by cold temperatures and/or emotional stress, the spasm can last a few minutes or go on for hours. Chronic Raynaud's can lead to skin changes, as well as sores on the ends of the toes and fingers.

Diagnosing and treating Raynaud's

Diagnosing Raynaud's is relatively easy, but distinguishing one form from the other is more problematic. Diagnosis and differentiation are made on the basis of symptoms and laboratory tests, such as the antinuclear antibody test and erythrocyte sedimentation rate. Much of the laboratory testing is designed to rule out other diseases.

Treatment for Raynaud's is sometimes as simple as teaching you what to do for yourself and monitoring the situation, or it may include taking powerful drugs. In very severe cases of Raynaud's, nerves to the afflicted areas are cut to provide temporary relief.

Raynaud's is usually here to stay, but you aren't a helpless victim. You can fight back in several ways:

✔ Stay warm all over. (Dress warmly, layer your clothing, and wear absorbent socks and underwear to draw perspiration away from your skin.)

✔ Immerse your fingers and toes in warm water to help keep them warm.

✔ If you smoke, stop. (Nicotine constricts blood vessels, a major problem with Raynaud's.)

✔ Speak to your doctor about switching medicines if you are taking drugs that constrict blood vessels. (Beta-blockers used to treat high blood pressure, and decongestants are common offenders.)

✔ Work on controlling your reaction to stress.

✔ Exercise regularly.

Sjögren's syndrome: Dry mouth, eyes, and maybe more

No one knows what causes *Sjögren's syndrome*, but the immune system is clearly involved. Sjögren's can occur alone or as a part of another autoimmune disease – most commonly RA. In fact, about 15 per cent of RA patients go on to develop Sjögren's. Other disease associations include lupus, dermatomyositis, and scleroderma.

Summarising the symptoms of Sjögren's

Characteristic dryness in the mouth and eyes occurs when those mainstays of the immune system, your white blood cells, invade and damage your salivary and tear glands. The same problem can also cause dryness of the trachea, vagina, the lining of the gastrointestinal tract, and other parts of your body.

About one-third of people with Sjögren's develop an arthritis similar to, but usually less severe than, rheumatoid arthritis.

Those with Sjögren's are more than 40 times more likely to develop *lymphoma* (a cancer of the lymph nodes) than people without the syndrome.

Diagnosing and treating Sjögren's

The combination of dry mouth, dry eyes, and joint distress makes the diagnosis of Sjögren's a simple matter. Tests can confirm that your production of tears and saliva is below par. Further clues are found in the abnormal blood tests.

Antibody abnormalities and possibly anaemia, fewer white blood cells, and an elevated *erythrocyte sedimentation rate (ESR)* – a sign of blood stickiness – are often found.

Symptoms of Sjögren's syndrome are usually readily improved, although a cure remains elusive. Chewing sugar-free gum (it must be sugar free, as lack of saliva associated with this condition causes severe dental cavities), sipping fluid, and using a mouthwash and artificial teardrops helps to keep your eyes and mouth moist. Frequent dental visits are also necessary. A drug called pilocarpine can increase your saliva production. Pain and swelling of the salivary glands and joints are treated with painkillers, but stronger drugs are needed to deal with any trouble arising from damage to your internal organs. For people with severe joint or salivary symptoms, NSAIDs, anti-malarials, or steroids are sometimes used.

The outlook depends upon which parts of your body are affected by Sjögren's. Most people manage reasonably well, but a small number succumb to kidney failure or other problems that arise when a key part of the body becomes too dry.

Polymyalgia rheumatica: The pain of many muscles

No one knows what causes *polymyalgia rheumatica (PMR),* which literally means *pain in many muscles.* PMR typically attacks people over the age of 50 and strikes more women than men. The older you are, the more likely you are to wake up one morning with the muscle pain and stiffness that are the hallmarks of this disease.

Summarising the symptoms of polymyalgia rheumatica

Typically, a woman goes to bed at night feeling fine. But she wakes up the next morning with tremendous pain and stiffness in her neck, shoulders, upper arms, lower back, hips, and/or buttocks. She may say, 'It feels like I worked out too much yesterday – but I didn't do anything!'

However, not everyone develops PMR overnight; sometimes it comes on gradually. In addition to the pain and stiffness, fever, weight loss, and a general under-the-weather feeling are common.

Although the pain can be severe and may seem to resemble that of RA, with polymyalgia rheumatica the muscles involved don't show signs of inflammation,

Seeing through the symptoms

Arthritis and arthritis-related conditions are often not diagnosed immediately. Many people are mistakenly told that their problems are due to stress, lack of sleep, or depression. Even when the disease is identified, the course is not always clear. You may spend money on one medicine after another and seek a number of professional opinions – both orthodox and complementary – in your quest for relief.

The following examples illustrate the experiences of some people just like you:

✔ Recurring chest pain sent a frightened 25-year-old Kristen to her doctor.

✔ Stricken by severe pain on the right side of his belly that suggested appendicitis, Frank found himself in hospital, about to undergo exploratory surgery.

✔ Middle-aged Janice has felt weak and tired for the past several weeks.

✔ After drinking too much at a New Year's Eve party, Rod woke early in the morning with excruciating pain in his big toe.

✔ Terry's fingers have a tendency to turn white, blue, and then red; they tingle, burn, and become numb.

✔ Fever, abdominal and joint pain sent 27-year-old Jennifer to her doctor's surgery.

What do these people, with such different and wide-ranging symptoms, have in common? They all have arthritis or an arthritis-related condition. These people's pain is not all in their heads, and it's not due to depression or psychological problems – their symptoms are absolutely real, and they need careful care.

and the joints rarely show any signs of arthritis. However, inflammation of the joint linings is sometimes present.

Diagnosing and treating polymyalgia rheumatica

With no characteristic joint damage, antibodies, skin rashes, or other obvious signs to look for, doctors must make the diagnosis of polymyalgia rheumatica by eliminating other causes for the pain and stiffness. The person's age is one clue, as most of those affected are over 50. The typically sudden onset of symptoms is another pointer to PMR. People with the disease may also have anaemia and a high erythrocyte sedimentation rate (a measure of blood stickiness), but these are not definitive clues as they can result from many other health problems.

Sometimes your response to the standard treatment, low doses of prednisone or other corticosteroids, clinches the diagnosis. Most people with PMR respond well to low doses of these drugs.

The pain of many muscles that is PMR often disappears on its own or improves dramatically with treatment. Many people do so well that they can start cutting back on their medication after a couple of years.

Fifteen per cent of those with polymyalgia rheumatica also have a life-threatening inflammation of the blood vessels called *giant cell arteritis* (GCA). Symptoms of GCA can include headaches, scalp tenderness, hearing problems, jaw pain, difficulty swallowing, and coughing. If you experience these symptoms, seek medical advice immediately; if left untreated, CGA can result in sudden blindness.

Paget's disease: Becoming too bony

Your bones grow throughout your life. Bones may not grow longer after a certain point, but they are constantly broken down and restored, right up until the end of life.

With *Paget's disease*, the normal break down/rebuild system shifts into overdrive, causing excessive destruction of your bone and poor-quality bone repair. As a result, your bones may become bulkier, softer, and weaker, with a greater tendency to fracture.

Summarising the symptoms of Paget's

Many people with Paget's have no idea that anything is wrong, whereas others suffer from gradual joint stiffness and fatigue. Sometimes your bones become enlarged, deformed, and painful. Secondary problems can also occur, such as pain, osteoarthritis, loss of height, and bow-leggedness.

Diagnosing and treating Paget's

Making the diagnosis of Paget's is fairly simple: X-rays of your bones show abnormal areas of growth, and laboratory tests detect elevated blood levels of *alkaline phosphatase*, an enzyme necessary for bone formation.

Treatment of Paget's depends upon the symptoms – if you don't have symptoms, perhaps nothing is needed. Surgery helps if nerves are pinched by abnormal bone growth, or if a joint no longer functions properly. In more severe cases of Paget's, your doctor may prescribe drugs that slow the disease and reduce pain, such as calcitonin, or drugs used to strengthen bones, such as alendronic acid.

Experiencing Arthritis as a Companion Condition

In these conditions, arthritis is centred in the structures that surround the joint (muscles, tendons, ligaments, and nerves) instead of in the joints themselves.

Although the joints are painful, these maladies don't begin in the joints and aren't classified as *true arthritis*.

Carpal tunnel syndrome: Nerve compression

You may have seen office workers or people working at supermarket check-outs wearing splints on their hands and lower arms to immobilise their wrists. Or perhaps you've noticed people rubbing and shaking their hands, complaining of pain and tingling in their thumbs and fingers.

These people may be suffering from *carpal tunnel syndrome*, a problem caused by compression of the nerve and tendons that pass through the *carpal tunnel* (a corridor between the ligaments and bones in the wrist).

Summarising the symptoms of carpal tunnel syndrome

Carpal tunnel syndrome causes pain, numbness, decreased sensation, and tingling in the thumb, index, and middle fingers that can sometimes spread all the way up to the arm and shoulder. If left untreated, carpal tunnel syndrome can cause the muscles on the thumb side of the hand to waste away, making it difficult to make a fist or grasp objects.

Diagnosing and treating carpal tunnel syndrome

Your doctor bases the diagnosis on your symptoms, medical history, and physical examination and looks for weakness and decreased sensation in your hand. An X-ray may provide helpful information, and nerve tests can confirm the diagnosis. Treatment of carpal tunnel syndrome often begins with a splint, followed by medication to reduce pain and inflammation. Corticosteroid injections into the afflicted nerve can help temporarily. If your problem is related to water retention, diuretics help rid your body of excess fluid. More advanced cases of carpal tunnel syndrome may need surgery to free the trapped nerve.

In addition to these medical measures, look for ways to cut back on – or completely eliminate – any repetitive motion that brings on the pain. Also, look for ways to relieve joint stress. For example, if you type a lot, consider getting an ergonomically designed keyboard or a voice-recognition program.

The outlook for people with carpal tunnel syndrome is generally good; most recover, and only a small percentage of those treated develop permanent nerve injury.

Fibromyalgia: The pain no one can find

An odd situation exists: You hurt, perhaps all over, but your doctor can't find any inflammation or damage to explain the pain. Someone may even imply, 'It's all in your head' and that you're stressed, depressed, or need more sleep.

Fibromyalgia is not all in your head; it's not an hysterical response to stress; and it's not a cry for help. Fibromyalgia is a real disease that happens to have an important psychological component – and that's good news, in a sense, because it means that you can begin doing something, right now, to help relieve your symptoms by controlling stress. (See Chapter 18 for methods of dealing with stress.)

Fibromyalgia affects 2 per cent of the UK population. Women are nine times more likely than men to suffer from this condition and it most commonly shows up between the ages of 45 and 60 years.

Summarising the symptoms of fibromyalgia

Pain and stiffness in the muscles, ligaments, and tendons are the primary signs of fibromyalgia. The pain and stiffness generally occur throughout the body, although they can begin in one area and spread (see Figure 5-2). Fatigue is also a major problem with as many as 90 per cent of people with fibromyalgia experiencing moderate to severe fatigue.

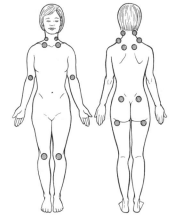

Figure 5-2: Common areas that are painful with fibromyalgia.

Symptoms of fibromyalgia may come and go, and are often associated with sleep disturbances; sufferers may also experience mood changes, numbness and tingling in the extremities, and headaches. No one knows what causes the disorder, but it's often triggered by stress, injury, lack of sleep, infections, and other diseases. Although fibromyalgia is painful, it's not life threatening or otherwise dangerous. However, for some people the symptoms are so severe that work is impossible.

Diagnosing and treating fibromyalgia

Diagnosis of fibromyalgia is often difficult as the symptoms are similar to those of other diseases. Finding the location and pattern of your pain helps your doctor make the diagnosis.

Increasing physical activity improves symptoms and is possibly the most important part of your therapy. Treatment may include medicines to kill pain, local anaesthetics injected directly into painful areas, and antidepressants, which have a beneficial effect on sleep patterns. Massage therapy, along with application of heat to affected areas, and relaxation techniques also help.

For immediate relief from the symptoms of fibromyalgia, try taking a warm bath or applying compresses to sore muscles. And you may have more luck sleeping with a different mattress, a white noise machine to block out disturbing sounds, blackout curtains, and a more comfortable pillow. (See Chapter 19 for the basics of good sleep.)

Overall, the outlook for people with fibromyalgia is good. Fibromyalgia causes no long-term damage to your joints or the rest of your body and is eased with medicine and stress reduction. Check out *Fibromyalgia For Dummies* by Roland Staud and Christine Adamec (Wiley) to find out more.

Polymyositis: A rare sapping of strength

An uncommon disease affecting less than one-tenth of one per cent of the population, *polymyositis* is an inflammation of the muscles that saps your strength.

Summarising the symptoms of polymyositis

In severe cases, those with polymyositis have trouble just lifting themselves out of a chair or brushing their teeth. The larger muscles closest to the torso – the muscles of the shoulders, upper arms, thighs, and hips – are usually the ones affected. But the neck muscles are sometimes also stricken, as well as those used to breathe and swallow. People affected with polymyositis may also experience fever, weight loss, pain in their joints, Raynaud's phenomenon, and feel generally rotten.

Polymyositis can strike at any age but usually hits adults between 30 and 60 and children aged 5 to 15. And once again, the disease prefers women to men, striking women about twice as often. No one knows what causes polymyositis – infections and immune system disorders are suspected, but for once, genetics is not.

Diagnosing and treating polymyositis

Lacking a quick-and-easy test that provides a definitive diagnosis, doctors look for identifying signs and symptoms. These pointers include unexplained muscle weakness, certain microscopic changes in the structure of muscle tissues, and changes in the level of certain enzymes in your blood.

A corticosteroid called prednisone, given to quell the inflammation and help strengthen the muscles, is a standard medication for polymyositis. But although some people respond quickly and dramatically to this medicine, other people don't. Ironically, when used over time, prednisone can cause muscle weakness itself, as well as a host of other unpleasant side effects. So your doctor may eventually prescribe other immunosuppressants, while gradually tapering off your steroid dosages.

Although many children who are stricken with polymyositis can stop their medication after a year or so, most adult patients with the disease continue taking their drugs for many years – or indefinitely. Some adults suffer from progressively more severe symptoms and eventually develop respiratory failure, pneumonia, or other problems, but most are able to keep the disease under control and live fairly normal lives.

Dermatomyositis: Polymyositis plus

With *dermatomyositis*, all the symptoms of polymyositis are present, plus rashes and other skin problems.

Summarising the symptoms of dermatomyositis

Signs of dermatomyositis include a reddish rash on the face, reddish-purple swelling about the eyes, and a rash elsewhere on the body. A violet-coloured rash on the knuckles, known as *Gottron's sign*, is an important diagnostic pointer suggesting dermatomyositis, as other skin conditions tend to produce more redness. The rash is initially raised, smooth, or scaly. With time, the rash fades but may leave behind areas with brownish pigmentation or no pigmentation at all, as well as scarred or shrivelled skin.

Diagnosing and treating dermatomyositis

Dermatomyositis is diagnosed and treated in much the same way as polymyositis. Doctors look for unexplained muscle weakness, certain microscopic changes in muscle tissue structure, and changes in your levels of certain blood enzymes.

To treat dermatomyositis, prednisone or other corticosteroids are used to decrease inflammation and suppress the autoimmune responses that are believed to cause the disease. Topical medicines (creams, ointments, gels, solutions, sprays, or foams) can bring relief to your skin.

Part II
Tests and Treatments: What to Expect

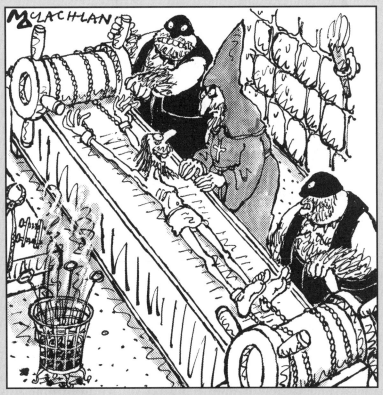

"No, no, carry on – I'm not ready to confess yet – this is doing my arthritis no end of good."

In this part . . .

1t would be great if a single test could tell you whether you had arthritis, which type, and which treatment is appropriate for your condition. Unfortunately, such a test doesn't exist. Diagnosis can be quick and easy, a long and drawn-out process, or anything in between. And making the treatment decisions can sometimes be difficult.

In this part, we explain how doctors go about diagnosing the many forms of arthritis and the high-tech and low-tech tests they may use. We also discuss the medicines they may prescribe and surgeries they may recommend. And, equally important, we show you how to work with your doctor to make treatment decisions, and then how to manage any pain you may suffer.

Chapter 6

Your Doctor and You: Allies Against Arthritis

· ·

In This Chapter

▶ Deciding what you need from treatment

▶ Choosing between NHS and private options

▶ Communicating effectively with your doctor

▶ Deciding if and when it's time to switch doctors

· ·

*N*ot long ago, doctors said, 'Jump,' and patients responded, 'How high?' Doctors were completely in charge, ordering tests as they saw fit, deciding how aggressively or conservatively to attack your problems, pushing you towards surgery or drugs, and generally taking a dim view of alternative approaches.

Fortunately, a real sea change has introduced a new approach to health care today: And although your doctor may not jump as high as you wish, they'll certainly be the one to jump. You and your doctor now work together as a team – with you, the patient, staying more in charge. Research shows that people who play an active role in their treatment tend to fare better than those stuck in helpless passivity. So selecting your doctor carefully, helping to draw up your treatment programme, and then following that programme to the letter, is important. Your odds of recovery improve if you believe in your treatment and pitch in with your recovery efforts, doing everything you can to get well.

Positioning Yourself for Treatment Success

Doctors are experts who are well-trained in diagnosis and treatment – and just as well, since you're putting your health in their hands. Still, doctors are only human, which makes them subject to limitations and foibles just like everyone else.

Although many people think of medicine as a science, it's often just as much an art. For example, doctors frequently follow hunches during their diagnostic work-ups. And although standard approaches, or guidelines, for treating most diseases exist, doctors know that everybody responds a little differently. Thus, most treatment programmes are individualised and change as time goes on – anywhere from slightly tweaked to radically altered.

Because everyone responds to treatment differently, physicians have some leeway when diagnosing and treating you – some wiggle room that also allows for the expression of personality. Some doctors are more aggressive than others; some like the idea of alternative approaches, and others are determined to stick strictly to Western medical techniques. Some doctors like telling you exactly what to do, but others are more willing to involve you in the decision-making process.

Although no degree certificate hanging on the wall is going to let you in on a doctor's treatment philosophy, these framed documents *can* offer some clues. Framed certificates of membership in medical or non-medical organisations dedicated to nutrition or exercise, for example, suggest that the doctor is open to alternative therapies, as do certificates stating that the doctor has attended lectures in chiropractic or herbal medicine. But the best way, by far, to figure out a doctor's philosophy about diagnosis and treatment, is simply to ask.

To help ensure that you get the best treatment, follow these three cardinal rules:

✔ **Select your doctor carefully.** Find someone who is not only thoroughly familiar with and experienced in treating your kind of arthritis, but who is up on the latest research and treatments. Finding such a doctor is often easier in the private sector, but is also important when signing on with a new general practitioner (GP) if you move to a different area.

If you feel that your relationship with your current National Health Service (NHS) doctor is not beneficial to your health, you have a right to request a referral to a specialist for a second opinion. You also have the right to change your NHS GP without giving a reason; however, it's not always easy to find a surgery accepting new patients. The Citizens Advice Bureau can provide guidance.

✔ **Work together with your doctor.** When you consult a doctor, regard him or her as the expert – your trusted advisor. Unless something feels wrong about the advice you're getting, follow it to the letter. Get behind your treatment and do all you can to make it successful – only then can you get the best possible results.

✔ **Research all you can about your condition.** How can you gauge whether your doctor is following correct procedure and doing everything possible to treat your condition unless you know something about the topic? Plenty of information about every type of arthritis, its symptoms, treatments, alternative healing methods, and so on is available from Arthritis Care (Freefone helpline: 0808-800-4050; Web site: `www.arthritiscare. org.uk`) and similar organisations. Appendix B provides more contact information.

Deciding between NHS and Private Care

When you need to see a consultant, naturally you want to have it happen as quickly as possible. Unfortunately, waiting lists are inevitable, as demands on the National Health Service (NHS) are high. Although you may strongly support the dear old NHS, private medicine offers an alternative that can speed-up your treatment process.

You can change to private medicine at any time – before or after you see an NHS consultant, and before or after you're added to an NHS waiting list.

Going private

Don't feel guilty if you choose to go private. Private health care is now an integral part of UK medicine, with private 'pay-beds' in many NHS hospitals and private facilities in many regions contracted to treat NHS patients. If you already have private medical insurance, check your policy to see whether the referral or operation you need is covered. If you don't have private health insurance, contact well-known care providers (such as BUPA and Nuffield Hospitals) who can answer your questions and send out information about treatments, operations, and payment plans. When you have all the information, then you can assess your options and make a fully informed decision about whether or not to proceed.

Only you can decide whether or not to go private, but it can help to discuss the possibility with family and close friends. Maybe people you know have already experienced private medicine themselves and can offer useful opinions.

Getting referrals

If you decide to go private, how do you choose your consultant? Your GP can usually recommend an arthritis specialist in your area who sees patients privately. You can also ring your local hospital (either NHS or private) and ask to speak with one of the secretaries working in the rheumatology or orthopaedic departments; they're usually happy to spill the beans about which consultants see arthritis patients privately.

If only one specialist performs the procedure you need at the private hospital you wish to attend, your choice is obviously limited. If two or more consultants are available, though, how do you choose between them? Many private consultants also work for the NHS for a fixed number of sessions each week and you may simply choose to see a private specialist you already know and trust, because you've already seen them on the NHS. Ultimately, though, your choice may come down to availability and which consultant can see you soonest – private medicine has waiting lists, too!

If you decide to go private, you still need a referral letter from your NHS GP – the good news is that you aren't usually charged for this service. This letter is important as your family doctor knows your full medical history and can provide the private specialist with all the relevant information about your symptoms and previous or current treatments.

If you have private medical insurance, contact your insurers as soon as your GP agrees to refer you. Your insurer foots your bills, so you need to know exactly what they're going to pay for!

Considering costs

You may not have considered private health care because you don't have private medical insurance and assume that costs are high. But you don't need to have private medical insurance, and treatment is often cheaper than you think.

When you're hurting with arthritis, it doesn't hurt any more to make a few tentative enquiries and request free, no-obligation quotations. After all, you don't have to take things further if the financial outlay is too high.

After you see a private consultant and are advised to have further treatment, you receive an estimate of the costs involved. Some conditions are suitable for a fixed-price fee, while others are paid for on an item-by-item basis.

Checking package prices for an operation

When exploring the possibility of a private operation, you need an accurate idea of all the costs involved. Always check what is included in any quotation you receive, such as:

✔ Initial consultation fees before your operation

✔ Overnight accommodation

✔ Diagnostic tests (for example, radiology and pathology)

✔ Surgeon's fees

✔ Anaesthetist's fees

✔ Operating theatre costs

✔ Drugs

✔ Dressings

✔ Nursing care

✔ Physiotherapy

✔ Follow-up consultations after your operation

Although most procedures go exactly as planned, complications can occur (any risks are fully explained to you in advance). If you have to stay in hospital longer than expected, you won't have to pay extra if you accepted a fixed-price option, but extra costs add up if you're paying on an item-by-item basis.

If you need more post-operative consultations than usual, you have to pay for any extra ones not included in your fixed-price quotation.

If you're claiming the cost of your treatment through private medical insurance, your GP usually has to fill in a section on the form. NHS doctors normally charge for this 'private' service, so check whether your insurers reimburse this cost.

Making the most of the NHS

The National Health Service (NHS) has changed a lot since it was first set up, with organisations like Strategic Health Authorities, Primary Care Trusts, Care Trusts, Mental Health Trusts, and Hospital Trusts all now working together to deliver health-care services in your area.

While the NHS offers excellent emergency health care, you often have to wait for non-urgent treatment. One thing the NHS is good at is providing information and advice on all aspects of health. As well as obtaining information from your GP's surgery, you can now also phone NHS Direct, a 24-hour, nurse-led advice service on telephone number 0845- 4647 in England and Wales, and 08454- 242424 in Scotland. For those with access to the Internet, the NHS sites www.nhs.uk and www.nhsdirect.nhs.uk provide information on common health problems and operations as well as pointing you towards health-care services in your area.

It's also nice to know that you're entitled to ask your GP for a referral to a specialist for a second opinion. If he or she agrees to refer you, your GP writes a referral letter to a specialist. However, your GP may suggest that you try various tests or treatment options first, to see if your condition improves.

Choosing when and where

As the government aims to increase the choices available to everyone – not just those opting for private health care – you now have more choice about when and where you receive health treatment. Major changes mean that, in the very near future, you may receive:

- A wider choice of service providers.
- The option to choose the time, date, and place of your first out-patient appointment. You can opt for an appointment that suits you and doesn't clash with your social diary.
- The opportunity to book your appointment yourself electronically. You can book from home or work, after you've thought through all your options – just like booking a holiday online!
- A choice of at least one alternative hospital for surgery, should you need it.

These innovations are rolling out according to a set plan, and it's possible that not all have reached your area. But, do ask about the choice of providers available when your GP refers you to a consultant, as you may find that you can choose between NHS trust hospitals, diagnosis and treatment centres, specialists operating from GP surgeries, and even private hospitals (but with the NHS footing your bills). If you don't ask, you may not get!

If you need surgery and face a wait that's longer than six months, you may be able to choose a different hospital in a different region if this means that you can get quicker treatment.

Tripping abroad for treatment

You may have an option to go abroad for NHS treatment, depending on a number of factors, such as the length of UK waiting lists for the particular treatment you need.

An Overseas Assessment Clinic may invite you for an examination and chat to see if you're eligible, and fit enough to travel. You're under no obligation to accept treatment, and you can turn down the offer and choose to stay on your current waiting list. But, if you agree to have treatment abroad, dates and transport are arranged for you – usually within a matter of weeks.

As this overseas treatment is funded by the NHS, you don't have to pay any of the treatment, travel, or accommodation costs. For more information about overseas treatment, ask your GP or consultant.

Working with Your Doctor

Nothing is quite as educating, enlightening, and reassuring as a long talk with your doctor about your condition. But, for many people, the time actually spent with the doctor seems all too short. Things you wanted to report can slip your mind, and you may miss the opportunity to ask important questions or clarify confusing explanations. A little advance planning helps you make the most of your doctor's time.

Before your first appointment, gather the information your doctor needs and bring the following information along with you to your initial meeting:

- ✔ Any medical records from other doctors, chiropractors, or health professionals.

- ✔ A log of your arthritis symptoms: Start a diary describing how each symptom feels, the intensity of your pain, when it occurs, and what you were doing when you noticed it. A couple of week's worth of information is enough for your doctor to assess how much arthritis is affecting your quality of life.

- ✔ A list of all prescription and non-prescription medications you're currently taking, plus all herbs, vitamins, minerals, and other supplements.

- ✔ A list of all the treatments you've used (including home remedies) to ease arthritis symptoms. Make a note of which treatments help and which do not.

- ✔ Questions you'd like your doctor to answer. For example:

    - How did you determine that I have this particular kind of arthritis?

    - What's causing my arthritis?

    - Do I have any joint deformity?

    - What kinds of treatment do you recommend?

    - What outcome can I expect?

    - Which non-medication treatments do you recommend?

    - Does physiotherapy help?

    - Do I need surgery? If so, how long can I wait before I have it?

    - What happens if I do nothing?

    - What's the cost of my treatment?

- ✔ A notepad: Take notes so you can review your doctor's answers at home when you have no distractions.

Seeing a GP versus a rheumatologist

Whether you need a specialist depends upon the kind of arthritis you have. If you have osteoarthritis (refer to Chapter 2), you may do well under the care of a GP or orthopaedic surgeon when the time comes to consider joint replacement. But if you have a more complicated kind of arthritis, one that involves entire body systems (such as rheumatoid arthritis – check out Chapter 3), you probably need to see a rheumatologist.

Rheumatologists specialise in diseases of the joints, muscles, and bones. They treat arthritis, musculoskeletal pain disorders, osteoporosis, and various autoimmune diseases. An important part of the rheumatologist's job is the proper diagnosis of the disease, because symptoms can point to many different conditions. After the rheumatologist pinpoints the disease, proper treatment can begin, so early and accurate diagnosis is crucial. If you don't have a clear-cut case of osteoarthritis, or if your GP seems baffled by your symptoms, ask to see a rheumatologist.

If, when you get home and review your notes, you find you don't understand an answer or you forgot to ask a question, try calling the doctor's office and asking for a quick phone consultation. The more you know, the better prepared you are to tackle your condition head-on.

Speaking Your Doctor's Language

Although you're not expected to know everything about arthritis terms and treatments (any more than an orchestra conductor has to play every instrument proficiently), you do need to know enough to communicate with your doctor(s) and the other members of your medical team. Knowing about your condition requires a certain amount of education. You needn't become an expert, and you don't have to stay up all night mastering arcane medical terms and memorising medical books. However, you should read all you can about the type of arthritis you have, as well as the medications that have been prescribed, to become informed about your disease.

Consider joining an arthritis support group. The other members understand what you're going through, so they listen sympathetically and can give you helpful advice. You can find support groups by asking your doctors, nurses, or the community support staff at your hospital. Some useful contact details are provided in Appendix B.

The Internet is a great place to find information – unfortunately, you can't treat everything you find there as gospel. Before accepting the validity of what you read, consider who's offering the material, who wrote the material and why, and when it was written. If the information is offered by well-known, reputable organisations, it's undoubtedly good information. However, if an organisation devoted to selling products mentioned in the literature prepares and posts the information you find, take what you read with a pinch of salt.

No matter where you find information, ask yourself who wrote it: A doctor or other health-care professional? A respected non-medical educator? Some guy off the street? Is the author qualified to present information or give advice? Ask yourself whether the article is offered to provide information or to sell a product. Selling products isn't wrong, and some pieces written with the idea of selling are packed with unbiased, useful information – however, others aren't. Do check the date that the information was posted, too. Even a well-researched article may contain erroneous information if it's several years old.

Working Out When to Find a New Doctor

Not every marriage is made in heaven, and not every patient–doctor partnership works out for the best. If you're wondering whether you ought to switch to a different doctor, take a look at the following list (adapted from the article 'Red Flags' by Doyt Conn, MD) and see if they ring any bells for you:

- **Feeling the progress of your treatment is too slow.** Finding the right treatment for you may take your doctor some time, and complete relief of your symptoms isn't always possible. If your doctor is still trying to adjust your treatment, you may want to stick it out a little longer. If not, find someone else.

- **Noticing that your treatment consists of medication only.** Treatment of arthritis is multifaceted and should include non-drug therapies, such as exercise, diet, joint protection techniques, rest, and so on.

- **Realising that your doctor relies solely on NSAIDs.** At one time, non-steroidal anti-inflammatory drugs (NSAIDs, such as ibuprofen, see Chapter 8) were the treatment-of-choice for arthritis, and they are better at relieving the pain of hip and knee osteoarthritis (OA) than paracetamol. But starting with paracetamol and escalating to NSAIDs, if necessary, is usually better because NSAIDs are notorious for causing stomach problems. For rheumatoid arthritis (RA), treatment may require the use of more aggressive drugs, such as methotrexate or sulfasalazine, in addition to

NSAIDs. In some cases, waiting too long to use these drugs can cause irreparable damage to affected joints.

✔ **Finding that your doctor gives you too many cortisone injections.** Injecting corticosteroids into an inflamed joint is a fast way of stopping an RA flare-up or decreasing the pain associated with OA. But over-use of injectable steroids (most experts recommend no more than three or four injections per joint per year) can have serious side effects including tendon rupture, destruction of the joint, and, occasionally, high blood pressure, diabetes, cataracts, and osteoporosis. As long as the injections aren't performed too frequently and are used in combination with other therapies, they are safe and effective.

The best advice is to go with your gut feeling. If something feels wrong or you and your doctor don't seem to click, try finding someone with whom you do feel comfortable. Having confidence in the type and quality of medical care you receive can make a positive difference in your recovery.

Chapter 7

Judging Joint Health with Low- and High-Tech Tests

iagnosing arthritis is sometimes as easy as 1-2-3; or it may take months or even years of following up on clues and running endless tests. With osteoarthritis (OA), the diagnosis is usually pretty clear: Those affected typically are over 40, have pain in a single joint but no swelling, and X-rays show narrowing of the joint space. But with other forms of arthritis, such as infectious arthritis, the symptoms are often more vague: Fatigue, chills, fever, rash, inflammation of the heart, meningitis, and joint aches that may come and go for years. However, doctors have access to many methods that can help narrow down the long list of possibilities and pinpoint a diagnosis. This chapter provides a low-down on the many tests available to diagnose your particular form of arthritis.

Checking In for a Check-up

No single test can determine for sure whether you have arthritis. Instead, your doctor goes through several procedures, such as taking a thorough medical history, examining you carefully, and requesting a series of tests. Together, these clues provide a pretty accurate picture of what's going on in your body.

Presenting the past: Your medical history

Your doctor needs to assemble a great deal of information about your overall health, as well as your specific complaints. The *medical history* includes any questionnaires you answer in your doctor's waiting room and questions your doctor asks you in person. Medical histories commonly include general information, such as your age, gender, and occupation, as well as specific information about

- ✔ Any accidents or injuries you've sustained
- ✔ Diseases that run in your family
- ✔ Illnesses you've had (especially recently)
- ✔ Other problems, including recent weight loss, depression, sleep disturbances, aches and pain, skin changes, and fatigue

The doctor also reviews your activities at work and at home. Knowing that you type eight hours a day may help the doctor connect your hand pain and tingling to carpal tunnel syndrome or discovering that you drink a lot of alcohol may point to the possibility of gout. You may guide your doctor to the diagnosis of Lyme disease by revealing that you went camping in the woods and discovered a rash on your back shortly before your joints began hurting. And of course, you should tell the doctor about any and all of your symptoms, including embarrassing ones like a discharge or pain when urinating.

Don't hold back information because you think it's not important. You may not mention that you have some difficulty in swallowing, because you don't think it's related to your joint and muscle pain. But if you have scleroderma or polymyositis (see Chapter 5 for information on both of these conditions), this symptom is an important piece of the diagnostic jigsaw puzzle.

Looking from head to toe: The physical examination

Even if you have pain in just a single joint, your doctor examines you from head to toe. Your GP is the doctor most likely to perform this initial examination. If you see a rheumatologist or other specialist, he or she probably won't look you over from stem to stern, but still carefully examines all affected and related areas.

How important is the head-to-toe examination? Well, urinary difficulties in men can result from reactive arthritis (Reiter's syndrome), gonococcal arthritis, or something totally different, such as an enlarged prostate gland. Without a thorough examination, the proper diagnosis is easily missed.

Tracing arthritis from dinosaur to tick

200,000,000 B.C.: A dinosaur is struck by osteoarthritis. Examination of dinosaur bones shows evidence of the disease.

2,000,000 B.C.: A prehistoric man develops chronic arthritis of the spine. He may not have been the first human to do so, but he's the oldest of those whose arthritic bones have been found.

8,000 B.C.: An Egyptian mummy has the evidence of his arthritis wrapped up with him.

440 B.C.: Hippocrates, the father of Western medicine, offers the first-known description of arthritis. He described gout as a 'violent attack on the joints'.

Circa 300 A.D.: Arthritis is so endemic in the Roman Empire that the Emperor Diocletian gives a tax break to citizens who are most afflicted with the disease. One reason the disease was so widespread was that ancient Romans used lead to clarify their red wines – lead poisoning in adults can produce arthritic symptoms.

Circa 400 A.D.: Colchicum, a poisonous extract from the Autumn Crocus from which the modern drug colchicine is derived, is introduced as a treatment for gout.

Circa 1600 A.D.: Guilaurne de Bailou introduces the term *rheumatism* and suggests it is a type of arthritis different from gout.

1907: X-rays are added to doctors' diagnostic arsenal, allowing them to further distinguish one type of arthritis from another.

1949: Rheumatoid factor, the antibody that plays a role in rheumatoid arthritis, is discovered. In the same year, cortisone is introduced as a treatment for this disease.

1951: Drugs are first used to suppress an errant immune system and modify the course of rheumatoid arthritis.

1960: Surgeons begin performing total joint replacement.

Early 1960s: The urate crystals that cause gout are identified, and new drugs to control the disease introduced.

1963: The introduction of indometacin, a new non-steroidal anti-inflammatory drug that blocks the action of the enzyme cyclo-oxygenase, takes the control of arthritic inflammation one step further.

1977: Lyme disease is recognised and named.

1998: A new class of drugs, the biological response modifiers (BRMs), takes arthritis treatment in a new direction by inhibiting certain components of the immune system, called cytokines, to ease stubborn cases of joint inflammation.

At some point, the examination focuses on your painful joint(s). Your doctor particularly wants to know:

- How many joints are affected?
- Does pain affect the same joints on both sides of the body?
- Is the joint red, swollen, warm, or tender to the touch?

The doctor may ask you to bend and straighten your affected joint(s) several times to determine the full range of motion. You can expect to have your joint(s) manipulated by the doctor and felt for joint cracking and pain upon bending and flexing. Your doctor also examines any related areas and checks your reflexes and muscle strength.

The doctor may ask you to walk, sit, rise from a chair, bend, and do other movements so they can assess the way you use your joints. You may be asked to reach for something or make a fist around a pencil so the doctor can estimate the way your condition affects your ability to perform daily activities. You and your doctor need to discuss in detail the kind and amount of pain you're experiencing, and you need to answer questions specifically geared to the pain itself. You may want to think about these issues before you see your doctor so you can have your answers ready. The following is a pain checklist that you can use to check-off symptoms, write in your own comments, and take with you to your doctor's appointment.

- ✔ Is it an ache, a burn, a throb, or a stabbing pain?
- ✔ Does the pain come and go, or is it constant?
- ✔ What activities or movements make your pain worse?
- ✔ What makes your pain recede?
- ✔ Are you stiff in the morning?
- ✔ Do your joints lock up?
- ✔ Is your pain more intense at certain times of the day?
- ✔ How does your condition affect your work and home life?

Rating your pain on a scale of one-to-ten, with ten indicating intolerable pain, may also be helpful.

Keeping a pain or symptom diary for several days or weeks before visiting your doctor helps you paint a more accurate picture of your pain and other problems.

Explaining X-rays and Scans

To understand what's making your knee hurt, your hip ache, or your finger swell, your doctor needs to take a peek inside the affected joint. Luckily, looking inside your joint is painless; several bits of sophisticated equipment are designed to do just that via X-rays and scans, while you just relax on a table.

Exposing the benefits of an X-ray

An X-ray is one of the first tools a doctor uses when gathering information to make a diagnosis. X-rays are useful in distinguishing between two of the most common forms of arthritis, osteoarthritis (OA) and rheumatoid arthritis (RA), and also help to diagnose gout, reactive arthritis, and ankylosing spondylitis.

X-rays are particularly helpful in confirming that cartilage and/or joint damage exist and can also confirm that ankylosing spondylitis and similar conditions are present.

In osteoarthritis, roughened bone ends, cartilage deterioration, uneven narrowing of the joint space, bony spurs, and thickened bone ends clearly show up on an X-ray. A joint afflicted with RA shows tissue swelling, decreased bone density, narrowing of the joint space in an even manner, and, possibly, bone erosion. In ankylosing spondylitis, X-rays reveal inflammation, small bony growths, and changes in your sacroiliac joints, of which you have two in your pelvis just beneath your spine.

X-rays are helpful in detecting rheumatoid arthritis, osteoarthritis, and reactive arthritis, but aren't so useful in diagnosing Raynaud's phenomenon or bursitis.

Seeing more with a scan

Sometimes a standard X-ray can't tell the doctor what he or she needs to know, because X-rays don't produce images of soft tissue or give a three-dimensional view. CT scans and MRIs come in handy at this point.

- ✔ **CT scans:** The CT scan (which stands for *computerised tomography*) is a marriage of X-rays and computer technology in which a series of X-rays of one area are taken from different angles. The computer builds these images into three-dimensional pictures, which are helpful for examining organs, such as the lung or gastrointestinal (GI) tract that are affected by diseases like lupus.

  Unlike MRIs, CT scans are completed in 15 to 30 minutes, make minimal noise and, because the machine isn't tunnel-shaped (CT machines are shaped more like doughnuts), they don't cause claustrophobia.

- ✔ **MRI scans:** MRI stands for *magnetic resonance imaging*. Magnetism, radio waves, and a computer are used to create detailed images of body structures. MRIs are especially helpful in diagnosing ailments that affect soft tissues and may detect OA even before symptoms are present. Some experts use MRI scans when they suspect a case of early RA, to detect erosions in the joints that are too subtle to see on X-rays.

For a traditional MRI scan, you lie on a narrow table that is wheeled inside a tunnel-like scanner. Unfortunately, you must lie perfectly still, you can feel claustrophobic while squeezed inside the tunnel, and the machine makes a great deal of noise – plus the scan can go on for as long as an hour and a half! The new open-MRI scanner is more comfortable, less noisy, and less likely to cause claustrophobia because it's similar to a tanning bed that's open on the sides.

Backing Up a Diagnosis with Biopsies and Blood Tests

Sometimes the best way to figure out what's going on inside your body is to take samples of blood or tissue for a close-up look. Doctors use blood tests and biopsies to develop a full picture of what's happening inside you.

Taking tissue for a biopsy

A *biopsy* is a sample of tissue taken from a diseased area of the body, which is analysed by a lab to help determine the cause of the problems. A joint biopsy, which involves taking a sample of the joint lining or synovial membrane, helps to determine why a joint is swollen or painful. A joint biopsy can diagnose gout, pseudogout, bacterial infections, lupus, reactive arthritis, and rheumatoid arthritis.

Diagnoses of some forms of arthritis may require samples of skin, muscle, kidneys, liver, and even arteries or nerves. For example, a muscle biopsy helps in the diagnosis of polymyositis, a skin biopsy is sometimes necessary to confirm diagnoses of psoriatic arthritis, lupus, or scleroderma, and a temporal artery biopsy helps to diagnose giant cell arteritis.

Testing your blood

Blood tests can help confirm a tentative diagnosis or rule out other causes of joint pain. Certain substances found in your blood can indicate inflammation, infections, muscle damage, or other signs of a particular type of arthritis. For example, the presence of RA factor suggests rheumatoid arthritis; certain antibody abnormalities can suggest lupus; and the presence of antibodies to *Borrelia burgdorferi* indicate Lyme disease. However, blood abnormalities can point to many different diseases, so these tests are usually used to supply diagnostic clues only.

Common blood tests for the various kinds of arthritis include:

- **Erythrocyte sedimentation rate (ESR):** During inflammation, your red blood cells *(erythrocytes)* clump together, becoming heavier than normal. When left to stand in a test tube, these heavy red blood cells fall faster than normal. The rate at which your red blood cells settle in a one-hour period is called the *erythrocyte sedimentation rate* or *ESR*. A high ESR indicates inflammation.

- **Plasma viscosity (PV):** Another test that assesses the level of inflammation in your body and measures the stickiness of your blood due to the presence of inflammatory proteins.

- **C-reactive protein (CRP):** A test used to assess inflammation in your body by measuring levels of a specific inflammatory protein.

- **Fluorescent antinuclear antibody (FANA):** More than 95 per cent of people with lupus have *antinuclear antibodies (ANA)* that attack the *nuclei* (command centre) of healthy cells. The fluorescent dye used in the FANA test shows these antibodies clinging to the cell nuclei. Besides those with lupus, up to 40 per cent of people with RA and even some healthy people test positive for ANA.

- **Anti-DNA and anti-Sm:** If the FANA test is positive, your doctor also looks for antibodies to *DNA* (your genetic material) and *Sm*, another substance found in the nucleus of your cells. Antibodies to either DNA or Sm or both are commonly found in those with lupus. Because these antibodies are rarely present in the blood of people who don't have lupus, this test is a reliable diagnostic tool. If the FANA test was negative, these tests are unnecessary.

- **Blood chemistries:** Abnormal amounts of various substances can indicate the possibility of certain forms of arthritis. A high level of *uric acid*, for example, is sometimes a sign of gout. High levels of *creatinine* indicate disturbed kidney function, which may point to lupus or another connective tissue disease.

- **Complement:** A group of blood proteins that are activated as part of the immune process, the *complement system* releases substances that kill bacteria and send white blood cells rushing to fight off invaders. A low complement level suggests your immune system is working in overdrive and that you may have a disease, perhaps lupus.

✔ **Complete Blood Count (CBC):** Although the presence of arthritis can't be confirmed by a CBC, it can be indicated. For example, a low red blood cell count (*anaemia*) is often a sign of chronic inflammation, and is found in rheumatoid arthritis, Sjögren's syndrome, and polymyalgia rheumatica. A high white cell count may signal some kind of infectious arthritis, such as Lyme disease or gonococcal arthritis. Low levels of blood platelets may be an indication of lupus.

✔ **Rheumatoid factor (RF):** About 80 per cent of people with rheumatoid arthritis have an antibody called *rheumatoid factor* (RF) in their blood. Like the chicken and egg, no one is quite sure which comes first – whether RF causes the disease or is the result of the immune system's reaction to the disease. Although rheumatoid factor is a pretty good indicator of rheumatoid arthritis, some people with RA don't have it, and some who do have the factor don't have RA. Like most blood tests, RF must be factored in with other symptoms before an accurate diagnosis is made.

These are not the only blood tests that your doctor may request, and the examples here are not the only reasons for using them; however, they are commonly used.

Taking Other Tests on the Road to Diagnosis

Doctors often have a good idea of what's wrong after listening to you describe your symptoms, examining you, and considering your medical history. With many forms of arthritis, your doctor may need nothing more than an X-ray or scan, a blood test, or a biopsy to confirm the diagnosis. However, sometimes more testing is necessary. If, for example, your doctor suspects that you have gout, you may have a sample of joint fluid examined in the laboratory. If your doctor feels that ankylosing spondylitis is likely, genetic testing is useful.

Joint aspiration

Your doctor may want to insert a needle into one or more of your affected joints to withdraw a small amount of fluid for examination under a microscope. Drawing out additional fluid also relieves pain and pressure inside your joint if swelling is intense.

Called *joint aspiration* or *tapping a joint*, the area is first sterilised, then numbed with a local anaesthetic before a needle is inserted to pull out a small amount of fluid (as little as a couple of drops or as much as a table-spoon or two), which is sent to a laboratory for analysis.

Healthy joints contain clear fluid; anything else probably indicates a problem. Blood in the fluid may result from a substantial injury to the joint. Cloudy fluid or the presence of large numbers of white blood cells can indicate infectious or inflammatory arthritis. Crystals in the fluid are probably due to gout or pseudogout. Bits of cartilage or bone in otherwise clear fluid usually indicate osteoarthritis.

Arthroscopy

An *arthroscope* (a fibre-optic camera about as big in circumference as a straw) is inserted into your joint through a small incision, allowing the doctor to view your joint's insides in all their glory. Your orthopaedic surgeon may use an arthroscope as a diagnostic tool or even as a way of performing surgery inside your joint to repair torn cartilage, cut away inflamed or diseased tissue, remove bits of bone or cartilage, or to reconstruct torn ligaments.

Recent studies have stirred-up controversy, as arthroscopic surgery did not produce any better effects on pain relief and joint function than placebo surgery, in which people had arthroscopic tools inserted into a joint with no corrections made. So although it's still used for diagnostic and surgical purposes, the exact role of arthroscopy remains uncertain.

Genetic testing

Scientists have discovered that certain genes are associated with certain types of arthritis. The genetic marker HLA-B27, for example, is often found in those with ankylosing spondylitis, and HLA-DR4 occurs in 80 per cent of adults with RA. Doctors can't rely solely on genetic testing, because many people who have these genes do not get arthritis, and many who have arthritis don't possess these genes. But genetic tests may show an inclination toward developing a particular kind of arthritis.

Urine testing

In this test, your urine is examined for protein, red blood cells, and other abnormal substances. Protein or red blood cells in the urine is an indication of kidney disease, which is often seen in lupus. Protein in the urine can also result from toxicity caused by certain medications used to treat arthritis, including gold therapy and penicillamine.

Chapter 8

From Aspirin to Steroids: Medicines for Arthritis

*M*any of the medicines doctors prescribe for arthritis are briefly described in this chapter. Naturally, whether any of these medications is right for you is a decision that you and your doctor can make together.

Talking to Your Doctor

Your doctor's job is to diagnose and treat you, but this important task needs your invaluable help. Your doctor has to be thoroughly familiar with all of your symptoms so that he or she can diagnose and treat your condition properly – and you're the only one who can supply that information. Your doctor needs to ask a lot of questions to build a 'knowledge database', but he or she probably won't think of everything, so:

✔ List everything that's bothering you. You should relate every little symptom and problem, whether physical, mental, or emotional.

✔ Tell your doctor about all of your allergies and any allergic reactions you've had to any medications over the years.

✔ List every prescription and non-prescription medicine you're taking, as well as any vitamins, minerals, amino acids, herbs, other supplements, weight-loss products, muscle builders, and so on.

✔ List every medicinal cream or ointment you're using.

- ✔ If you're pregnant, planning a baby, or are breast-feeding, make sure you mention this to your doctor.
- ✔ Inform the doctor if you're on hormone replacement therapy.
- ✔ Tell the doctor what chemicals, liquids, or fumes you're exposed to at work and at home.
- ✔ Explain the tasks you handle at work and home, and tell your doctor about your hobbies and recreational activities.

Tell your doctor all about yourself, your job, your habits, and everything you're ingesting. Tell him or her about your previous experience with medicines, even if it was good. (Knowing that you tolerated a certain drug well may help your doctor choose a new medicine for you, or it may persuade them to stick with the same one.) The more your doctor knows about you, the better off you are. If you're not asked for the information, volunteer it.

The following questions are good ones to ask your doctor concerning any medications prescribed for you:

- ✔ How do I take this drug, exactly? (With or without food, in the morning, with fluid, after shaking the bottle, and so on.)
- ✔ What activities are unsafe while I'm taking this medication? (For example, can I drive? Take other medicines? Take my vitamins?)
- ✔ Are there any drugs, supplements, foods, or anything else that I should avoid while I'm taking this medicine?

Doctors love to use big words, especially when talking about drugs. When you talk to your doctor, you're likely to hear words like *analgesic*, *antimalarials*, *NSAIDs*, and *immunosuppressants* tossed around. If your doctor uses any word that you don't understand, ask for a definition. You may also want to ask your doctor to spell the word for you.

Uncovering Specific Medicines for Specific Types of Arthritis

Before deciding exactly which drug to prescribe, doctors first consider which class of medication is best. Doctors can choose from five main classes, each of which is explored in the following subsections.

It's not just gulp and swallow

Medicines are tricky. Some medicines are best absorbed on an empty stomach, so are taken between meals. Others can irritate the stomach, and are best taken with food. You take some long-lasting medicines once a day; others only work for a brief period of time and are taken two, three, or even four times a day. Sometimes, having a constant level of the drug in your body is necessary, so you need to take it according to a rigid schedule. Other drugs are taken whenever you feel they're necessary. Some medicines mix well with others, and some don't.

Taking medicines involves more than gulp and swallow. Ask your doctor for precise instructions on taking all your medicines: When, how (for example, with or without food), how often, and so on. Ask what to do if you forget to take a dose – do you take it when you remember, miss it out, or take a double dose when your next one is due? Ask what side effects you can expect, which of them are dangerous, and which are not. If your doctor doesn't tell you all about the medicine(s), don't be afraid to ask!

New classes of drug are under development all the time, however, and the list is undoubtedly set to expand. Doctors may also prescribe muscle relaxants, sleeping pills, anti-anxiety drugs, or opiate painkillers. And, when treating certain forms of arthritis and related conditions, doctors may prescribe drugs that deal with problems extending beyond the joints. For example, people with Raynaud's phenomenon are often treated with drugs normally thought of as heart medications, such as *vasodilators*, to open up (dilate) the blood vessels and increase circulation to the extremities.

No matter what medication you take, get complete instructions from your doctor, and follow those instructions carefully. If anything seems amiss or if you have any questions, ask your doctor!

If you have difficulty remembering to take tablets at a set time of day, try setting the alarm on a digital wrist-watch (or your mobile phone) to help you remember.

Fighting pain with analgesics

If you have arthritis pain without inflammation (that is, without heat, redness and swelling, as is often the case with osteoarthritis or fibromyalgia), your doctor may recommend an *analgesic* that fights pain but does not interfere with the inflammation process.

Generic name, brand name, generic equivalent: I'm so confused!

A *generic name* is a medication's official chemical moniker. A *brand name,* on the other hand, is a proprietary name given to the medication by the pharmaceutical company that owns it. When a drug is first launched, it is available only in the branded version. After the patent (which has a limited timespan) runs out, other companies can start making the generic equivalent of that drug, too (and may even give it their own brand name!).

Generic names often tell you something about the drug's structure or chemical formula and they tend to be dull and unpronounceable. But brand names are often chosen with an eye toward prescribing sizzle. For example, a fictional drug with the generic name of codswallop sulphate may have a brand name such as Painstop.

You can quickly distinguish generic from brand names by looking at how they're written: Generic names begin with lowercase letters;

brand names start with capitals. (This rule doesn't apply when the drug name appears at the beginning of a sentence, or is written on a product's packaging, of course, where it is nearly always capitalised.)

A *generic equivalent* is a drug whose active ingredients are chemically identical to the drug your doctor prescribes under its brand name, but the inactive ingredients (binders, fillers, and so on) may vary.

In the UK, most doctors prescribe the generic name of a drug, and it's up to the pharmacist to supply the cheapest version available to help save money for the NHS. Therefore, you may receive a different version of the drug when you fulfil a prescription, if that drug is no longer under patent. You may find being prescribed a different drug confusing – if you are concerned that you don't have your usual medicine, check with the pharmacist.

Paracetamol

Paracetamol is the most commonly used first-line treatment for osteoarthritis pain. This analgesic works through a direct effect on the brain to kill pain (and also to lower a fever). Paracetamol does not reduce swelling or stiffness and does not irritate the stomach lining.

Side effects of paracetamol are rare but include rashes and blood problems. Liver damage is possible when large amounts of paracetamol are consumed, especially with alcohol. Never exceed the stated dose.

Don't take more than one product containing paracetamol at a time. If in doubt, ask your pharmacist for advice.

Codeine

Codeine is an opiate analgesic prescribed for short-term, mild-to-moderate pain. This analgesic works directly on the nervous system to reduce the transmission of pain signals. Codeine also changes the way you feel pain so, although you still have pain, it doesn't seem to matter any longer.

Codeine is highly constipating. To avoid bringing your bowels to a grinding halt, codeine is best reserved for short-term use.

A combination of paracetamol plus codeine may work better than either alone. The name for this blend is co-codamol and low doses are available over the counter.

Dihydrocodeine

Dihydrocodeine is codeine's older brother – it works in a similar way, shows more strength, but is more likely to induce nausea. This analgesic is often combined with paracetamol to treat rheumatic pains.

Do not take dihydrocodeine regularly over the long term as it is both highly constipating and potentially addictive.

A combination of paracetamol plus dihydrocodeine, called co-dydramol, is useful for more intense pain. Low doses of co-dydramol are available over the counter, but stronger doses require a prescription.

Fentanyl

Fentanyl is an opiate analgesic prescribed to relieve chronic, intractable pain. This analgesic commonly comes in the form of a skin patch, through which the drug is slowly and continuously released into the body. Each patch is designed to last for 72 hours before it is removed and replaced. The effects of the first patch may take a day or so to feel.

Some possible side effects of fentanyl include nausea or vomiting, constipation, drowsiness, breathing problems, dry mouth, sweating, headache, flushing, dizziness, palpitations, mood changes, and difficulty urinating. The patches can also cause local effects such as rash, redness, and itching.

Buprenorphine patch

The buprenorphine patch is the latest weapon in the arthritis-painkilling armoury. This patch is especially helpful for those who cannot take other painkillers or who forget to take their medication.

The patch contains buprenorphine, an opiate analgesic related to morphine. You apply the patch to intact, relatively hairless skin – often on the upper outer arm, upper chest, upper back or the side of the chest. If no hairless skin is available, hair should be cut with scissors, not shaved. The maximum painkilling effect is achieved within three days. The patch is replaced every seven days. The patch site may develop redness, rash, or itching. If you develop a skin reaction, tell your doctor who can advise on whether or not you should stop using the patches.

The buprenorphine patch affects your ability to drive and use machines.

Possible side effects of the buprenorphine patch include headache, dizziness, constipation, dry mouth, nausea, loss of appetite, sweating, confusion, insomnia, nervousness, anxiety, depression, and shortness of breath.

Swallowing non-steroidal anti-inflammatory drugs (NSAIDs)

NSAIDs (pronounced EN-seds) block an enzyme called _COX_ (_cyclo-oxygenase_). Blocking the COX enzyme interferes with the way that the body produces inflammatory substances and helps to reduce pain, swelling, and inflammation.

To complicate matters, there are two main COX enzymes in the body, named imaginatively: COX-1 and COX-2. Some NSAIDs are _non-selective_, and block both enzymes, while others are _highly selective_ and block mainly COX-1 (for example, aspirin) or COX-2 (celecoxib, for example).

Widely used for many forms of arthritis, NSAIDs are mainly only available on prescription, but you can buy ibuprofen over-the-counter.

Although over-the-counter versions have lower dosages and are generally well-tolerated, all NSAIDs are associated with numerous side effects that include: Nausea, diarrhoea, peptic ulceration, rashes, breathing problems, headache, dizziness, nervousness, depression, drowsiness, insomnia, tinnitus (ringing in the ears), and blood disorders. Rarely, kidney and liver problems can occur as a side effect, too.

NSAIDs are not prescribed for people with active peptic ulcers, and are best avoided in those with previous peptic ulceration. If you are at risk for a peptic ulcer, ask your doctor if an NSAID is really the best medicine for you.

Recent NSAID concerns

Because NSAIDs can cause stomach upsets, there was a trend for doctors to prescribe the newer COX-2 inhibitors, which are less likely to irritate the stomach. Unfortunately, a recent study published in the *British Medical Journal* showed an increased risk of heart attack in people taking some NSAIDs, especially the newer COX-2 inhibitors. As a result, one COX-2 inhibitor, rofecoxib, has been voluntarily withdrawn from the market. Another, valdecoxib, is now also unavailable due to an increased risk of serious skin reactions.

Doctors are now increasingly wary of prescribing NSAIDs, and guidelines suggest that the lowest possible dose is given for the shortest possible time. COX-2 inhibitors are best avoided in people with existing coronary heart disease.

Aceclofenac

Aceclofenac is licensed to treat pain and inflammation in people with rheumatoid arthritis, osteoarthritis, and ankylosing spondylitis.

Acematacin

Acemetacin is derived from indometacin (see the upcoming section) and, as well as its ability to relieve the pain and inflammation of rheumatic and other muscle-and-joint problems, is also used to treat post-operative pain.

Aspirin

Although usually thought of as a pain reliever, aspirin is actually an NSAID used to reduce the pain, inflammation, and even fever of some forms of arthritis.

Some possible side effects of aspirin include indigestion, heartburn, nausea, and bleeding stomach ulcers. Aspirin can also lead to tinnitus (ringing in the ears) and, as it has a blood thinning action, may mean that you bleed longer after a cut. Aspirin is not given to children under the age of 16 years.

Azapropazone

Azapropazone is restricted for use in people with rheumatoid arthritis, ankylosing spondylitis, and acute gout – and only when other NSAIDs have been tried and failed. Azapropazone has a tendency to cause rashes and people taking it also need to avoid direct exposure to sunlight (or use total sunblock) as it increases skin sensitivity to ultra-violet light.

Only low doses are given to people aged over 60 years to reduce the risk of peptic ulceration.

Benorilate

Benorilate is an interesting combination of an analgesic (paracetamol) and an NSAID (aspirin) chemically joined together. Two grams of benorilate supplies just over 1 gram of aspirin and just under 1 gram of paracetamol. Benorilate reduces mild-to-moderate pain and its possible side effects are the same as those of both aspirin and paracetamol.

Celecoxib

Celecoxib is a selective COX-2 inhibitor. This drug is used to relieve the pain, inflammation, and stiffness of osteoarthritis and rheumatoid arthritis with fewer of the gastrointestinal side effects seen with standard NSAIDs.

Although designed to have fewer side effects, celecoxib may cause flatulence, insomnia, sore throat and mouth, sinusitis, constipation, palpitations, fatigue, pins and needles, muscle cramps, and, rarely, taste alteration and hair loss (alopecia). Although this seems like a long list, most people tolerate cele-coxib well.

Dexketoprofen

This NSAID is used for short-term treatment of mild-to-moderate pain, and is especially helpful for women with painful periods.

Diclofenac sodium

Diclofenac sodium (also available as diclofenac potassium) is used to treat the joint pain, swelling, inflammation, and stiffness of osteoarthritis, rheuma-toid arthritis, juvenile arthritis, and ankylosing spondylitis.

Diclofenac sodium is sometimes prescribed in a formula that includes the anti-ulcer medication, misoprostol. This combination may help to protect the stomachs of people who are likely to develop an ulcer if they take an NSAID alone.

Diflunisal

Diflunisal is derived from aspirin, but its effects last for such a long time that you take it only twice a day. This drug is useful for relieving pain and inflam-mation in rheumatic disease and other musculoskeletal problems, including sports injuries. Diflunisal is also used to treat other forms of mild-to-moderate pain, especially period pain.

Etodolac

Etodolac is used to reduce the joint pain, swelling, inflammation, and stiff-ness seen in osteoarthritis and rheumatoid arthritis.

See your doctor regularly to monitor for possible internal bleeding or stomach ulcers.

Etoricoxib

One of the COX-2 inhibitors, this NSAID is prescribed to treat pain and inflammation in osteoarthritis, rheumatoid arthritis, and acute gout. Among etoricoxib's possible side effects are changes in appetite and weight, chest pain, muscle pains, and an influenza-like syndrome.

Fenbufen

Fenbufen is a fairly standard NSAID used to reduce pain and inflammation in people with rheumatic disease and other musculoskeletal disorders. However, this drug carries a higher risk of rashes than normal, especially in people with seronegative rheumatoid arthritis (those who do not have auto-antibodies aimed against body tissues), psoriatic arthritis, and women.

If rashes occur, stop taking the drug immediately and contact your doctor.

Fenoprofen

Fenoprofen is a typical NSAID used to reduce mild to moderate pain, especially in rheumatic conditions and other muscle and joint problems.

Flurbiprofen

Flurbiprofen is used for osteoarthritis and rheumatoid arthritis. This drug reduces joint pain, swelling, inflammation, and stiffness. A modified-release once-daily version of flurbiprofen is available.

Flurbiprofen is also used to ease migraines, relieve post-operative pain, and treat sore throats.

Ibuprofen

Ibuprofen is an NSAID with anti-inflammatory, analgesic, and anti-fever actions. This drug has fewer side effects than other NSAIDs, which is a trade-off as its anti-inflammatory actions are also weaker. Ibuprofen is great for relieving the pain and swelling seen in osteoarthritis, rheumatoid arthritis, juvenile rheumatoid arthritis, and carpal tunnel syndrome.

Some brands of ibuprofen are available over the counter without a prescription.

Indometacin

Indometacin is used to reduce the joint pain, swelling, inflammation, and stiffness seen in osteoarthritis, rheumatoid arthritis, bursitis, ankylosing spondylitis, gout, and tendonitis. This drug is available as a suppository, which you insert night and morning, if required. The suppositories can occasionally trigger localised irritation and bleeding.

Indometacin has a high incidence of side effects, including headache, dizziness, indigestion, nausea, and stomach pain and upset.

See your doctor regularly to monitor for possible internal bleeding and stomach ulcers.

Ketoprofen

Ketoprofen is used to treat the joint pain, swelling, inflammation, and stiffness seen in osteoarthritis and rheumatoid arthritis. One of ketoprofen's major advantages is that it's licensed for use after orthopaedic surgery.

Ketoprofen can be given as a suppository or injection to reduce the pain and stiffness that can accompany surgery. This drug is also available in an extended-release form used for long-term treatment of osteoarthritis and rheumatoid arthritis.

Make sure your doctor monitors you for possible internal bleeding and stomach ulcers.

Mefenamic acid

This NSAID is used for mild-to-moderate pain in rheumatoid arthritis, including juvenile arthritis, osteoarthritis, and related conditions. Mefenamic acid is also licensed for post-operative pain, painful periods, and heavy periods.

Mefenamic acid can cause skin rashes. If you develop a rash, stop taking this drug and seek medical advice.

Meloxicam

This NSAID is used for pain and inflammation in rheumatic disease, ankylosing spondylitis, and, short-term, for flare-ups of osteoarthritis pain.

Nabumetone

Nabumetone is a standard NSAID used to reduce the joint pain, swelling, inflammation, and stiffness seen in osteoarthritis and rheumatoid arthritis.

Naproxen

Naproxen is used to treat the joint pain, swelling, inflammation, and stiffness seen in osteoarthritis, rheumatoid arthritis, juvenile rheumatoid arthritis, bursitis, tendonitis, gout, and ankylosing spondylitis. Naproxen is also available in slow-release forms, and in a combination pack also including a drug (miso-prostol) designed to help reduce risk of peptic ulcers.

Some possible side effects of naproxen include difficulty breathing, drowsiness, skin eruptions, bleeding in general, stomach ulcers, itching, abdominal pain, bruising, and constipation.

See your doctor regularly to monitor for possible internal bleeding, ulcers, and stomach ulcers.

Piroxicam

Piroxicam is used to reduce the joint pain, swelling, inflammation, and stiffness seen in osteoarthritis and rheumatoid arthritis, including juvenile arthritis plus acute gout. This drug's long-lasting effects means that you take it just once a day.

Possible side effects of piroxicam include abdominal pain, anaemia, dizziness, nosebleeds, elevated blood pressure, sweating, stomach ulceration, the blahs, headache, itching, and nausea.

See your doctor regularly to monitor for possible internal bleeding or stomach ulcers.

Sulindac

Sulindac is used for osteoarthritis, rheumatoid arthritis, bursitis, tendonitis, gout, and ankylosing spondylitis. This drug reduces joint pain, swelling, inflammation, and stiffness.

An unusual side effect associated with sulindac is possible discolouration of urine.

Tenoxicam

Tenoxicam is prescribed to treat pain and inflammation in most rheumatic disorders. This drug lasts so long, you take it only once a day.

Tiaprofenic acid

Although tiaprofenic acid is a fairly standard NSAID used to treat rheumatic disorders, reports have occurred of severe *cystitis* (bladder inflammation) associated with its use. Therefore, your doctor may avoid prescribing this drug if you have a urinary tract problem. It is important to stop taking it immediately, and let your doctor know, if you develop urinary symptoms such as increased frequency, urgency, pain on urinating, blood in urine, or urinating at night (*nocturia*).

Taking corticosteroids

Corticosteroids are used to treat severe rheumatoid arthritis, lupus, polymyositis, polymyalgia rheumatica, and other forms of arthritis. These drugs are synthetic versions of certain natural hormones that your body produces in times of stress to help your body recover. And just like the natural hormones, corticosteroids are powerful in both good and bad ways.

Injected directly into inflamed joints, these powerful anti-inflammatories can quickly reduce damaging inflammation of the joints or organs, relieve pain, increase mobility, and reduce deformity. Full anti-septic precautions are needed to keep the area sterile and avoid introducing infection. Occasionally, an acute inflammatory reaction develops after an injection into soft tissues or a joint, which shows itself with redness, swelling and heat in the affected joint. This acute inflammation may represent a reaction to the drug used, but it is important to rule out an infection at the site of the injection.

Corticosteroids have more warnings attached to their use than just about any other type of drug. Therefore, it's important that every person prescribed an oral corticosteroid drug receives the manufacturer's patient information sheet so they can study these warnings in detail.

✔ Repeated injection of steroids into a joint, especially a weight-bearing joint, is not recommended as it can lead to joint degeneration. A joint is not usually injected more than three or four times in one year. Unfortunately, regular treatment with high doses of corticosteroids can produce significant side effects, including increasing your risk of infections, diabetes, high blood pressure, skin thinning, easy bruising, increased weight, loss of muscle, osteoporosis, and glaucoma. Because of these side effects, doctors look for the lowest effective dose when prescribing these medicines, especially by mouth, and use them for the shortest possible time. Wherever possible, local treatment with an injection into the affected joint is preferable to oral treatment, as this reduces the amount of drug that reaches the circulation – and puts it to use exactly where it is needed.

✔ A prolonged course of corticosteroid drugs is always tailed off with reducing doses. This is because long-term treatment damps down adrenal gland function, and suddenly stopping the tablets can lead to collapse. Therefore, those taking steroids long term (more than three weeks) must carry a steroid treatment card with them at all times. This card warns against stopping treatment suddenly, and is important information for doctors treating you if you're involved in an accident, for example, and are unconscious or otherwise unable to tell the doctors yourself.

✔ If you are taking oral steroids and come into contact with anyone who has an infectious disease, consult your doctor promptly. If you have never had measles or chickenpox and come into close contact with someone who has measles, chickenpox, or shingles it's especially important to consult your doctor urgently. These infections are often very severe in people whose immune system is damped down with corticosteroids, and your doctor can give you an antibody injection to help protect you.

✔ For one year after stopping treatment with oral steroids, you must tell any health-care professional (nurse, doctor, pharmacist, dentist) that you've recently had steroid treatment, in case this affects their intended treatment.

Dexamethasone

Dexamethasone is mainly given as a local injection to reduce inflammation of joints and soft tissues, especially in people with rheumatoid arthritis and lupus. Injections are repeated at intervals of 3 to 21 days according to how well (or badly!) you respond to the treatment.

Dexamethasone tablets are sometimes given to suppress inflammatory and allergic conditions.

Hydrocortisone

Hydrocortisone is usually given through an injection into a joint or into the synovial joint lining. Injections are repeated at intervals of 21 days, when necessary, and no more than three joints are treated on any one day.

Methylprednisolone

Injections of methylprednisolone help reduce the inflammation seen in rheumatoid arthritis, gout, and lupus. Injections are repeated at intervals of 7 to 35 days according to response.

Prednisolone

Prednisolone is the most commonly prescribed oral corticosteroid. This drug is used to reduce inflammation in rheumatoid arthritis, lupus, and many other conditions. As with all oral steroids, to minimise side effects, the smallest dose is given for the shortest possible time. Often a short, sharp course is prescribed in which the dose is quickly tailed off, then stopped.

Prednisolone acetate is a corticosteroid injection used to reduce joint and synovial inflammation seen in rheumatoid arthritis, gout, lupus, and other conditions. No more than three joints are treated on any one day.

Triamcinolone acetonide

This compound is almost insoluble, so it sticks around in the place where it's been injected and has a long-acting, slow-release effect. A drug that has this long-acting effect is often referred to as a 'depot' as it provides a storage depot inside you, and it's for this reason that tiamcinolone acetonide is often preferred for injection directly into a joint. Injections are repeated at intervals of one-to-two weeks as necessary.

Dealing with disease-modifying antirheumatic drugs (DMARDs)

DMARDs alter the way the immune system works and slow or halt its disastrous attack on the body. DMARDs take time to work – in some cases, months – so they are often prescribed along with an NSAID, or a corticosteroid, to ease inflammation in the meantime.

DMARDs are generally reserved for serious forms of arthritis – such as rheumatoid arthritis, psoriatic arthritis, and ankylosing spondylitis – that aren't helped with other medicines. But because these diseases are so destructive, many doctors prescribe DMARDs early on to try to prevent inflammation-related joint damage. DMARDs include several wildly different types of drug, including gold injections, methotrexate, some anti-cancer drugs, and even some otherwise used to treat malaria!

Azathioprine

Azathioprine is used for rheumatoid arthritis and lupus. This drug works on the immune system to decrease the body's response to infections and interferes with the action of white blood cells, which, if not stopped, worsen the symptoms of rheumatoid arthritis and lupus. Azathioprine is also used with other medications to prevent the rejection of kidney transplants.

Some possible side effects of azathioprine include infection, suppression of the bone marrow, loss of appetite, liver damage, hair loss, skin rashes, diarrhoea, nausea, and vomiting.

If you take azathioprine, you need to have regular blood tests to check that the drug isn't damping down activity of your bone marrow too much.

Azathioprine may promote the development of shingles by reducing the body's immunity against the chickenpox virus lying in hibernation in nerve roots.

Ciclosporin

Ciclosporin is used to treat severe cases of rheumatoid arthritis where conventional second-line treatment is ineffective. This drug's suppression of the immune system is what modifies the disease's progress. Ciclosporin appears to slow the rate of disease progression and to improve symptoms in people who have only partially responded to methotrexate.

Some possible side effects of ciclosporin include elevated blood pressure, kidney damage, growth of the gums, tremor, convulsions, coughing, acne, tumour of the lymph system, difficulty breathing, and joint or muscle pain.

Because ciclosporin suppresses the immune system, you face the possibility of increasing your likelihood of developing other diseases, including cancer.

The amount of cyclosporin absorbed from a dose varies from person to person, so your doctor may check your blood levels regularly. Blood tests to check kidney function are also advised, along with liver-function tests if you are also taking an NSAID. Regular blood pressure checks are also needed.

Chloroquine and hydrochloroquine

These antimalarial drugs are also used to treat moderate rheumatoid arthritis, including juvenile arthritis, and mild lupus but are not used for psoriatic arthritis as they can make psoriasis worse. Chloroquine and hydrochloroquine are slow-acting drugs that may take several weeks to bring about beneficial effects. In general these drugs are better tolerated than gold or penicillamine.

During treatment, your eyesight is monitored as visual acuity is sometimes affected. If you develop visual changes or blurring, stop treatment and seek immediate advice from your doctor.

Some possible side effects of chloroquine and hydrochloroquine include headache, skin rashes, changes in eye pigmentation, blind spots, difficulty focusing the eyes and other eye problems, decreased muscle co-ordination, hair loss, and changes in skin and hair colouration. Rarely, mental changes, blood disorders, and convulsions have occurred in people taking these drugs.

Chloroquine and hydrochloroquine pass into breast-milk and women who have a baby while using one of these drugs are advised not to breastfeed.

Cyclophosphamide

Cyclophosphamide is an anti-cancer drug that is sometimes also used for very serious cases of rheumatoid arthritis and lupus. This drug apparently kills some of the white blood cells that bring on arthritis symptoms.

Some possible side effects of cyclophosphamide include severe nausea and vomiting, damage to the bladder or bleeding from the bladder, loss of appetite, loss of hair, mouth ulcers, darkening of skin and fingernails, low blood counts, and abdominal pain. This drug can also cause irreversible sterility, bone marrow suppression, and an increased risk of cancer.

As cyclophosphamide is toxic, regular blood counts are needed in case the bone marrow stops producing enough blood cells and platelets (needed for clotting).

Gold

One of the few advantages of having rheumatoid arthritis is that you can tell people that you're worth your weight in gold – well, almost. Gold given by injection (sodium aurothiomalate) or by mouth (auranofin) sounds glamorous, but can cause severe side effects – occasionally fatal – in up to 5 per cent of people who take it. Reactions from gold include skin problems (including irreversible pigmentation in sun-exposed areas); blood disorders; kidney problems; inflammation of the colon, nerves, lungs, and liver; as well as conjunctivitis and hair loss. The most common side effect with oral gold treatment is diarrhoea (which is often improved with bulking agents such as bran).

Tell your doctor immediately if you are receiving gold treatment and develop sore throat, fever, infection, non-specific illness, unexplained bleeding or bruising, breathlessness, cough, mouth ulcers, a metallic taste, or rashes.

Leflunomide

Leflunomide slows the growth and reproduction of white blood cells and attempts to reduce the symptoms and tissue damage seen in rheumatoid arthritis. Interfering with white blood cells, which are involved in the inflammation process, means that leflunomide may help to relieve joint pain and swelling and can slow the progression of tissue damage.

Leflunomide doesn't cure rheumatoid arthritis, but it can help relieve symptoms and reduce the rate at which the disease progresses. This drug produces the same kind of relief as methotrexate. In fact, leflunomide often works for people for whom methotrexate and other medications are not helpful, or those who can't tolerate methotrexate's side effects or who have preexisting kidney failure.

Don't expect rapid results. Improvements usually start after four-to-six weeks' treatment, and can continue for a further four-to-six months.

Some possible side effects of leflunomide include nausea, diarrhoea, vomiting, loss of appetite, abdominal pain, weight loss, raised blood pressure, headache, dizziness, hair loss, blood disorder, and liver problems. Careful monitoring is required in people who have elevated blood pressure, problems with the immune system, or kidney disease. Liver function is closely monitored in those taking leflunomide as serious liver toxicity has occurred in some people.

As with most of these powerful DMARDs, it is important to use a reliable method of contraception. With leflunomide especially, it is important that neither men nor women taking it are involved in conceiving a child. Contraception is advised for at least two years after treatment in women, and for at least three months after treatment in men.

Methotrexate

Methotrexate is an anti-cancer drug also used for moderate-to-severe rheumatoid arthritis when drugs such as NSAIDs don't work. This drug helps to slow the immune system reactions that cause many of the problems seen in rheumatoid arthritis. But in the process, methotrexate may lower your body's overall resistance, so a chance for infection exists. Avoid getting any live vaccines while taking methotrexate, because you may contract the disease you're trying to avoid. Note that methotrexate is taken once a *week*, not once a day.

Besides a greater susceptibility to infections, some possible side effects of methotrexate include liver toxicity, lung toxicity, bone marrow suppression, mouth ulcers, the blahs, dizziness, fatigue, abdominal pain and distress, impotence, and may trigger diabetes.

You need to have regular blood tests to check your liver, kidneys, and blood count. You should have a blood test before starting treatment, then weekly until therapy is stabilised. Monitoring continues every two-to-three months. Seek immediate medical attention if you develop signs suggesting an infection (such as sore throat or fever) or lung problem (such as a cough or shortness of breath).

Penicillamine

Penicillamine is used to treat rheumatoid arthritis. This drug has a similar effect to gold, but is better tolerated even though side effects are frequent. The exact way that penicillamine works is not fully understood, but it may interfere with the action of certain white blood cells that inadvertently damage joints.

Penicillamine is a slow-acting drug that may take two-to-three months to bring about beneficial effects. If and when penicillamine works, it reduces joint pain, swelling, and tenderness.

Some possible side effects of penicillamine include nausea, loss of taste sensation, lack of appetite, fever, swollen lymph glands, diarrhoea, skin rashes, alopecia, blood disorders, and protein in the urine, which your doctor tests for using a urinary dipstick.

A blood count and urine test are important before starting treatment, then every week or two for the first two months of treatment, then monthly (plus a week after any dose increase).

Mineral supplements are not recommended when taking penicillamine, as some minerals bind to penicillamine and reduce its effectiveness.

Sulfasalazine

Sulfasalazine is an anti-inflammatory (and antibiotic) DMARD used to treat rheumatoid arthritis and ulcerative colitis. Sulfasalazine is not active in its ingested form, but is broken down by bacteria in the colon to form two other products: *5-aminosalicylic acid* (related to aspirin) and sulfapyridine. Which of these two products are most responsible for sulfasalazine's beneficial actions in arthritis is not certain. Sulfasalazine is mainly reserved for those who haven't responded well to other medications. People with rheumatoid arthritis usually take this medication in its time-release form.

Some possible side effects of sulfasalazine include hives, nausea, vomiting, loss of appetite, rashes, headaches and blood disorders. One unusual side effect of this drug is that treatment may result in staining of contact lenses!

Taking sulfasalazine may put you at risk of several nasty problems. Heed these warnings:

- ✔ Avoid sulfasalazine if you are allergic to *sulfa* drugs, para-aminobenzoic acid (PABA)-containing sunscreens, or local anaesthetics. Sulfasalazine may cause increased sensitivity to the sun or to bright light. Use sunscreen and wear sunglasses and protective clothing.

- ✔ Make sure your blood counts and liver and kidney functions are monitored before treatment and at monthly intervals for at least the first three months of treatment, in case the treatment adversely affects your bone marrow, liver or kidneys.

- ✔ Report any unexplained bleeding, bruising, sore throat, fever, or malaise to your doctor.

Benefitting from biologic response modifiers (BRMs)

For people who don't respond to DMARDs, a new class of drugs, the *biologic response modifiers (BRMs)* – also referred to as *cytokine inhibitors* – are sometimes the answer. First introduced in 1998, BRMs inhibit certain components of the immune system, called *cytokines*. As the cytokines play a part in the inflammation seen in rheumatoid arthritis, ankylosing spondylitis, and psoriatic arthritis, BRMs are often effective in reducing stubborn inflammation.

Currently, only four BRMs are available in the UK. Adalimumab, etanercept, and infliximab suppress a cytokine called *tumour necrosis factor (TNF),* a substance that causes arthritis-related swelling and joint damage. The fourth BRM, anakinra, blocks a cytokine called *interleukin-1*, a cytokine that causes arthritis-related swelling and joint damage.

The BRMs are mighty expensive (one of them costs almost £400 per injection, although it's given only every two weeks; another costs more than £20 per day), although researchers are working on less expensive oral versions.

Possible side effects of BRMs include redness, pain, swelling, itching or bruising at the injection site, and infections of the upper respiratory tract. Some BRMs may increase your risk of developing serious infections, such as tuberculosis or pneumonia. Tell your doctor if you have tuberculosis, pneumonia, a current infection, a history of serious infections, or asthma.

Treatment with BRMs is usually stopped if there is no response after three months.

Adalimumab

Adalimumab is usually prescribed together with methotrexate to reduce the pain, swelling, and difficulty in moving seen in moderate-to-severe rheumatoid arthritis. This drug is used alone if methotrexate is inappropriate for any reason. Adalimumab blocks the activity of tumour necrosis factor. This drug is given in the form of injections, usually every other week, and is only given to those for whom other rheumatoid arthritis medications have proved unhelpful.

People needing adalimumab are screened for tuberculosis before treatment. Rarely, symptoms of lupus occur with treatment with this drug. Tell your doctor if you develop symptoms suggestive of tuberculosis (TB), such as persistent cough, weight loss, or fever.

Anakinra

Anakinra is used alone or with other medications to reduce the pain, swelling, and joint stiffness seen in rheumatoid arthritis. This drug blocks the activity of *interleukin-1*. Anakinra is given in the form of daily injections and is given only to those for whom other rheumatoid arthritis medications are unhelpful.

A low white blood cell count often develops in people receiving anakinra. Therefore, blood counts are checked before treatment, then every month for six months, then every three months.

Anakinra may increase your risk of developing a serious infection, including pneumonia. Tell your doctor if you develop fever, sore throat, or other signs of infection.

Etanercept

Etanercept is used to reduce the pain and swelling seen in rheumatoid arthritis, juvenile rheumatoid arthritis, psoriatic arthritis, and ankylosing spondylitis in people who have not responded to other treatments. This drug works by blocking the activity of tumour necrosis factor. Etanercept is given – usually twice a week – in the form of injections in the thigh, stomach, or upper arm. Though rare, symptoms of lupus have occurred with treatment with this drug.

Etanercept may increase your risk of developing a serious infection, including tuberculosis and chickenpox. Tell your doctor if you develop any signs suggesting an infection. If you are in contact with someone who has chickenpox or shingles, you may need immunoglobulin treatment to help boost your immunity against the Herpes zoster virus.

Infliximab

Infliximab treats highly active rheumatoid arthritis in adults who have failed to respond to at least two other standard DMARDs, usually including methotrexate. This drug is also used to treat ankylosing spondylitis in people who have not responded adequately to conventional therapy. Infliximab helps to slow the progression of joint damage, relieves pain and stiffness, and improves joint function. Infliximab is infused intravenously every two months and is often used in conjunction with the drug methotrexate.

People are observed carefully for one to two hours after infusion with infliximab as hypersensitivity reactions can develop, including fever, chest pain, blood pressure changes, itching, shortness of breath, hives, and even collapse. People needing this drug are screened for tuberculosis (TB) before treatment.

As infections can develop during treatment with infliximab, it is not used if any infections are present. Tell your doctor if you develop symptoms suggestive of TB, such as persistent cough, weight loss, or fever.

Infliximab is not recommended if there is an interval of more than 16 weeks since the last treatment, as this interval increases the chance of developing a delayed hypersensitivity reaction.

Looking at Other Drugs

Several other types of drug are also used to treat other forms of arthritis, including gout and joint problems linked with infections such as Chlamydia or gonorrhoea. These drugs are looked at in the following sections.

Going for drugs for gout

Gout is usually treated with high doses of NSAIDs (but not aspirin) such as diclofenac, indometacin, ketoprofen, naproxen, piroxicam, or sulindac (see the previous 'Swallowing non-steroidal anti-inflammatory drugs (NSAIDs)' section). The NSAID azapropazone is used only when other NSAIDs are ineffective.

Make sure you take in a lot of fluid if you have gout, especially if you are taking anti-gout treatments.

Colchicine

Colchicine is a yellow alkaloid originally derived from the poisonous corms of the Autumn crocus, or meadow saffron. Colchicine binds to a protein (*tubulin*) found in white blood cells to literally hobble them, stopping them migrating into areas of inflammation, where they would have released enzymes and chemicals to further hot things up.

Colchicine is used for acute gout, and for short-term 'cover' when people start taking a longer-term treatment to prevent gout (such as allopurinol; see the next section). Although it is as effective as NSAIDs in reducing the pain and inflammation of gout, colchicine's use is limited due to side effects at higher doses. Possible side effects of this drug include nausea, vomiting, and abdominal pain. Large doses may cause profuse diarrhoea, intestinal bleeding, rashes, and kidney or liver damage.

Colchicine is useful for older people who have both acute gout and heart failure, as it does not encourage fluid retention, as some NSAIDs can. Colchicine is also suitable for people taking blood-thinning drugs.

Allopurinol

Allopurinol is used for the long-term prevention of gout. However, this drug does not stop an acute gout attack that has already begun, and, in fact, can worsen an attack. Instead, allopurinol is used after an acute attack subsides to lower the production of uric acid, which helps stop crippling, frequent attacks. Treatment is continued indefinitely, once per day. Colchicine is given with allopurinol for one month after starting treatment to ensure that gout doesn't occur before allopurinol kicks in.

Allopurinol is usually well tolerated, but possible side effects include chills, fever, diarrhoea, rashes, itch, stomach pain, headache, and joint pains. The most serious side effect of this drug is a life-threatening allergic reaction, which, although very rare, requires immediate medical attention because it is fatal in about 25 per cent of cases. The allergic reaction symptoms include a skin rash, fever, and liver and kidney failure.

Sulfinpyrazone

Sulfinpyrazone is an anti-gout medication that also helps to lower uric acid levels. However, unlike allopurinol, which reduces uric acid production in the body, sulfinpyrazone pushes more uric acid out into the urine, which is rather clever, really. Unfortunately, pushing more uric acid out into the urine does mean that treatment is unsuitable for those with a tendency towards kidney stones. If you are taking this drug you must, *must*, **must** drink lots of water to discourage formation of uric acid crystals in your urinary tract. As an extra precaution, your doctor may also suggest that you take something to ensure your urine is alkaline rather than acid.

Some possible side effects of sulfinpyrazone include nausea, itching, redness, rash or other signs of skin irritation, salt and water retention, and kidney and liver problems. Blood disorders are rare, but regular blood counts are advisable.

Avoid aspirin, which cancels the effects of sulfinpyrazone.

Fighting bacteria with antibiotics

Antibiotics are drugs that either kill bacteria outright, or which disable them so your immune system can finish them off. There are several different classes of antibiotic drug, but only a few are needed to treat the bugs associated with some arthritic conditions.

Penicillins

Penicillin and amoxicillin are penicillin antibiotics used to treat Lyme disease and gonorrhoea. These antibiotics work by punching holes in bacterial walls so their insides leak out, water floods in, and they explode and die. Shame.

Some possible side effects of penicillins include nausea, allergic reactions (such as rashes, tongue swelling, itching), diarrhoea, and acute kidney failure.

If you have asthma, hives, hay fever, or other allergies, make sure that your doctor knows this before you take penicillins, as you may have a mould allergy, in which case penicillin (which is derived from a mould) is best avoided.

Cephalosporins

Cephalosporins, such as cephalexin hydrochloride, are broad-spectrum antibiotics used for bacterial infections, including those found in infectious arthritis. These drugs work in the same way as penicillins by interfering with bacterial cell wall synthesis.

If you have an infected joint, your doctor may prescribe a two-week course of a related, intravenous form of this drug as a first-line treatment then switch you to the oral version.

Some possible side effects of cephalosporins include upset stomach, diarrhoea, vomiting, mild skin rash, colitis, yeast infections, fatigue, fever, hallucinations, joint pain and inflammation (which is rather ironic if this is why you're taking them in the first place).

About 10 per cent of people with a penicillin allergy also react against cephalosporins.

Tetracyclines

Tetracycline antibiotics are used to treat Lyme disease and Chlamydia. Several variations of these antibiotics exist, including oxytetracycline and doxycycline. Tetracyclines work by inhibiting bacterial protein production so they can't go forth and multiply.

Some possible side effects of tetracyclines include allergic reactions causing swelling of the face, difficulty swallowing, inflamed tongue, pain in the chest, sore mouth, nausea, vomiting, abdominal pain, faintness, and skin sensitivity to sunlight.

Chapter 9

Cuts That Cure:
Surgeries for Arthritis

. . . .

In This Chapter

▶ Deciding whether you're a candidate for joint surgery

▶ Getting to know the different types of joint surgery

▶ Preparing for surgery and its aftermath

. . . .

*T*he idea of having surgery is always scary. Any time you allow a surgeon to rummage round in your body, you're taking certain risks, some great, and others small. But under the right conditions, surgery performed on a diseased joint can bring results that are nothing short of miraculous. Pain is reduced or eliminated, range of motion restored, deformities corrected, and joint function vastly improved. Still, surgery isn't for everyone and whether it's right for you depends on many factors.

If you're considering surgical treatment for your arthritis, you need to consult an orthopaedic surgeon or orthopod (the kind of doctor who specialises in treating diseases of the muscles, bones, and joints). An orthopaedic surgeon is trained in both surgical and non-surgical methods. Non-surgical treatments consist of casting, splinting, and joint injections. Surgical treatments include removal of the joint lining, cutting and resetting a bone, bone fusion, and joint reconstruction. Arthroscopic surgery, a special technique that has gained great popularity in recent years, is one of many techniques in the orthopaedic surgeon's repertoire.

Knowing What to Ask Your Doctor Before Undergoing Surgery

Because surgery is a drastic and (at least somewhat) risky option, don't consider it until all other measures are exhausted. Only resort to surgery once you and your doctor use up all the many non-surgical options available, such as medication, diet, physiotherapy, pain-management strategies, exercise, and a wide range of complementary approaches. Most people don't actually need surgery to manage their arthritis.

In some cases, though, surgery is a godsend. When rheumatic finger joints render your hands nearly useless, or when a painful, osteoarthritic hip makes walking to the postbox a major feat, certain surgical procedures can give you a new lease of life.

Whether surgery succeeds depends on two things: The condition itself and the body in question – yours! Some disease states respond wonderfully to surgery, though others show little or no improvement. People's responses are like that, too. One person may come through a surgical procedure with flying colours, zip through recovery, and remain thrilled with the results. Another person, equally affected and undergoing an identical operation, may feel trapped in a long, drawn-out recovery period that garners less-than-optimal results. Thus, surgery is a highly individual matter and may or may not suit you. To find out if surgery is an option for you, begin by asking your orthopaedic surgeon the following questions:

- **Do my symptoms and my test results go hand-in-hand?** That is, can your doctor confirm your diagnosis? You certainly don't want to undergo surgery for a problem that isn't definitely confirmed.

- **Does my kind of arthritis respond well to surgery?** Surgery is most often performed on those with rheumatoid arthritis or incapacitating osteoarthritis; on the other hand, surgery is rarely the treatment-of-choice for gout, scleroderma, or lupus. Those with ankylosing spondylitis are iffy candidates for surgery: Sometimes surgery is used to straighten their spines or replace joints, but excessive bone growth can complicate the recovery process. (Refer to the Contents page for chapters dealing with the conditions listed above.)

- **How do I know if I need surgery?** In most cases, surgery for arthritis is not an emergency – it doesn't absolutely have to take place at a certain time. The decision to undergo surgery, and the timing of the operation, is usually dictated by pain levels, your overall health, and your degree of disability. Although a few arthritis-related problems need surgery immediately (for example, a ruptured tendon), most can wait. But delaying an optional operation (for example, a hip replacement) for too long can lead to a more difficult procedure, poor surgical outcome, the irreversible contraction of certain muscles supporting the joint, and increased post-operative pain. Therefore, timing your operation properly is something of an art, but usually comes down to waiting lists and local resources. Ask your doctor about the possibility of irreversible damage or disability brought about by waiting too long for an operation.

✔ **What results can I expect from this operation?** That is, what is surgery going to do for you? How may it affect your pain, your range of motion, and the stability of your joint(s)? What kind of activities can you enjoy again after you recover? What limitations can remain?

✔ **What risks are involved?** Make sure that your doctor explains all the complications that can result from the operation (for example, infection, nerve damage, and so on), as well as the risks involved in undergoing surgery itself (such as those relating to the anaesthetic).

✔ **What is involved in the post-surgery rehabilitation?** Rehabilitation is often a long, painful process that requires your utmost dedication and hard work. Make sure that you know what lies ahead before consenting to surgery. If you're not willing to do the work, your surgical outcome is compromised.

✔ **Am I physically able to withstand the operation?** A full physical examination is usual before surgery to make sure that you and your body are up to the procedure. The condition of your heart, lungs, blood, and overall health are taken into account when assessing whether you can withstand the rigors of a major operation.

✔ **What does the future hold if I don't have surgery?** If you are already in great pain, finding out that it may get worse unless you have surgery can influence your decision in favour of the procedure. If arthritis is not reducing your quality of life too much, your doctor may suggest that postponing surgery isn't going to compromise its eventual effectiveness. However, sometimes, waiting too long can result in muscle wasting, a decline in joint function, or permanent deformities, all of which can make future operations less successful. Find out which category of urgency you're in.

Looking At Different Kinds of Joint Surgery

Because joints are intricate pieces of machinery, and many different things can go wrong with them, joint surgery is complex and wide-ranging. Joint

Finding out if you're (mentally) prepared for surgery

Although your doctor can tell you all about what goes on inside your body, only you know what's going on inside your head. Do a little soul-searching to determine whether you really want and need the surgery by asking yourself the following questions:

✔ Is the pain interfering with my ability to lead a productive and satisfying life?

✔ Do I rely on pain relievers, taken at the maximum allowable dosage, to get me through the day?

✔ Have I tried all other pain-relieving methods (physiotherapy, exercise, pain-management strategies, and so on) without success?

✔ Are my expectations of surgery results realistic?

✔ Will I participate fully in my post-surgery rehabilitation?

If you can answer 'yes' to all of these questions, you may be mentally and emotionally ready to undergo joint surgery.

surgery can involve flushing the joint with water, resurfacing rough bone ends or cartilage, cutting away inflamed membranes, growing bone where it didn't previously exist, and even taking the whole joint out and starting from scratch with a new one.

Synovectomy: Removing a diseased joint lining

People who have rheumatoid arthritis may benefit from having a *synovectomy*, in which the surgeon removes an inflamed, overgrown joint lining (*synovium*).

In rheumatoid arthritis, the inflamed, thickened synovium can overgrow to the point of invading the joint's supporting structures – bones, cartilage, muscles, and ligaments. Synovial overgrowth can cause progressive damage to a joint. At the same time, the synovium releases enzymes that cause bone and cartilage to break down. Removing the offending lining stops the synovial invasion and reduces the amount of destructive enzymes released.

The surgeon may make a large incision that exposes the entire joint. Or, in the case of *arthroscopic surgery*, he or she makes tiny incisions just large enough to accommodate insertion of an arthroscope. The *arthroscope* is a flexible tube, about the diameter of a pencil, which has a camera on the end. It's used for diagnostic and surgical purposes. In either procedure, the joint lining is cut away, leaving just enough behind to produce lubricating fluid. This type of surgery isn't a permanent cure, as – rather like pond weed – the synovium eventually grows back. However, pain relief and protection against joint destruction can last for a couple of years, so more radical treatments, such as joint replacement, are happily postponed.

Osteotomy: Cutting and resetting the bone

To perform an *osteotomy*, the surgeon removes a section of bone to correct joint alignment. (*Osteo* is the Greek word for *bone*; *tomy* means *to cut*.) People suffering from osteoarthritis (especially of the knee, see Chapter 2) and ankylosing spondylitis (discussed in Chapter 4) often benefit from this surgery. Osteotomy is also helpful for joints that are wearing improperly but still have a healthy area.

A misaligned joint can cause uneven wearing on the bones and cartilage as well as general joint pain. After proper alignment is restored, the force exerted on the joint is distributed more evenly. Excess pressure is released from cartilage and bone, worn spots have the chance to repair themselves, and pain is reduced.

Typically, in someone with osteoarthritis (OA), a slice or wedge of bone is surgically removed, allowing the joint to realign. The raw edges of the bone are then connected with screws and eventually knit together again. If someone has ankylosing spondylitis (or bamboo spine), the damaged tissue and bone that lock the spine into its unnatural, bent-over position are removed so that they can return to a natural, upright position.

The main benefits of osteotomy are: Pain relief, improved joint function, increased range of motion, and greater joint stability. Absolute bliss. Recovery from osteotomy may take anywhere from 6 to 12 months, but the possibility exists that joint function may not improve. Alterations in joint alignment can make future joint replacements difficult and, for many people, the benefits last only a few years.

Arthrodesis: Fusing the bone

People with rheumatoid arthritis may benefit from having certain bones fused. The surgeon positions the joint into its most functional alignment and then permanently 'locks' it in place.

Arthrodesis helps to stabilise and relieve pain in highly unsteady and painful joints. This surgery is primarily performed on the spine but is also used on the thumb, hip, knee, and wrist when replacement is not feasible or has already proved unsuccessful.

Although fusion of the hip joint is no longer a common operation, this procedure remains an option for those who need a total hip replacement but can't have one; usually because their bones aren't healthy enough, or because they're too young or too active. (Hip replacements typically last about 10 to 15 years, and second replacements often don't work as well.) Although a fused hip has no movement, it is locked into a position that allows maximum mobility of the body. Usually, the thigh is slightly flexed and slightly rotated so that the foot points outwards a little. This position minimizes excessive movement of the lumbar spine and opposite knee during walking, helping to avoid future pain in these areas.

Fusion of the thumb joint can make grasping possible. Fusion of the knee is sometimes performed when a knee replacement is infected and won't 'take'. The wrist is another candidate for fusion, as it's a highly unstable joint and very difficult to replace.

The surgeon removes cartilage from the opposing bone ends along with a thin surface layer of bone. The joint is then aligned in the position of greatest functional use, and the raw bone ends joined using pins, rods, or screws. Splinting or casting helps to keep the joint stable while new bone growth fuses it permanently into place – like superglue.

Arthrodesis helps to relieve pain and can increase the ability to use a joint, albeit in a limited way. Although joint movement is forfeited with arthrodesis, joint function improves. A person with a fused hip, for example, *can* walk, even if it is with a limp, which is a fantastic advance for someone who is otherwise confined to a wheelchair. However, recovery from this surgery can take several months.

Arthroplasty: Replacing the joint

Sometimes a joint degenerates to the point where pain is severe or constant and joint function is seriously impaired. Surgically removing the old, diseased parts of the joint and replacing them with new, synthetic ones means that pain is usually relieved, and mobility restored. This procedure is called *arthroplasty*, or joint replacement surgery, and it has revolutionised the treatment of hip and knee arthritis.

Hip and knee arthritis routinely disabled people in the past (especially the elderly), but today replacing old worn-out joints with artificial parts can offer relief from excruciating pain, loss of mobility, and disability.

Surgery can help stabilise a wobbly joint, realign a joint to improve function, and in some cases even make cosmetic improvements. Many people undergoing hip or knee replacements feel they have a new lease of life – suddenly they can walk, ramble, cycle, and just move around without pain! Hip replacement is one of the most common orthopaedic procedures in the UK, with 43,000 operations carried out each year. The knee is the next most commonly replaced joint, followed by the ankles, shoulders, elbows, and knuckles.

Getting surgery earlier, instead of waiting, is probably the best plan. A study of 222 OA patients undergoing total hip or knee replacement surgery found that those who delayed surgery, until joint function had severely declined and pain was severe, had the worst surgical outcomes; they were most likely to need assistance with bathing, dressing, and other daily tasks afterwards.

People with the best surgical outcomes are usually older, have arthritis-related pain, loss of movement, or stiffness that hasn't responded to other forms of treatment, and are otherwise in good health. In addition, these people are highly motivated to help themselves and willing and able to participate in an exercise regimen after they receive their new joint.

You have a much better chance of enjoying a successful hip or knee replacement if you exercise, stay away from high-impact sports and activities, and maintain your ideal body weight.

Joint replacement surgery involves the use of artificial parts as well as some existing natural tissues. With the patient under anaesthesia, the surgeon opens the joint and detaches the tendons and ligaments from the bone. Then, the surgeon dislocates the joint, and cuts away the diseased or weakened parts of the bone. The surgeon uses plastic and/or metal prostheses to replace the missing parts of the joint and may cement them into place. Finally, the surgeon fits the joint parts together, reattaches the ligaments and tendons, and closes the incision. (See Figure 9-1 and the sidebar 'Looking at the total hip replacement procedure'.)

Figure 9-1:
The hip socket is replaced with a poly-ethylene cup, and the head of the femur is replaced with a metal ball.

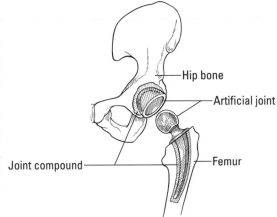

Hip bone

Artificial joint

Joint compound

Femur

Although called 'joint replacement surgery', a more accurate description of this procedure is 'joint rebuilding surgery'. The surgeon tries to maintain the integrity of your natural joint as much as possible, and may simply resurface certain areas and cut away diseased tissue. The surgeon may replace just part of the joint, for example the socket of the ball-and-socket joint in the hip, while leaving the ball intact; or they may reconstruct the entire joint using artificial parts.

In the majority of cases, joint replacements provide pain relief, restored mobility, and improved joint stability. In the case of the weight-bearing joints, such as the hip or knee, this improved function can restore not only a person's independence but also their overall outlook on life.

Looking at the total hip replacement procedure

Total hip replacement surgery gives you a good idea of how joint replacement (arthroplasty) surgeries are performed. The ball-and-socket joint in the hip must provide a secure anchor between the pelvis and thigh bone (femur) to do its job properly. In a total hip replacement, the ball and the socket are separated, removed, and then replaced with artificial structures. The surgery is completed in several stages:

✔ The tendons and ligaments that are connected to the femur's ball-shaped end are carefully detached.

✔ The hip joint is dislocated, in order to separate the pelvis and femur.

✔ The ball-shaped end is cut away from the femur.

✔ A special tool is used to hollow out the socket to make it large enough to hold the new socket, a cup-like structure made of high-density, polyethylene plastic.

✔ The plastic socket is cemented into place using joint compound.

✔ A shaft is cut down the centre of the femur. A metal ball with a rod attached (it looks like a door knob with a root) is slotted down the shaft. Some prostheses are fixed in place with a strong bone cement, while others are designed as cementless.

✔ The metal ball is inserted into the plastic socket, the ligaments and tendons repaired, and the wound is closed.

Recovery from a total hip replacement can take time. People usually stay in hospital for at least 4 to 5 days after surgery and may need to stay for 8 to 12 days or more. (For the latest on joint replacement surgery techniques that are cutting times spent in hospital, see Chapter 23.)

A walking stick, frame, or crutches are usually needed for the first 6 weeks after total hip replacement surgery. After that time, most normal activities are resumed – walking, cycling, driving, golfing, and so on. Some doctors estimate that 80 per cent of a patient's recovery occurs within the first 10 to 12 weeks after surgery, and the last 20 per cent occurs during the following 3 to 6 months.

Complications exist, however. Infection at the site of the operation may require removal of the implant, the prosthesis can loosen, or the joint may dislocate. Replacements of weight-bearing joints can wear out – traditional artificial hips typically last only 10 to 15 years, knees may last as long as 20, but a shoulder replacement can last a lifetime as it doesn't have to prop up your whole weight when walking. If and when joint replacements wear out, you need to go through surgery again. Other complications of joint replacement include blood clots (especially in the leg), damage to nerves surrounding the replacement, and ending up with legs that are unequal in length.

Until recently, total hip replacement was thought of as a last resort, because replacement parts (implants) tended to wear out or loosen with the passage of time. People needing this kind of surgery were asked to hold out as long as possible, as most implants needed replacing within 10 to 20 years. So, people aged 40 didn't want to have joint replacement surgery unless they were absolutely desperate, as they knew they'd have to undergo further surgery by the age of 60, if not sooner!

However, recent advances in the durability of implant materials (for example, prepared polyethylene and metal or ceramic surfaces) now make it more likely that a joint replacement lasts longer. As a result of this increased durability, earlier total joint replacement surgery is now an option – great news for baby boomers or young adults with arthritic knees and hips! And joint replacement surgery doesn't have a cut-off age: A study released by the Mayo Clinic found that even those 90 years old and up can undergo safe and effective hip replacements as long as their heart and lungs are sound.

If you're planning to have a knee replacement, you may think that replacing both knees at once is a good idea to save both time and money. But studies show that those undergoing double-knee replacements are more likely to suffer from serious complications (dislocation, inflammation, nerve damage, and so on) than those who take it one step (or one knee) at a time. Healing is also easier when you have one good leg to put your weight on, while allowing your newly-replaced knee to heal.

Although the risk of developing an infection in a joint replacement is relatively rare (1 in 100), this complication can require more surgery and the removal of joint replacement parts. Any infection in your body can spread to your joint replacement, so be scrupulous about taking antibiotics as prescribed – both before and after surgery. Also, during the months or even years after surgery (infection can occur years later) you need to take antibiotics if you develop a skin or bladder infection, undergo more than just a simple dental treatment, or have another operation. These examples are all high-risk times for bacteria to enter the bloodstream and travel to the site of your joint replacement, where they can settle in and cause an infection.

With cement or without?

Over time, the cement used in hip replacements can crack and break into little pieces, causing the prosthesis to loosen. These wayward little pieces of crud can take fragments of bone with them as they fall away, weakening and degrading the overall bone structure. Some surgeons opt for *cementless* hip replacements to avoid this problem. The ball-and-stem part of the cementless prosthesis has a rough, bumpy outer skin, like that of a toad, which causes bone to grow into the spaces between the bumps, securing the real bone to the artificial part.

Advantages of cementless replacements:

✔ This type of replacement may last longer, because you don't have any cement to crack and break away.

✔ Revision surgery is often easier.

Disadvantages of cementless replacements:

✔ Recovery can take a long time, with activity limited for as much as 3 months while bone grows into the replacement part of the joint.

✔ Soft or porous bones may not bond tightly enough to the prosthesis to allow a successful cementless hip replacement.

✔ A perfect fit is hard to achieve – 10 to 20 per cent of people experience pain in the thigh, which is sometimes severe.

Autologous chondrocyte implantation: Transplanting cartilage

Osteoarthritis sufferers (especially those under 40 years old who have experienced trauma to the joint) benefit from a cartilage transplant.

During this procedure, the surgeon takes healthy cartilage cells from one part of your body and transplants them into a joint with damaged cartilage. These transplanted cells continue to grow, producing new cartilage that eventually replaces the old.

When a joint suffers trauma, the *chondrocytes* (cartilage-producing cells) can change the way they act. Chondrocytes may make smaller amounts of certain cartilage components *(proteoglycans* and *collagen),* while churning out more of the enzymes that break down the cartilage. This decrease in the building-up of cartilage, plus an increase in cartilage destruction, adds up to damaged, poor-quality tissue. But if the old chondrocytes are replaced with new chondrocytes that work properly, production and maintenance of healthy cartilage is restored.

The surgeon harvests healthy cartilage cells from another area in your body (not the damaged joint, obviously!) and mixes them together with a special solution that includes some of your own tissue fluids. The cells are then carefully cultured in a laboratory for a few weeks, and cosseted so that they grow and multiply. Then these cells are injected into your damaged joint, where they take hold and begin to grow new cartilage. Because the cells and fluid come from your own body, your immune system is much less likely to recognise them as foreign and attack them. Transplanting cartilage helps to relieve pain and restore mobility using a relatively non-invasive method. Because this is a new approach, which is not yet widely available, no one knows how long the new cartilage lasts.

Getting Ready for Surgery

If you decide to undergo surgery, you need to plan ahead for the event, starting with taking excellent care of your health. Ask your doctor or pharmacist to review your medications, vitamins, minerals, herbs, and other supplements and tell you which ones to stop taking prior to surgery. (Certain drugs and supplements can thin the blood and increase the risk of bleeding.) You may also want to explore how to donate some of your own blood so you can receive it back during or after surgery, if necessary. Making plans for your post-operative care, working out any financial and insurance angles, and arranging for someone to handle your daily responsibilities ensures that you can relax while convalescing and concentrate on getting well!

Getting yourself into the best possible physical shape

Prepare for surgery like an athlete training for a competition. Eat highly nutritious meals, exercise regularly (if you're up to it), get plenty of sleep, and stay away from alcohol or unnecessary drugs. Surgery is done carefully, utilising every precaution, but it is still a major assault on your body. The better your health is going in, the better your body can withstand the trauma and the faster you recover coming out.

Your doctor can undoubtedly give you several pre-surgical instructions. You may need to wash with a special soap or take a course of antibiotics. Most certainly, you need to avoid taking certain drugs and supplements that can thin the blood and increase bleeding time – seek advice about this from your doctor and/or pharmacist.

Arranging adequate post-operative care

You need someone to take you home from hospital, someone who can take care of you for the next several days, and someone who can help around the house for at least a week or two, depending on the extent of your surgery. You may have an angel in your life who can play all three roles, or you may have to call on a variety of friends and family members. One thing is sure: You can't recover alone.

Finding someone to handle your responsibilities

After undergoing major surgery on a weight-bearing joint, you are at least partially out of action for several months. Driving, shopping, taking care of children, doing housework, or going to work are impossible for quite some time. You must have a solid support system in place. The last thing you need is to feel you have to do things that are beyond your capabilities.

Resolving financial and insurance matters

Before your operation, find out exactly what your insurance company covers (if you have any private medical or sickness insurance policies). If undergoing private surgery, make sure that you know exactly how much of the tab you have to pick up, if any. The stress of unexpected medical expenses is extremely disruptive mentally and emotionally and is a major hindrance to anyone's recovery.

Making a recovery plan with your doctor

Although no one can predict exactly when you'll pass certain milestones on the road to recovery, it may ease your mind and give you something to look forward to if you have a list of the progressive steps of healing. Ask your doctor to help you construct a recovery plan that maps out these steps – many doctors have leaflets on the subject to hand out. Studies show that people recover better and faster if they have a good idea of what to expect both during and after surgery.

Your recovery begins while you're still in hospital, where you undergo physiotherapy beginning the day after surgery. If you're doing well after four-to-five days, you can often go home. But if you need more help, you may require more rehabilitation to get you going.

After you're home, you need to continue your physiotherapy exercises and liaise with your general practitioner (GP) and out-patient clinic. The success of your joint replacement depends heavily on your doing the required exercises and following the treatment plan. The rehabilitation process involves a lot of work, but your health is worth it.

Chapter 10

Overcoming the Ouch: Strategies for Pain Management

*T*rying to feel happy when you hurt is not easy. Pain has a way of enveloping your mind, hijacking your brain, and making it difficult to concentrate on work, family, hobbies, or anything else. You desperately want to fully involve yourself in life, but the pain distracts, worries, irritates, and depresses you to the point where you think of little else. The things that you used to do with ease can suddenly seem difficult or even impossible to accomplish. Living with long-standing, chronic pain wears you down, is exhausting, depressing, and makes you feel as if life isn't worth living. Fortunately, plenty of strategies (both physical and mental) can help you to cope with pain. So, even if your pain isn't completely banished, you *can* release its stranglehold on your life.

In this chapter, we focus on physical strategies for managing the pain. (See Chapter 14 for mental pain-management strategies.)

Understanding Arthritis Pain

Arthritis pain comes in many forms: Stabbing, aching, twisting, burning, pressing, stretching, and crushing. Some people describe the pain as 'killing', 'a fire', 'a knife that someone keeps jabbing into me', 'a continual car crash', and 'something I wouldn't wish even on my worst enemy.'

Several things cause the pain of arthritis. For example, the pain may result from something about the disease process itself:

- ✔ **Inflammation:** Swollen, hot, inflamed joint tissues.

- ✔ **Joint damage:** Bones grinding against each other, tendons that have slipped, joint misalignment or loosening, invasion of the synovium (joint lining) into the underlying bone, and so on.

Your arthritis pain may also relate to your body's response to the disease:

- ✔ **Muscle tension:** Tensing up as you react to your pain can spread pain to your muscles and make everything feel worse.

- ✔ **Strained muscles and supporting tissues:** When over-compensating for an injured area, you can unintentionally put excessive stress on a different area.

- ✔ **Fatigue:** Feeling worn out due to illness can make your pain even more intense and difficult to cope with.

Of course, when you're hurting, whether your pain is related to your arthritis doesn't matter much. You just want the pain to stop! But for many people, the pain just seems to go on and on – and on.

Differentiating between Acute Pain and Chronic Pain

The kind of sudden pain you feel when you touch a hot cooker, called *acute pain*, is absolutely vital to your wellbeing. Acute pain is a warning that you've injured yourself and need to do something about it – now! Acute pain is episodic, meaning that it comes on quickly, builds rapidly to a crescendo, then tapers off and disappears. Suppose, for example, that you fall down and graze your knee: It really hurts! But, by the time you wash, disinfect, and put a plaster on the area, your pain is already receding and soon disappears entirely. The acute pain has served its purpose – it got you to address the source of the pain and attend to the damage caused. Although acute pain is sometimes excruciating, at least it has a purpose and an end.

However, *chronic pain* is another story. Like a barrage of telegrams repeating the same message over and over, chronic pain is not a useful warning, but an agonising, debilitating tirade. More resistant to medical treatment than acute pain, chronic pain is like a constantly tormenting drumbeat underlying your every activity, day and night. Bam! Bam! Bam! The pain won't let up. And what's the number-one cause of chronic pain? You've guessed it: Arthritis.

Breaking the pain cycle

Many people with arthritis feel extremely frustrated and depressed by their pain and the decline in their physical abilities. Unfortunately, stress and depression can, and do, make pain worse. The physical pain from arthritis causes stress and upset about the loss of physical abilities. This stress, in turn, can trigger muscle tension that worsens the pain and further limits physical activities, causing even more stress and depression; thus, the cycle continues.

Happily, many things can help to break the pain cycle so you live more comfortably, even if your pain is chronic. The key is to block the pain signals moving through your nerves and spinal cord so your brain doesn't register them. Medicines can eliminate a little or a lot of your hurting (refer to Chapter 8 for more on drugs that can help).

With medication and the pain-management methods described in this chapter and the next, you can block many of your pain signals and manage your arthritis pain more comfortably. The key word here is *manage*. Managing chronic pain means reducing its severity and decreasing it to the point where you can get on with your life, not eradicating the pain completely.

Dealing with chronic pain

You usually don't have to worry much about dealing with acute pain. This type of pain certainly hurts, but it often responds well to medicine and doesn't wear out its welcome. Getting rid of acute pain is typically your doctor's job. However, dealing with chronic pain is a different matter.

The goal in chronic-pain management is to block pain messages before they reach the brain. You can try several natural things, apart from using drugs:

- Exercises appropriate to your condition
- Hot or cold treatments
- Water therapy
- Massage
- Magnets
- Topical pain relievers
- Relaxation
- TENS (transcutaneous electrical nerve stimulation)

However, several 'natural' things can make your pain even worse, all of which we discuss in Chapter 14:

- ✔ Anxiety
- ✔ Depression
- ✔ Fatigue
- ✔ Focusing on your pain
- ✔ Physical overexertion
- ✔ Progression of the disease
- ✔ Stress

Understanding the role of your treatment team

Chronic pain is a complex phenomenon that involves the original or ongoing disease process, the way your body deals with the problem mechanically, and your mental and emotional responses. A team of professionals, each with their own expertise, best handles this multifaceted problem. Your treatment team may include:

- ✔ **Your doctor** who guides your treatment and prescribes medication, if necessary.
- ✔ **A physiotherapist** who helps you to build strength and restore your range of motion. (See the sidebar 'What does a physiotherapist do?' later in this chapter.)
- ✔ **An occupational therapist** who teaches you how to place less strain on your joints when performing daily activities, overcome limitations, and prevent further damage.
- ✔ **A psychologist, behavioural therapist, or other mental-health professional** who helps you to cope with depression, anger, and/or other emotional issues.
- ✔ **A pharmacist** who offers advice on the proper use of medication.
- ✔ **A social worker** who recommends support groups or other special services and can also tell you about the welfare benefits and allowances to which you are entitled.

Pain-management clinics also exist and specialise in treating 'pain' that has not responded to the usual treatments your doctor and other consultants have to offer.

Controlling pain the natural way

Your body makes certain substances that can decrease or even block pain sensations, as well as others that can increase your pain. The pain blockers include *endorphins* and *enkephalins*, substances that can slow or stop nerve cells from sending pain messages to the brain. These chemicals are so powerful that their effects are often compared to morphine. Naturally, you want to produce more endorphins and enkephalins when you're in pain. You also want to have plenty of the brain hormone *serotonin* and other substances that play a role in manufacturing and releasing these internal painkillers.

Natural irritants – substances that increase a nerve cell's sensitivity to pain – are the flipside of the body's natural pain blockers. These irritants include *lactic acid, potassium ions, substance P,* and the stress hormone *noradrenaline* (also known as *norepinephrine*). Most of the pain-control process revolves around increasing your production of pain blockers while decreasing your production of pain intensifiers. For example, massage increases your production of endorphins while helping your body dispense with excessive amounts of lactic acid. Meditation, deep breathing, and a good belly laugh also do much to increase endorphin levels, while transcutaneous electrical nerve stimulation (TENS, described later in this chapter) decreases *substance P.*

Relieving Pain with Non-invasive Therapies

Remember being ill as a child? Your mother probably had a whole bag of tricks to make you feel better: A cool cloth on your forehead, a warm bath, letting you lie in her bed to watch television, drinking chamomile tea, and so on. Although simple little things, your mother's methods really *did* make you feel better.

Your mum's methods were *non-invasive*, which means that they didn't intrude on, or cause harm to, your body. Non-invasive methods include physical or psychological approaches and are the least traumatic forms of pain management.

The ins-and-outs of useful non-invasive physical treatments are included here; mental strategies for pain relief, such as psychotherapy, self-hypnosis, deep breathing, progressive relaxation, creative imagery, and biofeedback, are covered in Chapter 18.

At best, non-invasive approaches to pain management are very helpful; at worst they're probably harmless. With no side effects, incisions, blood loss, addiction potential, or other hazards, these techniques are worth exploring thoroughly before you move on to the harsher, and potentially more dangerous, methods of pain relief.

Many people are surprised at just how much relief the following simple physical strategies provide from arthritis pain. Although these techniques don't *cure* your arthritis (the relief is temporary), any respite from pain is more than welcome! So, next time your arthritis flares-up, try some of the following methods.

Applying heat

Warmth encourages your blood vessels to expand, bringing more blood to the painful area and stimulating the healing process. Heat also helps your muscles to relax, which is just what you need if your pain makes you tighten up. You can use hot packs, heating pads, heat lamps with infrared bulbs, electric blankets, or hot paraffin wax treatments to rev up your circulation, encourage overall relaxation, and make you feel better.

Another way of applying heat is to wrap yourself in a flannelette sheet or a blanket that you've just popped into the tumble-drier for a few minutes. Although the heat won't last long, it's very cosy!

Ultrasound is a more high-tech way of utilising heat, and can penetrate more deeply into your muscles and joints. High-frequency sound waves are aimed at the affected area, producing deep-tissue heat, which increases circulation and promotes muscle relaxation. Ultrasound is typically performed in a physio department or rehab centre, although your physiotherapist may have a portable machine to bring for home visits. Ultrasound machines are available for sale on the Internet but are pretty expensive.

Take care not to damage your skin when applying heat. Follow these rules to protect yourself:

- ✔ Limit heat applications to no longer than 30 minutes in one area.
- ✔ Wrap the hot pack or heating pad in towels as insulation; don't place the source of heat directly on your skin.
- ✔ To avoid steam burns or skin reactions, make sure that your skin is dry and free from lotions or cream (particularly deep-heating creams).
- ✔ Inspect the area every five minutes for purplish-red skin, hives, or blisters, which are signs of skin damage.
- ✔ Allow your skin temperature to return to normal before reapplying heat.

Heat may make some conditions worse. Check with your doctor in advance to see if heat treatments are appropriate for you.

Applying cold

Cold packs are used to reduce inflammation, ease muscle spasms, and block pain signals by numbing the affected area. Although blood flow to the chilled area is temporarily reduced, cold applications eventually *increase* circulation, acting much like hot packs (perhaps because the body senses the need to warm the area). Ice is the usual medium used to numb painful areas, but you may find it more convenient to use cold packs containing chemical mixtures that thaw slowly and don't drip.

A bag of frozen peas makes a good cold pack, because you can mould it round any shape, unlike a block of ice or bulky cubes. But make sure that you put the bag inside a watertight plastic bag and wrap it in a towel, because it does drip through condensation.

Protect your skin and other tissues when using cold packs by following these steps:

- ✔ Limit treatment to no longer than 20 minutes.

- ✔ Remove the cold pack once the area is numb.

- ✔ Be on the lookout for skin damage – redness, white patches, and so on.

- ✔ Avoid cold packs if you have Raynaud's, poor circulation, sensitivity to cold, nerve damage, a lack of sensation, or heart problems.

In general, if inflammation is present, use cold; if not, use hot, although many doctors recommend that you use whatever feels good to you. Best advice is to consult your doctor before using either method.

Washing away pain with water therapy

Ah, what feels better than easing your stiff, sore body into a nice warm bath? The ancient Romans evidently agreed, building several health resorts throughout their wide-ranging empire for the express purpose of bathing. Most notable was the Romans' spa in the town of Bath, where people with arthritis came from far and wide to 'take the waters'.

Warm showers, baths, and whirlpools can help to ease your stiffness and make you feel better. Warm-water therapy is also a good way to warm up your muscles before an exercise session, relaxing them and making movement easier.

Hot paraffin wax treatments

Hot paraffin wax treatments are a nice, comfortable way to warm up painful joints in your hands and feet. These treatments sustain their warmth because they use wax as insulation. A physiotherapist usually applies hot paraffin wax treatments, but you can also do it yourself at home.

How do hot paraffin wax treatments work? Your painful hand or foot is repeatedly dipped into a blend of comfortably warm, melted wax plus mineral oil and allowed to cool between immersions so the wax can harden. When the build-up is thick enough, your hand/foot is wrapped in plastic and covered with towels to preserve the heat. The locked-in warmth is very soothing for stiff, painful fingers or toes. After 20 minutes or so, the wrapping comes off, and the wax is peeled away.

As if pain relief weren't benefit enough, hot paraffin wax treatments leave your skin wonderfully soft!

Don't use this treatment if your hand or foot shows any signs of skin damage (excessive redness, blisters, and so on).

Cool water can also help, especially when inflammation is present. Immersing a painful, swollen joint in cool water or using cool compresses is a milder, less jolting version of applying an ice pack.

Pool exercises are another extremely effective form of water therapy. Because water supports your body, exercising in a pool is like exercising in a weightless environment. With the tiresome pull of gravity greatly reduced in water, your joints can rest, even as your muscles are put through a real workout. Because water provides resistance, your muscles also have to work harder to perform a movement in water than they do on land. This combination adds up to more effective exercise, with less wear and tear on your joints. (See Chapter 14 for more on water exercise.)

Whether warm or cool, water can be used in a variety of ways to help ease your pain:

- Cool hand or foot baths
- Cool moist compresses
- Drinking warm tea
- Warm full-body baths
- Warm hand or foot baths
- Warm, moist compresses
- Warm showers
- Whirlpool baths

Trying topical pain relievers

Many topical creams, lotions, rubs, and sprays can help with chronic arthritis pain. Topical applications typically contain one or more of the following ingredients:

- ✔ **Capsaicin** is a substance derived from chilli peppers that decreases the nerves' concentration of substance P in the painful area, thus reducing pain. See the sidebar 'Controlling the pain the natural way' for more on substance P.

- ✔ **Irritants** include menthol, camphor, and other substances that produce feelings of heat, cold, or itching. These feelings distract you from the sensation of pain.

- ✔ **NSAIDs** are topical versions of some non-steroidal anti-inflammatory drugs (ibuprofen, felbinac, and ketoprofen, for example) that sink through your skin to relieve deeper pain in muscles and joints.

- ✔ **Salicylates** are aspirin-like compounds that desensitise nerve endings.

Topical pain relievers are usually safe and at least somewhat effective. Make sure that you don't apply these topical applications to broken skin, you wash your hands immediately after use, avoid contact with your eyes, and watch for signs of skin irritation. Check packs for warnings to avoid during pregnancy or breast-feeding, if appropriate.

Manipulating the joints

Joint manipulation is also known as *passive movement*, because something other than your own energy is moving your joints for you. That 'something' is usually a physiotherapist. During joint manipulation, the physiotherapist moves your joints through their range of motion. Then, by applying pressure (stretching) or simply moving the joint back and forth or around and around (depending upon the joint type), the therapist also loosens up your joints. Joint manipulation is carried out with care, and never overdone. Otherwise, your joints may complain with even more irritation and pain.

If you don't move your joints, you may lose the ability to do so. In most cases some joint movement is *absolutely necessary*. People with arthritis have a tendency to guard their stiff, sore joints by moving them as little as possible – unfortunately, this is the worst thing for those joints. When joints are held still, they aren't lubricated or nourished; their supporting muscles become weaker, circulation decreases, and ligaments and tendons tighten up, losing their resilience. Over time, an immobile joint can actually freeze into position. To avoid this freezing, you must keep moving your joints, whether they hurt or not. Even splinted joints are moved, at least a little, every day.

What does a physiotherapist do?

Described as a combination of friend, drill-sergeant, cheerleader, and work-out partner, a physiotherapist works with you to help increase your range of motion, reduce your pain, build strength, and decrease any disability. The hardest part is getting you to do the exercises that remind you that you can't move like you used to. This makes some people more angry and depressed than their pain, but a good physio keeps pushing you, because that's the only way to help you feel better.

A physiotherapist takes you through a series of exercises designed to get your joints lubricated and stretch your range of movement. Joint manipulation and massage are also important parts of a physiotherapy session. Perhaps most importantly, the physiotherapist helps you stamp out procrastination and get to work!

Helping the joints with splints and supports

Splints are designed to support and immobilise an injured or inflamed joint, and are nothing more than a moulded piece of metal or plastic that's strapped to the affected area and then wrapped with elastic bandages. You can find splints for your wrists, fingers, hands, ankles, knees, back, and neck. Splints are widely available in off-the-shelf varieties or are produced, custom-made, from an impression of your joint moulded with heat-sensitive material to replicate your shape. Splints help by

- ✔ Providing support, stability, protection, and rest for injured or inflamed joints
- ✔ Immobilising a joint after surgical fusion (arthrodesis) and allowing healing
- ✔ Easing pain during arthritis flare-ups, although they're only temporary measures
- ✔ Keeping inflammation under control
- ✔ Correcting or preventing deformities (in certain cases) by correctly positioning the joint

Supports (sometimes called *braces*) are strong, elasticised tube bandages rather like a footless sock, which you slide over a certain body part, such as your wrist, knee, ankle, and so on. Their tight fit lends stability to the joint, while their elasticity allows movement and blood circulation.

Supports are used in two ways: To support and stabilise an injured joint or to protect a weakened joint from injury. Use supports in conjunction with a good exercise programme, so your muscles and supporting structures also become strengthened and don't rely solely on the elasticated tube to do the trick.

Magnetising the pain

Magnets are everywhere these days, in pharmacies, health-food shops, via mail-order catalogues and even in supermarkets! Magnets used for pain relief are generally embedded within a belt or wrap – a strip of material designed to fasten round a specific body part (your neck, knee, ankle, wrist, and so on). You can also buy magnets in patches to tape wherever your pain settles.

The magnets used for pain relief are much like the horseshoe-shaped toys you played with as a child, except they're small, flat discs. Just like your old toys, these magnets exert a pull – a magnetic field that can attract or repel certain elements in the environment. Some researchers propose that this magnetic field produces calming effects on the body, which promote healing and help normalise body function. More important, the magnetic field helps to block pain signals to the brain, causing a release of endorphins (the body's natural morphine). Like many other pain-relieving techniques we discuss in this chapter, magnets also increase blood flow to the painful area.

The strength of therapeutic magnets is measured in hundreds or thousands of *gauss*. By way of comparison, the earth's natural magnetic field is approximately 0.05 gauss and fridge magnets weigh in at about 60 gauss. The actual amount of gauss delivered to the skin is much less than that listed on the magnet's packaging, however. For example, a 6,000-gauss magnet may transmit only 1,800 gauss to your skin. And, the more wrapping or distance between the magnet and your skin, the weaker the magnetic effect. If possible, find a physiotherapist or other health professional well-versed in magnetic therapy to advise you.

The beneficial effects of magnets are still largely unproven, so mainstream medicine has yet to fully embrace their use as a valid therapy. Still, magnets are safe for most people, and many have found that they help to relieve pain. Consult your doctor before you try magnetic therapy; and if you're pregnant or have a pacemaker or other electronic implant, you should not use this treatment.

Transmitting a tingle with TENS

Transcutaneous electrical nerve stimulation (TENS) is a mild electrical buzz that overrides pain signals in tender areas. The process may sound scary, but it really isn't, and TENS is easy to apply. Electrodes are attached to your skin with a small amount of gel, and then a mild shock (from a battery-powered unit connected to the electrodes) is transmitted to the painful area. As a result of these shocks, the production of endorphins is supposed to increase. The physiologic basis for TENS is the Gate Theory of Pain (discussed in Chapter 18). TENS helps to 'close the gates', thus inhibiting pain impulses.

TENS is usually used to treat back and spine problems that don't respond to other treatments. This process offers welcome temporary relief for many people but isn't a cure.

You can purchase your own TENS unit and give yourself treatments at home. Knowing how to operate the TENS unit properly is important; some people don't benefit from TENS simply because they use the equipment incorrectly. Because the units are very expensive, consider renting one before committing yourself to a purchase.

Don't use TENS if you have a pacemaker or are pregnant. Also, don't use TENS on open wounds or near sensitive parts of the body, such as the eyes.

Taking Pain Relief to the Next Level

When non-invasive techniques don't work and your pain interferes with your ability to live a comfortable and productive life, looking into medications or, in more serious cases, surgery is necessary.

Medicating the pain away

From mild aspirin to powerful DMARDs (refer to Chapter 8), medicines are beneficial but risky. The most commonly prescribed painkillers for most forms of arthritis are *NSAIDs (non-steroidal anti-inflammatory drugs*, like aspirin or ibuprofen) and *analgesics* (drugs that reduce pain without reducing consciousness, like paracetamol).

If a joint is particularly painful and not responding to painkillers, your doctor may recommend injecting substances like *corticosteroids* (high-powered anti-inflammatory agents) right into the afflicted area. *DMARDs (disease-modifying antirheumatic drugs,* like methotrexate) alter the way the immune system works and are reserved for serious forms of arthritis – rheumatoid arthritis, psoriatic arthritis, and ankylosing spondylitis. And *BRMs (biological response modifiers,* like etanercept and infliximab) also target your immune system, and are used for aggressive, debilitating forms of arthritisthat have not responded to one or more of the DMARDS.

All medications, from aspirin to joint injections have side effects. Although they may help initially, these drugs' long-term use can cause problems ranging from stomach upsets to drug dependence. And, over time, medications' effectiveness can wane. So taking medication exactly as prescribed and seeing your doctor regularly to monitor its effects on your body are important.

Undergoing surgery

Surgery, which involves making incisions and manipulating the inner workings of your body, is always a risky and traumatic procedure.

Undergoing surgery to relieve pain can produce dramatic results for some people, but always carries serious risks and side effects, ranging from infection to death. Consider surgery only as a last resort. (Refer to Chapter 9 for a complete discussion of the operations available for arthritis.)

Part III

Is Complementary Medicine for You?

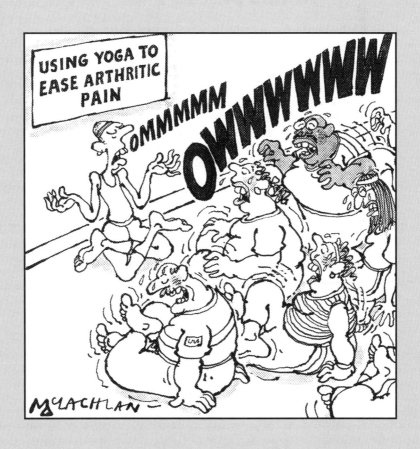

In this part . . .

*I*f the treatment of arthritis were as straightforward and effective as, say, getting rid of a mild headache (that is, take two aspirin and forget it), complementary therapies might not be so popular. But because medical doctors don't offer a real "cure" for arthritis, up to 60 percent of those who suffer from this disease turn to complementary medicine. Some feel that traditional methods just aren't working, others want help with pain relief and additional symptoms, while still others believe that they really can find a cure if they just look hard enough.

In this part, we discuss the most popular complementary therapies for arthritis, from herbs and homeopathy to "hands on" healing methods, and everything in between.

Chapter 11

Exploring Complementary Medicine

- -

In This Chapter

▶ Defining complementary medicine

▶ Examining the various approaches

▶ Finding an alternative healer

▶ Talking with your doctor about complementary healing methods

▶ Making decisions about complementary medicine

- -

*C*omplementary medicine is going mainstream – well, sort of, and only a tiny step at a time. But there has been a major change in the way that those who are firmly entrenched within the world of traditional Western medicine view therapies generated by anyone outside their realm. In the early decades of the 20th century, Western medical doctors positively vilified other therapies and crusaded to make practising other approaches illegal. In fact, well into the 1960s, talking to a chiropractor was considered unethical for a medical doctor!

Fortunately, the attitude that everything Western medical doctors do is great and that other therapies are, by definition, evil, is falling by the wayside. As a society, we've figured out that medical doctors don't have the cures for all our ills, and that other approaches have a lot to offer. During the late 1980s and 1990s, doctors and alternative therapists started working together, using a variety of treatments to complement conventional medical care. Physiotherapists, midwives, and even general practitioners (GPs) using acupuncture or homeopathy with their patients, is now relatively common.

But complementary approaches aren't perfect. In fact, many alternative theories and practices aren't backed by any scientific proof, and some things that alternative healers do are downright dangerous (although both arguments can apply to aspects of Western medicine, too!). Regardless of the debates surrounding these therapies, complementary medicine is now extremely popular. Countless testimonials exist for the effectiveness of almost all types of alternative therapies, and an increasingly impressive number of studies indicate that some of these approaches work as well as standard medicines – and sometimes even better.

Understanding the Many Faces of Complementary Medicine

Alternative, complementary, holistic, unorthodox, integrative, and preventive medicine: Many similar terms are used to describe the various different approaches to treatment. But what do these terms mean?

The most recent term used to describe non-orthodox approaches to wellbeing is *complementary and alternative medicine*, or CAM for short. CAM incorporates a variety of healing approaches that are, generally speaking, not taught in many medical schools, not used in many hospitals, and not covered by many private insurance policies.

The following list sets out the common terms and their definitions:

- **Conventional** or **allopathic medicine** is modern Western medicine – the drugs-and-surgery approach used by medical doctors.
- **Unorthodox medicine** is anything that's not conventional.
- **Alternative medicine** is an approach used in place of conventional medicine.
- **Complementary medicine** works together with conventional therapies. This approach is the one most widely accepted in the UK.

    The concept of **holistic medicine** is an important part of complementary approaches. Instead of focusing only on symptoms or the damaged part of the body as conventional doctors tend to do, the idea behind holistic medicine is to examine and treat the entire person, including the body, mind, emotions, and spirit.
- **Integrative medicine** combines the best of all worlds, using only those conventional medical treatments and complementary approaches for which there is high-quality scientific evidence of both safety and effectiveness.
- **Preventive medicine** aims to close the door on disease and keep it from striking in the first place. Education, lifestyle changes, and buffing up the body, mind, emotions, and/or spirit are all parts of this pre-emptive campaign.

CAM you dig it?

Although numbers are difficult to assess, estimates suggest that at least half of all Brits have used at least one kind of complementary alternative medicine (CAM) at one time or another – sometimes to complement and sometimes to replace standard treatment. If you include those who buy their own herbal or homeopathic supplements and special diets, the number is significantly higher.

One recent survey found that 68 per cent of people think complementary approaches – which included naturopathy and nutritional medicine – are as valid as conventional medicine. In fact, the survey found that 81 per cent of the population preferred natural therapies, with 35 per cent claiming

that they *don't* see their GP for problems such as tiredness, headaches, skin rashes, or allergies.

Who sees CAM healers? Most CAM in the UK is paid for privately, although the NHS does provide some, and there are, in fact, five homeopathic hospitals in the UK (see Chapter 12). However, CAM is used mostly by those who can afford it, and in general, it's those who are better educated, aged between 40 and 60, and female.

Ethnic communities tend to use techniques such as acupuncture, t'ai chi, and Ayurveda, which are considered complementary in this country but are traditional in their home cultures, and tend to use traditional remedies such as herbs rather than consulting a GP.

The practitioners of many complementary therapies, such as chiropractic, are now regulated, which has gone a long way towards their acceptance by orthodox practitioners.

Easing Arthritis through Complementary Approaches

Look into the medicine cabinet of just about anyone with arthritis and you're bound to find at least a few bottles of herbs, vitamins, or other supplements that promise to relieve arthritis symptoms. Because there's no real cure for arthritis, alternative approaches to treating this disease are wildly popular and run the gamut from bee venom to prayer. And in most cases, they work – at least to some extent.

In Chapters 12, 13, and 14, we discuss some of the most popular alternative approaches to treating arthritis-related pain, inflammation, and joint dysfunction. We also touch on a few approaches in Chapter 18 – positive thinking, prayer, and spirituality.

Check out the following overview of the alternative techniques most often used for easing arthritis pain:

- **Acupuncture/acupressure:** Inserting fine needles or exerting pressure with the fingers, hands, or special tools on specific areas of the body to release energy blockages and pain.

- **Aromatherapy:** Using fragrant essential oils to calm the mind and body.

- **Bee venom therapy:** Alleviating arthritis pain with venom from bee stings.

- **Chiropractic:** Realigning the spine to relieve pressure on the nerves that may be increasing arthritis pain.

- **Herbs:** The roots, stems, or leaves of plants that can act as anti-inflammatories, antirheumatics, sedatives, muscle relaxants, or pain relievers.

- **Homeopathy:** The 'like cures like' method of showing the body what's gone wrong so that it can correct itself.

- **Hydrotherapy:** The use of hot or cold water, ice, and steam to stimulate or soothe the body and ease pain.

- **Food intolerance testing:** Measuring levels of specific anti-food antibodies belonging to the protein class known as immunoglobulin G (IgG); avoiding foods against which your IgG levels are raised may reduce joint symptoms.

- **Massage:** Rubbing, stroking, or kneading the muscles to ease muscular tension and pain.

- **MSM:** An odourless crystalline powder, taken in capsule or tablet form or applied to the skin in a lotion or cream to ease arthritis pain (see Chapter 14).

- **Polarity therapy:** Balancing the body's energy systems through touching that ranges from light to firm.

- **Prolotherapy:** Injecting an inflamed joint, or the area surrounding a joint, with dextrose (sugar) water, which promotes the proliferation of new ligament tissue.

- **Reflexology:** Applying pressure to specific reflex points on the soles of the feet, palms of the hands, or even on the ears, to relieve pain in a corresponding part of the body.

- **Reiki and touch therapy:** Two ways of channelling healing energy from the hands of the practitioner to the body of the patient, without actually touching.

Finding a Reputable CAM Practitioner

Select a CAM practitioner with the same care that you give to finding the right medical doctor. You can find the names of practitioners of various alternative forms of health care in several ways:

- ✔ Ask for recommendations from friends or complementary therapists you're already seeing, whose opinions you trust.

- ✔ Get names from the various societies to which practitioners belong. (See Appendix B for the names of some of these organisations.)

- ✔ Ask your doctor or check with your local hospital. A small number of medical doctors practise one form of alternative medicine or another, and those who don't may make recommendations.

- ✔ Look for listings in the phone book.

When you've compiled a selection of possible practitioners, put together a list of questions to ask them, such as:

- ✔ Where did you study?

- ✔ What are your qualifications and experience?

- ✔ What is your treatment philosophy?

- ✔ What does treatment consist of?

- ✔ What benefits can I expect from your treatment?

- ✔ What are the possible side effects and how do you recommend handling them?

- ✔ How will I know whether your treatment is working?

If you feel your questions aren't answered forthrightly, or that you're getting the run-around, run out of the door!

Checking credentials and qualifications

Complementary and alternative medicine has a lot to offer, and it can fill in some of the gaps in conventional medical care. Unfortunately, CAM suffers from a lack of standardisation. Herbs, for example, may vary greatly in purity and potency. Likewise, although some CAM healers are incredibly knowledgeable and skilful, others are not.

Before selecting a complementary or alternative healer, make sure you do the following:

- ✔ **See a medical doctor to get an accurate diagnosis.** Some forms of arthritis are easy to recognise; others aren't. You need to know exactly what you're dealing with before undergoing any kind of treatment – conventional or CAM.

- ✔ **Educate yourself.** Gather and study all the information you can about any given CAM therapy before subjecting yourself to it. Read books and articles, get information from the Internet, talk to people, and contact the professional organisations associated with the particular CAM that interests you.

Take all information with a grain of salt until you consider its source carefully. Is the person or group that offers this information knowledgeable? Does the therapist have a solid educational background and/or practical experience? Is the therapist an unbiased source or a salesperson? Is he or she genuinely trying to help, or just trying to flog you 'natural' pills and potions?

- ✔ **Ask for credentials.** Ask the CAM therapist where he or she studied, whether he or she's registered, accredited, has professional indemnity insurance, and so on. Don't be shy or afraid to ask questions. Any healer – conventional or CAM – who won't happily review their background with you isn't a good prospect. And ask for the name and phone number of the school or society that issued the credentials, too, so you can investigate that organisation.

- ✔ **Ask for references.** Ask the CAM therapist for the names and phone numbers of people they've already worked with. Contact these people; ask them what they were suffering from, what the CAM practitioner did for them, how well the therapy worked, what the side effects were (if any), and so on.

- ✔ **Ask about the price.** Health insurance doesn't cover most CAM therapies.

Identifying false claims

Everyone wants a miracle pill to cure their ills. And everyone would like it even better if that pill were tiny and easy to swallow, worked instantly with a single dose, and didn't cost more than a packet of chewing gum.

Unfortunately, such a cure doesn't exist for arthritis, although this hasn't stopped some people claiming they have miracle cures for your aches and pains. Most alternative practitioners are honest and sincere, but charlatans happily tell you tales to take your money. So, to safeguard your health and your wallet, watch for the following warning signs.

✔ **The secret formula trap:** If the cure offers no list of ingredients or is based on a secret formula, pass on it. Claiming that something is secret is an easy way for quacks to avoid admitting their 'cure' doesn't contain anything remarkable. Reputable healers, on the other hand, are happy to tell you exactly what they're asking you to take. And knowing what you're taking is important, for even if the stuff in the secret formula is helpful, it may interact dangerously with a medicine or supplement you're already taking. Or perhaps you're allergic to the secret stuff, or it's just not right for you.

✔ **One-study wonders:** Proceed with caution if the therapist bases all the claims for treatment on just one study. Although all evidence has to start with one clinical trial, it's better if the therapy is studied many times, with different patients and under different conditions. A therapy may work in one study with, say, elderly and bedridden osteoarthritis patients, but not work so well when tested again with younger, more active subjects. The more studies, the better – and preferably of the gold standard, which are randomised, placebo-controlled, and double-blind (so neither the researchers nor participants know whether they're taking the active or placebo treatments). Reputable healers know this, which is why they want to cite as many studies as possible for their therapies.

✔ **Catch-all cures:** Avoid cures that purport to work for all types of arthritis – and other diseases as well. No therapy is a cure-all and the many different forms of arthritis have widely different causes and symptoms. How could one remedy work for them all?

✔ **The case-history game:** Be wary of any therapy if its proof of effectiveness is made up entirely of anecdotal case histories. Even if the case histories are absolutely genuine, they aren't as valid as large-scale, long-term, carefully controlled scientific studies. After all, the patients in the case histories may not have the same form of arthritis as you, they may have mild (or complicating) conditions, and they may not have taken uniform doses of therapy. The *placebo effect* can account for good results in many case histories – that is, some of the patients get better primarily because they *believe* in the therapy.

A lack of studies doesn't mean that a therapy is bad, and good study results don't guarantee that a treatment or therapy works for you. Having a combination of both studies and case histories to review is often best.

✔ **Miracle cure myths:** Steer clear of practitioners who promise their approach is the long-awaited *miracle cure*, the magic potion that erases all your problems. Some standard and alternative cures are amazingly effective, but no one has yet developed a miracle cure that eases all your ills.

✔ **Shady demands:** Avoid practitioners who tell you to throw away your crutches, stop taking your medicine, or ignore your doctor's advice. Likewise, steer clear of those who demand large sums of money in advance or who don't want you to tell your doctor what they're doing for you. In general, trust your instincts and don't do anything you don't feel good about.

Working with Your Doctor

Of all those people who use complementary therapies, it's estimated that three-quarters of them don't tell their doctors what they're doing. Many people don't confide in their doctor because they're afraid they may pooh-pooh their ideas, tell them they're foolish, try to talk them out of it, or even refuse to continue working with them if they insist on using CAM.

Try not to keep what you're doing a secret from your doctors. Telling your doctors everything that you're doing, from taking herbs to using bee venom therapy, is important, because you may inadvertently try something that clashes with your medical treatments. For example, combining St John's wort with antidepressants can cause severe central nervous system depression.

Talking to doctors about alternatives is often difficult. Doctors have the weight of medical authority on their side; they've gone to medical school and can speak a language that you may not understand. But doctors are there to help you, and work with you. You have the right to ask questions and receive complete answers. To practise medicine effectively, a doctor must practise good communication. Any doctor who closes their ears throws away an important tool for understanding what their patients need. (For more information about finding a doctor with great qualifications – and great ears – turn to Chapter 6.)

Try these tips for discussing CAM with your doctor:

✔ **Begin with the assumption that your doctor is supportive.** If you open your conversation with a challenge or disparaging remark, you probably won't get very far. Make it clear up front that you're not challenging or rejecting your doctor's ideas, but that you're simply looking for more information and help.

✔ **Ask your doctor what they know about the CAM that interests you.** Ask them whether the CAM is appropriate for your ailment, whether you need to watch out for anything while participating in the alternative therapy, and so on.

✔ **If your doctor doesn't know about the CAM that interests you, offer them information.** Go online and get studies about the CAM, copy pages from articles and books, ask the CAM's professional organisations to supply you with information, and then help your doctor to find out more about the CAM you're considering.

✔ **If you don't have time to discuss CAM during this visit, ask for another appointment.**

✔ **If your doctor gives you trouble, ask why.** Do they know that this CAM is dangerous? Have they had a bad experience with it? Have they seen patients in which the CAM had negative or dangerous results? Is their objection based on knowledge or simply a feeling that anything unconventional is bad?

✔ **If your doctor refuses to discuss CAM with you or refuses to work with you if you're using a CAM, get a new doctor.** Closed-mindedness is a terrible trait in any healer and may limit your road to recovery.

Remain as open-minded as your ideal doctor. Take into consideration any bad reports about the CAM that interests you, as well as the good reports. No healing art, conventional or unconventional, is perfect. Each therapy has its strengths and weaknesses, and it's best to know what your CAM can do for you – and what it can't.

Figuring Out whether Complementary Medicine Is for You

Deciding whether to experiment with complementary therapies is a very individual matter and depends on many things: How dissatisfied you are with traditional Western therapies, how adventurous you are, how willing you are to try unproven or controversial methods, what your inner voice tells you, and how your body responds.

If you opt for alternative treatments, always remember that many of them aren't supported with reams of scientific studies, so you're taking a chance. Always research any therapy you may want to try, find yourself the most qualified and highly recommended practitioner, consult your doctor before and during treatment, and make sure that your doctor monitors your progress. But perhaps the most important thing you can do is to listen to your body: Are you feeling better? Does this approach work for you? Sometimes even the most scientifically sound method won't help you, whereas something strange and virtually inexplicable does. Your body possesses its own brand of wisdom – when it speaks to you, make sure you listen.

Chapter 12

Discovering Herbs and Homeopathy

*U*nderstandably, many people are frustrated by the inability of standard Western medicines to cure their arthritis or relieve their symptoms completely. Luckily, some of the older, more natural approaches, such as herbal medicine and homeopathy have much to offer.

Herbal medicine uses plants and plant parts to help the body return to a state of internal balance. Herbs used to treat arthritis generally fall into the classes of anti-inflammatories (which damp down inflammation), antirheumatics (which are immunosuppressive and, as their name suggests, damp down overactivity in the immune system), sedatives/muscle relaxants, and pain relievers.

Homeopathy is a system of medicine based on the ideas that 'like cures like' and 'less cures more'. Tiny, tiny amounts of a substance that produces similar symptoms to the disease itself are given, which prompts the body to get to work on healing itself. Homeopathic remedies for arthritis usually target the swelling and tenderness caused by inflammation.

Digging into Medicinal Herbs

Ever since humans started roaming the earth, healers have used herbs to cure or at least alleviate common ailments. Essentially, a *herbal medicine* is any part of a plant – leaves, roots, bark, sap, fruit, seeds, or flowers – that can be used for medicinal purposes.

Investigating herbal applications

Some herbs are eaten in their natural form. Other herbs are harvested, dried, and ground to produce a powder that can be made into a watery *infusion* (a tea or tisane), a *tincture* (an alcoholic solution) or packed into tablets or capsules. The active ingredients of herbs can also be extracted using a dissolving substance (a solvent such as alcohol, or even water), which is then removed to produce a more concentrated extract for making into tablets or capsules. Herbs can also be boiled or mixed to form a paste and applied as a poultice or, if pressure is applied, as a compress – for example around a swollen ankle or knee.

Not all herbs are taken as pills or capsules; some are taken in the form of teas or, more accurately, *infusions*. (The only true tea is one made from tea leaves, or the leaves of the *Camellia sinensis* bush.) To make an infusion, the herb is submerged in water that is just slightly cooler than boiling, and then left to steep so its health-promoting ingredients can diffuse into the water. After a few minutes, the herb is skimmed out, and the liquid is ready for drinking.

Try infusions of any one of these or a combination of a couple, as they suit your mood:

- **For a pick-me-up:** Basil, borage, ginseng, Hawthorne berry, bilberry, cinnamon, yarrow

- **For depression, stress, or tension:** Borage, catnip, jasmine, hops

- **To strengthen the immune system:** Elderflower, green tea, goldenseal

- **To promote sleep:** Chamomile, orange flower, valerian

Solid extracts are produced by dissolving the herb in a solvent such as alcohol or water, then collecting the fluid and evaporating it to leave a solid residue. These solid extracts are described according to their concentration. For example, a 10:1 extract means that ten measures of raw or dried herb results in the production of one measure of the extract; so, for a product with this concentration, 1 kilogram (just over 2 pounds) solid residue is produced for every 10 kilograms (22 pounds) of herb used. The more concentrated the extract, theoretically the stronger it is, although substances may become lost through evaporation, so that the concentration does not always reflect the level of potency. Because of these differences in concentration, you're better off selecting a standardised preparation whenever possible.

Standardisation is a method that helps to ensure consistency so that each batch of a product provides consistent amounts of selected active ingredients and provides the same benefit. Standardised remedies are also more likely to have good quality clinical trials supporting their use.

Exploring the difference between a herb and a drug

Drugs are often just highly refined versions of herbs. About one-quarter of all modern medicines come from herbs. To turn herbs into drugs, pharmacological researchers need to home in on the main, active ingredient that produces the herb's medicinal effect. This ingredient is then separated from the rest of the plant and usually modified in some way, before being concentrated and standardised so that each dose delivers an exact amount. The drug is then tested in a number of clinical trials to prove its safety and efficacy before it's ready to be sold.

The good part about this drug-making approach is that it makes use of the special part of the herb that cures a particular ill, treating it like a great soloist in an orchestra. The bad part is that refining the herb allows only that soloist to shine, casting aside the rest of the orchestra.

Doctors say drugs are better than herbs because the active ingredient is isolated, drugs are modified and pure, they're served up strong, and they work much faster than herbs.

Herbs: Everything old is new again

No one knows exactly when people began using herbs, or who realised that eating certain leaves could help to stop a headache, and drinking liquid from boiling roots could help to promote sleep. But once the connection was made, people undoubtedly gathered whatever they could find and started experimenting. Some results worked well, and others sent them back to the drawing board – hopefully without any unwanted Dr Jekyll and Mr Hyde effects.

Herbs were a vital part of ancient medicine, with the Egyptians using garlic and other herbal medicines as early as 1800B.C. Hippocrates, the Greek father of medicine, even developed a way to classify herbs based on their healing qualities. Herbs were the backbone of Western medicine until the development of modern pharmaceutical-based drugs in the 19th and 20th centuries. Herbs are still the mainstay of present-day Native American, Ayurvedic, and Eastern medicines.

Although herbs, like homeopathic remedies and other therapies, were swept aside by the tidal wave of pharmaceutical drugs pouring out of laboratories during the 20th century, they were certainly never forgotten. Indeed, herbs still serve as the source of one-fifth of all modern drugs. Even today, pharmaceutical companies scour the world (especially the tropical rainforests), looking for previously unknown plants that may have medicinal properties. These companies also routinely ask herbalists and traditional healers about herbs in their quest for new sources of drugs – a process that has been given the posh name of *ethnopharmacology*.

Herbalists (those who practise the medicinal and therapeutic use of plants) say that herbs are better than drugs because the so-called active ingredient is only one of many substances that work in concert to relieve or cure ailments. Unfortunately, modifying and purifying the active ingredient makes that ingredient overly strong, dangerous, and more likely to cause side effects. Herbalists point out that some of the alleged impurities in herbs can actually modify their effects to make them gentler and safer. And although speed is sometimes necessary, it's not always essential for effective treatment. In fact, drugs that work too fast may even be overly harsh.

Although many pharmaceuticals are more potent and potentially more dangerous than most herbs, you need to consider all herbs as drugs and treat them with respect. Herbs provide a concentrated source of active ingredients that can change or modify the way the body works. Just because something is natural does not guarantee that it's safe – otherwise your doctor might still be prescribing arsenic!

Getting the Low-down on Herbs for Arthritis

Which herbs have medicinal value? How much of each herb do you use? Which herbs are good for osteoarthritis and which for rheumatoid arthritis and gout? Do you take herbs in powder form, rub them on as ointment, or sip them in the form of tea? The answers to these and many other herbal questions depend on whom you ask, and whether that person is a doctor of Eastern medicine, a herbalist, a naturopath, a chiropractor, or an assistant in a health-food shop. The advice you receive about herbs to treat arthritis undoubtedly varies from one healer to another based on their personal experience and preferences. A variety of herbs may be prescribed, some specifically for your type of arthritis, others for joint problems in general, and still others for pain, depression, or to help strengthen your immune system.

Bear in mind that although some herbs have scientific studies to support their effects on arthritis, others do not. The following herbs are proven to ease the symptoms of arthritis and are usually used as a first-line treatment:

Even though many people consider that herbs are safe, it's best not to self-medicate. You could do more harm than good, as:

- ✔ You may have an allergic reaction.
- ✔ The herb may interact with another medicine that you're taking, which can increase the intended effect of either, create the opposite effect, produce a toxic effect, or otherwise affect your body in harmful ways.

  ✔ You may have a medical condition that makes it dangerous for you to
     take a particular herb.

  ✔ The herbal concentration is too strong, too weak, or the herb is mixed
     with other ingredients that your body cannot handle.

Avoid potential risk by checking with a pharmacist or herbalist before taking
any herbs. Even if he or she isn't an advocate of complementary medicine,
you must still let your doctor know that you are taking herbs or planning to
take them, in case there are any interactions or contra-indications with any
drugs you are taking.

In addition to the herbs in the following sections, your herbalist may suggest
black willow, caraway seed, cinnamon, clove, couch grass, dandelion, juniper
berries, oats, nutmeg, poke root, prickly ash, skullcap, spearmint, star anise,
wintergreen, wormwood, yarrow, and more. Herbalists can draw from a
lengthy list of herbs when recommending treatment for arthritis pain, inflammation, anxiety, depression, insomnia, skin rashes, muscle pains, and other
symptoms!

Peeking inside the herbalist's toolbox

Herbal medicine is used to treat just about anything that can go wrong with the human body –
from glaucoma, to liver disease, to cancer. A
tremendous number of herbs are at home in the
herbalist's little black bag, including:

  ✔ **Agrimony** for allergies

  ✔ **Cayenne pepper** to strengthen the immune
     system

  ✔ **Celery** for arthritis

  ✔ **Elderberry extract** for 'flu'

  ✔ **Feverfew** for migraine

  ✔ **Fringe tree bark** for liver disease

  ✔ **Garlic** for elevated cholesterol and blood
     pressure

  ✔ **Ginger** for nausea

  ✔ **Ginkgo biloba** for problems with memory
     and circulation

  ✔ **Goto kola** for varicose veins

  ✔ **Hemp** for glaucoma

  ✔ **Hyssop** for asthma

  ✔ **Linden** for tension

  ✔ **Skullcap** for asthma

  ✔ **St John's wort** for insomnia and depression

  ✔ **Turmeric** for inflammation

  ✔ **Valerian** for asthma

  ✔ **Vervain** for headaches

Applying anti-inflammatories

Inflammation, a condition in which a part of the body becomes reddened, hot, swollen, and painful, is a major problem in several forms of arthritis and related conditions. Doctors have powerful anti-inflammatory drugs, including painkillers and corticosteroids, but many people prefer the gentle relief offered by herbs such as those listed below. Anti-inflammatory herbs don't suppress inflammation on their own as much as they help the body to reduce the inflammation naturally.

Alfalfa

Rich in minerals, alfalfa is a folk remedy for arthritis favoured in the Middle East for its ability to reduce swelling and inflammation. Alfalfa is scientifically known as *Medicago sativa*.

Angelica

Angelica, or *Angelica archangelica*, is a heaven-sent remedy used to treat the inflammation associated with rheumatism. This herb is also believed to purify the blood and protect against contagious diseases – a property worth bearing in mind if bubonic plague ever makes a comeback in your area.

Black cohosh

Scientifically known as *Cimicifuga racemosa*, black cohosh is a Native American remedy taken to reduce the inflammation and pain of rheumatoid arthritis.

Bladderwrack

Rest assured that bladderwrack is named after its bulbous floatation devices rather than any harmful effects on your waterworks. Rising to prominence in the early 1800s, bladderwrack was originally used as a source of iodine. Today the herb, known by the unwieldy scientific name of *Fucus vesiculosus*, is used in compresses to help reduce arthritis inflammation.

Boswellia

Known scientifically as *Boswellia serata*, boswellia comes from India, where its gummy resin has been used for thousands of years as an anti-inflammatory. Substances in boswellia, called *boswellic acids*, are believed to reduce inflammation and help relieve the pain of osteoarthritis and rheumatoid arthritis. Boswellia has also been used to treat psoriasis, ulcerative colitis, and allergies, and may also help to lower high cholesterol and high triglyceride levels. Boswellia is used as an extract, cream, or ointment.

Cat's claw

Cat's claw (also known as uña de gato) is derived from the bark of a South American vine native to the Peruvian rainforest. Cat's claw was used for generations by the Ashanica Indians of South America to treat colds, tumours, and cold sores. Known scientifically as *Uncaria tomentosa*, the herb helps to combat arthritis symptoms by reducing inflammation and boosting the immune system. Cat's claw is taken in the form of tea or capsules. The herb may also be used to help counteract gastrointestinal damage caused by NSAIDs (which are discussed in Chapter 8).

Centaury

Also known by its scientific name, *Erythrina centaurium*, centaury was used by the ancient Egyptians to reduce high blood pressure, and later by German herbalists for anxiety and melancholy. Today, centaury is often recommended for cases of gout and rheumatism because of its ability to help relieve inflammation.

Devil's claw

Devil's claw, or *Harpagophytum procumbens*, is named after the sharp hooks that develop on its fruit. Devil's claw is a South African desert plant whose tap root contains a variety of compounds, such as harpagoside, whose inflammation-reducing qualities have been compared to cortisone and phenylbutazone. An infusion made of devil's claw is a folk remedy for arthritis, rheumatism, and gout.

Sarsaparilla

With the official name of *Smilax officinalis*, sarsaparilla originated in the New World and was brought to Europe in the 1600s. There, the herb was used to treat inflammation due to rheumatoid arthritis. Herbalists still use sarsaparilla today to relieve the pain and swelling of arthritis and to enhance overall wellbeing. As a bonus, some consider sarsaparilla to have an aphrodisiac action, too.

Wild yam

Known scientifically as *Dioscorea villosa*, wild yam is perhaps most famous as a traditional female remedy, used for menstrual ailments and to prevent miscarriage. Wild yam also has anti-inflammatory properties, which is why some herbalists recommend it for rheumatoid and other forms of inflammatory arthritis.

Reining in rheumatoid arthritis with antirheumatics

Antirheumatics help to damp down the pain, swelling, stiffness and other symptoms of inflammation that accompany rheumatic conditions. Several herbs are especially helpful in reducing the symptoms of rheumatoid arthritis (joint inflammation in a majority of joints, swelling in two matched joints such as two wrists, fever, fatigue, and so on) and related conditions. The better-known antirheumatics include the herbs listed below.

Bogbean

This herb, with a less than delightful name, was once used to prevent scurvy as it is rich in vitamin C. Despite its moniker, this pretty wild flower is renowned for its ability to relieve the pain of rheumatism. Known to scientists as *Menyanthes trifoliata*, bogbean has mild sedative properties.

Be careful – large doses of bogbean may cause vomiting. Don't use bogbean if you have inflammatory bowel disease.

Celery seed

Celery seed (botanical name *Apium graveolens*) was used by Eastern healers to reduce elevated blood pressure. Today, celery seed and celery juice are used to rid the body of excess water and aid digestion. The seed is also believed to ease both rheumatoid arthritis and gout.

Chinese Thunder God Vine

Used medicinally in China for over 400 years, an extract from the root of the magnificently named, yet toxic, Thunder God Vine *(Tripterygium wilfordii)* can ease pain and inflammation safely and effectively in people with otherwise treatment-resistant rheumatoid arthritis. The extract helps to 'turn off' an overactive immune system and tone down the activity of certain inflammatory genes. Researchers believe that Chinese Thunder God Vine also has potential as a treatment for lupus, although more study is needed.

Don't use this on your own without medical supervision; as mentioned, the herb can be toxic.

Meadowsweet

Meadowsweet *(Filipendula ulmaria)* contains a substance with aspirin-like properties. The herb has been used for hundreds of years to relieve arthritis pain and help combat rheumatic conditions.

Sedatives and muscle relaxants

Sleep is often a major problem for people with arthritis. How can you sleep if moving hurts, turning over is difficult, or if you're worried and stressed? The herbs in this category can help you to relax and sleep better.

Lemon balm

Lemon balm *(Melissa officinalis)* is an aromatic herb native to the Mediterranean whose leaves contain a variety of aromatic essential oils. Lemon balm has been used since ancient times as a healing, soothing herb with calming, sedative, and anti-spasmodic actions. Traditionally known as the Scholar's Herb because it helped students suffering from exam stress to sleep, lemon balm can help to promote a good night's rest for anyone needing it.

When combined with valerian (see the next section), the two herbs work together to reduce symptoms of tension, stress, and mild depression.

Valerian

Known as *Valeriana officinalis*, valerian comes from the roots of a perennial herb. Valerian is recommended for arthritis patients because it helps ease pain and tension, and it also encourages sleep. In Germany, valerian is used as a mild sedative, and one study shows that it works as well as a standard sedative drug with the added advantage of being non-addictive.

Don't take more than the recommended dosage of valerian – very high doses can cause a weakened heartbeat and even paralysis. Check with your physician to see how much valerian you can take.

Pain relievers

Pain is one of the worst symptoms of arthritis. Dull or sharp, constant or intermittent, achy or gripping, pain usually makes your life miserable. Here are some of the better-known herbs that can help relieve pain.

Aloe

Used internally or externally, aloe is a popular herbal cure for pain associated with wounds, burns, and arthritis. Aloe boasts more than 200 different species, of which only three or four are used medicinally, the most useful being *Aloe vera* and *Aloe barbadeni*. As well as relieving arthritis pain, aloe is used to treat gastrointestinal problems and ulcers, as first aid for wounds and burns, and as a mild laxative.

Taken internally, aloe may hamper or increase the action of certain medications, and cause uterine contractions or miscarriage in pregnant women.

Burdock

Burdock *(Arctium lappa)* is an ancient remedy that has been used to treat snakebites, dog bites, and a variety of other conditions thought to leave impurities in the blood. Today's herbalists have found that burdock has a diuretic effect and may ease arthritis pain as well as skin irritation due to psoriasis, eczema, and aphthous ulcers (sores in the mouth). Dandelion and Burdock is a popular traditional drink.

Capsaicin

Capsaicin, which comes from chili peppers, is the ingredient that makes spicy cayenne so hot. Capsaicin is believed to prompt the release of endorphins, the body's natural, built-in pain relievers, and to interfere with substance P, which helps transmit nerve signals through the nervous system. Known scientifically as *Capsicum frutescens*, capsaicin is used to treat pain. Your doctor can even prescribe a capsaicin-containing cream on the NHS to treat the pain of osteoarthritis if they think that it may help you.

Fennel

Well-known among chefs, fennel is also used to relieve stiff, painful joints. Herbalists and folk medicine healers often suggest that their patients apply fennel oil directly to their distressed joints and rub it in. This herb's scientific name is *Foeniculum vulgare*, which, as it's a bit of a mouthful, is worth promptly forgetting.

Ginger

The aromatic root of a tropical herb, ginger has been used by the Chinese to treat indigestion, stomach cramps, and stomach upset for over 2,000 years. Scientifically known as *Zingiber officinale*, ginger is recommended by modern herbalists for people with arthritis. Studies show that taking ginger supplements or eating fresh ginger can help ease the pain, morning stiffness, and inflammation associated with some forms of arthritis, while increasing flexibility and range-of-motion.

Ginger is typically taken as a powder, capsule, extract, tea, or tincture. It can also be freshly grated and added to food or eaten as a side dish. Ginger compresses may be applied to painful joints.

Mustard (black)

A preparation of mustard, or *Brassica nigra*, has long been a favourite remedy for painful joints. Sometimes black mustard is taken internally (often with honey), and sometimes it's applied directly to the joint. (Mustard oil plus rubbing alcohol can be applied to the skin to increase circulation to the affected area.) Black mustard is generally considered stronger and more effective than white mustard.

Stinging nettle

A prickly plant with stinging hairs that 'inject' an irritant into the skin, stinging nettle has traditionally been used to treat allergies, insect bites, and wounds. Today stinging nettle may be recommended to relieve joint pain and swelling; laboratory studies suggest that it can counteract at least some part of the inflammatory response. A German study found that stinging nettle plus a small amount of an NSAID to be as effective as the full dose of the NSAID in relieving symptoms of osteoarthritis. In addition, stinging nettle contains boron, a mineral important for bone health. Known scientifically as *Urtica dioica*, stinging nettle is typically taken as a capsule or extract. A poultice of cooked leaves may be applied to the painful area.

Stimulating Your Body to Heal Itself with Homeopathy

No one has proven why or how homeopathy may work, and though some studies suggest that homeopathic remedies are significantly more effective than a placebo, others have found the results unimpressive. Although all the evidence is not yet in, many people are convinced that homeopathy is right for them.

Before drugs and surgery came to dominate Western medicine, healers called *homeopaths* flourished in Europe and the United States. Their guiding philosophy was *homeopathy*, which means 'similar suffering'.

The idea behind homeopathy, which was created by the German doctor, Samuel Hahnemann in the 18th century, is to stimulate the body's natural healing mechanisms by 'showing' it a piece of what's wrong. This idea may sound odd; after all, you're accustomed to modern Western medicine killing disease with strong medicines. But Dr Hahnemann believed that like cures like. If large amounts of a substance could cause the symptoms of a disease in a healthy person, Dr Hahnemann reasoned, that very small amounts of the same substance should be able to help the body eliminate the same ailment. These small doses would act something like vaccines and gently stimulate the body to heal itself.

Homeopathic remedies are not highly concentrated; in fact, they're diluted again and again until only minuscule amounts of the original substance are left. This method is counter-intuitive to practitioners of Western medicine, who believe that medicines should have more of the active ingredient, not less. But remember, homeopaths argue that smaller portions are better, because larger portions can actually cause the problem being treated. The tiny portions, homeopaths insist, help the body to heal itself.

For example, suppose that a large amount of Substance X caused constipation in healthy people. According to Dr Hahnemann's homeopathic theory, a very tiny dose of the same Substance X would unlock the bowels in people who were already constipated. This idea was codified as homeopathy's *Law of Similars*.

Determining remedies according to your symptoms

Although medical doctors try to suppress symptoms, doctors of homeopathy look upon symptoms as helpful signs that the body is trying to heal itself. To the homeopath, symptoms are more than simply indicators that a certain disease is present, they're the body's way of describing what has gone wrong on a physical, mental, and emotional level. Probing beyond the symptoms (where Western medicine stops), homeopaths look for the essence of their patients. Thus, they ask what their patients like to eat and drink, when and how well they sleep, whether they're day or night people, what they wish for and what they fear, what kind of weather they prefer, how they respond to stress, and so on.

If you complain of pain, a good homeopath looks beyond its location, intensity, and number of occurrences and asks additional questions, such as:

- When does it hurt?
- What are you doing when it starts to hurt?
- How are you feeling, emotionally, before the pain strikes?
- What does the pain feel like? Is it sharp? Throbbing? An ache? Does it radiate? Is it constant? Does it come and go?
- What makes the pain feel better? A warm bath? Eating certain foods? Going to work?
- What makes the pain feel worse? Movement? Cold temperatures? Stress? Work? Family get-togethers? Holidays?

These kinds of questions are designed to get to the essence of the patient's problem – the physical and emotional state that allowed the disease to take hold and grow.

After the homeopath identifies the essential problem, it can be treated – but not with a medicine designed to destroy anything. Instead, the homeopath looks for the single best remedy (homeopathic medicine). What remedy is most effective depends mostly on the individual. If a patient has joint pain, for example, not just any remedy for pain will do – it has to be the remedy that best matches the patient's *constitutional make-up*. Every one of the 2,000 or so homeopathic remedies closely matches a particular temperament – a person's fears and hopes, likes and dislikes, and sleep and behaviour patterns.

In *classical homeopathy*, only the absolute minimum dose of a remedy is given, and only one remedy is prescribed at a time. If the right remedy is given, the patient's symptoms begin to clear up in a few days. If the symptoms are not affected, a different remedy is selected. No new remedies are used after the body has begun to heal itself. However, practitioners of *complex homeopathy* prescribe more than one remedy at a time.

Discovering homeopathic remedies

Homeopathic remedies are derived from a variety of sources: Leaves, berries, fruits, bark, roots, minerals, and sometimes animals – including snakes and spiders! But no matter where they come from, all homeopathic remedies are processed in a very special way.

In keeping with the idea that small amounts are best, the remedies are diluted over and over again in solutions made of water and alcohol, lactose, or other diluents. And each time they're diluted, these remedies are shaken and struck in a special way. The more diluted, shaken, and struck, so the theory goes, the stronger the remedy becomes. Indeed, a finished remedy may only contain one part per million of the active ingredient. Critics charge that very little or even none of the active ingredient remains after these successive dilutions, so the remedy can't possibly work. Supporters believe that either what's left over is enough to do the trick; or that the fluid retains a molecular memory of the medicinal substance and acts accordingly.

Remedies are rated according to their potency. When one drop of the medicinal substance is shaken and struck into 99 drops of diluent, the remedy has a potency rating of 1 c. (This mixture is sometimes written as 1CH.) If one drop is taken out of this mixture and added to 99 drops of new diluent, the new remedy has a potency rating of 2 c. If one drop of the 2 c remedy is then diluted with 99 drops of a new diluent, the potency rating rises to 3 c, and so on. How potent the remedy is depends on the state of the disease. Here are the general guidelines used in many countries:

✔ **Low potency:** Up to 6 c, used typically at the start of treatment, especially if only physical symptoms exist.

✔ **Medium potency:** From 12 c to 30 c, used when physical and mental/emotional symptoms exist.

✔ **High potency:** Up to 200 c or greater, used when the problem is long-standing or acute, or the symptoms are mental/emotional.

Another, very similar rating system is based on 10 drops of diluent rather than 99. Instead of shaking and striking one drop of substance into 99 drops of diluent, you use only 9 drops of diluent. In this method, based on 10 drops, potencies are rated 1 x, 2 x, 3 x, and so on.

Determining how to take a remedy

Although it's best to see a trained homeopath who can assess your constitutional type, personality, lifestyle, family background, likes and dislikes, as well as your symptoms before deciding which treatment is right for you, remedies can be self-chosen according to your symptoms. Many books and charts are available to help you select an appropriate remedy.

Self-medicating is never a good idea and can lead to unintended consequences, interactions with other substances, and possible damage to your health. No matter how much you may have heard about the safety of homeopathic remedies, working with a medical doctor or doctor of homeopathy is essential when you're using them. If you are using any homeopathic remedies, be sure that your doctor knows exactly what and how much you're taking, even if he or she doesn't believe in homeopathy. Although interactions with prescribed drugs are unlikely, it is good to let your doctor know that you're using homoeopathic medicines, so they can monitor their usefulness; you never know you might help convert a sceptic!

Dr Hahnemann believed that only a single homeopathic remedy should be given, for the shortest possible time, to stimulate the body's own healing powers. However, some modern remedies contain a number of homeopathic substances – these are known as *combination* or *complex remedies*.

In most cases, start with a 6c potency. Apply the treatment two or three times a day for up to a week. If you experience partial relief but the symptoms return when you stop taking the remedy, you can increase the effect by taking a 30c potency.

Ideally, you take homeopathic medicines on their own, without eating or drinking at least 30 minutes before or afterwards. Don't handle tablets as this may interfere with their energy. Instead, tip tablets into the lid of the container or onto a teaspoon to transfer them to your mouth. Then suck or chew the tablets so you absorb the benefits through your mouth; don't swallow them whole as stomach acids may neutralise their effects.

When taking homeopathic remedies, it's recommended that you avoid drinking strong tea or coffee as these may interfere with the homeopathic effect. Similarly, it's best to avoid using certain powerful essentials oils such as lavender, rosemary, and peppermint.

Occasionally, symptoms get worse before they get better – a reaction known as *aggravation*. Although aggravation is uncommon, try to persevere as it is a good sign that the remedy is working.

After completing a course of homoeopathy, you can usually feel much better in yourself, with a greatly improved sense of wellbeing that lets you cope with any remaining symptoms in a more positive way.

Homing in on homeopathic remedies for arthritis

The purpose of the homeopath is to find the best match between remedy and patient. The remedy that the homeopath selects depends as much on the patient's constitutional make-up as it does on the symptoms, which is why you can't just pull any old arthritis remedy off the shelf. The following are some of the homeopathic remedies used for arthritis:

- ✔ *Actea spic:* May be indicated when the joints are swollen and pained, and the focus of the arthritis is in the hands and feet or the smaller joints.

- ✔ *Aconitum napellus:* May be indicated for gout under conditions in which the pain grows worse at night or when temperatures rise, and gets better when the patient rests or gets fresh air. May be useful if the patient is anxious and imagines terrible things are happening.

- ✔ *Ammonium carbonicum:* May be indicated when poor circulation to the hands exists, as in Raynaud's phenomenon (refer to Chapter 5).

- ✔ *Apis mellifica:* May be indicated when the joints are stiff and swollen, when pressure makes the pain worse, and when the skin over the swollen joints feels stretched and tight.

- ✔ **Arnica montana:** May be indicated when the patient has rheumatoid arthritis linked to cold and dampness, and soreness and bruising are problems. May be useful if the patient is nervous and extremely sensitive, prefers to be alone, and denies that anything is wrong.

- ✔ **Belladonna:** May be indicated for sudden, sharp pain, and red, swollen joints. May be useful in cases where getting wet or chilled makes the pain worse, and the patient usually avoids any kind of stimulation.

- ✔ **Benzoic acid:** May be indicated when rheumatoid arthritis settles in the smaller joints, and nodular swellings exist.

- ✔ **Bryonia alba:** May be indicated for gout with greatly swollen joints and in conditions in which heat, movement, or touch makes the pain worse; cold, rest, and pressure help.

- ✔ **Calcarea carbonica-ostrearum:** May be indicated for rheumatoid arthritis in the shoulders and upper back. May be useful in cases in which wetness and dampness worsen the pain, and fear and perhaps confusion engulf the patient.

- ✔ **Causticum:** May be indicated when arthritic joints are stiff and tight, when lying on the afflicted joints increases the soreness, and when the patient is restless at night.

- ✔ **Chamomilla:** May be indicated for severe pain when anger and restlessness are present.

- ✔ **Cimicifuga racemosa:** May be indicated when pain is centred more in the muscles than the bones and when restlessness, talkativeness, and an unstable mood often accompany the pain.

- ✔ **Ledum palustre:** May be indicated when pain is primarily in the smaller joints and travels up the body, with little or no swelling, and the pain is worse when the patient is in a warm bed.

- ✔ **Ruta graveolens:** May be indicated when the patient suffers from bursitis (refer to Chapter 5).

- ✔ **Sabina:** May be indicated when the patient is suffering from gout, and the gouty joints have nodules. May be useful if the pain worsens with heat and movement, feels better with cool air, and is usually accompanied by depression.

- ✔ **Sambucus:** May be indicated when the patient is suffering from poor circulation to the hands, as in Raynaud's phenomenon. May be used in conditions in which the hands are blue and cold, and the patient sweats excessively while awake but not while sleeping.

Finding homeopathic help

Homeopathy is practised by a variety of healers in the UK: Naturopaths, chiropractors, osteopaths, herbalists, dentists, acupuncturists, and even certain medical doctors – especially GPs. However, the level of training and skill varies from healer to healer, so be forewarned!

You are entitled to homeopathic treatment on the National Health Service (NHS), and if your doctor decides it is appropriate, they can refer you to an NHS doctor at one of the five NHS homeopathic hospitals, or at an NHS homeopathic clinic. If your doctor refuses to refer you, they can discuss the decision with you to explain why they don't feel homeopathic treatment is appropriate. You can then request a second opinion. The British Homeopathic Association publish a useful guide called 'How to get Homeopathic Treatment on the NHS', which you can request by phone 020-7566-7800, e-mail: info@trusthomeopathy.org, or by visiting www.trusthomeopathy.org.

Homeopathic remedies may be prescribed by a medically-trained homeopathic doctor on the normal NHS prescription form and dispensed by homeopathic pharmacists for the usual prescription charge or exemptions. Alternatively, you can consult a private homeopathic practitioner or buy remedies direct from the pharmacist.

Chapter 13

Making the Most of Hands-On Healing Methods

*F*or thousands of years, healers have known the 'laying on of hands' has a powerful therapeutic effect on the body. And why wouldn't it? Human beings are made for touching. Babies fail to thrive if they're not touched enough. Huddling together against the cold was undoubtedly a survival technique for scores of our ancestors, and lovemaking is perhaps one of life's most fulfilling, restorative activities. So, looking to hands-on methods for healing your body when it's ill or in pain makes sense. This type of therapy doesn't necessarily cure the disease, but it can help to relieve pain, increase vital circulation, ease mental stress, relax tensed muscles, increase overall relaxation, and help your body in its struggle to rebuild itself.

The various methods of hands-on therapy, from ancient acupressure to the relatively new trigger point therapy, are explored in this chapter. However, keep in mind that if you decide to engage in any of these therapies, you must use them in addition to – not in place of – standard medical treatment, and discussing your preferred therapy method with your doctor first is also a good idea (although he or she may not necessarily know much about it).

Unblocking the Energy Flow: Eastern Hands-On Healing Methods

Eastern therapies are rooted in either Chinese or Japanese medicine, and are designed to remove blockages and restore balance in your body's energy flow. After balance is restored, the body can begin to heal itself.

Pinpointing the pain with acupuncture

Acupuncture is an important part of traditional Chinese medicine, with thousands of years' worth of history showing its success in preventing and treating disease.

In traditional Chinese medicine, disease is thought to result from an imbalance or blockage of energy, or *chi* (pronounced 'chee'), in one or more parts of the body. (Air and food supply energy, while the stresses and strains of living diminish this energy.) *Acupuncture* is the practise of manipulating specific points on the body to unblock the energy flow and restore the body's balance.

According to traditional Chinese medicine theory, energy flows through your body along invisible channels called *meridians*. Twelve major meridians run through your body to deliver energy and sustenance to your tissues. When these channels become obstructed, the obstructions act like tiny dams, blocking or slowing the flow of energy and serving as a major cause of pain and disease. Luckily, the meridians touch the surface of your skin at some 300 different points called *acupuncture points*, and acupuncturists manipulate and stimulate these points to remove obstructions and re-establish a healthy flow of energy throughout your body.

During your first visit, an acupuncturist interviews you extensively about your symptoms, level of pain, medical history, diet, bowel habits, quality of sleep, and so on. Usually, your eyes, tongue, skin, or fingernails are also examined. The acupuncturist takes your pulse and listens to your voice, breathing, and bowel sounds.

During your visit, you either lie or sit on a padded table for the treatment, but you don't have to remove all your clothing, just loosen it and uncover the treatment areas. Your acupuncturist then stimulates and manipulates certain acupressure points, but just a few – not all 300 of them! The following list explains the various methods your acupuncturist may use to stimulate and manipulate acupressure points:

✔ **Inserting fine needles:** Your acupuncturist may insert anywhere from 2 to 15 hair-thin needles into certain points and leave them standing for a period of time (usually 20 to 40 minutes). He or she may not necessarily insert the needles directly into the area that's bothering you, but rather along the meridian that affects that area. So don't be surprised if your feet are manipulated to ease your back or neck pain! The needles are so fine, you may not feel them, but if you do, you usually feel just a moderate sting that disappears quickly. Your acupuncturist may insert needles shallowly (just under your skin) or as deep as an inch or more.

✔ **Adding a low-level current (electro-acupuncture):** Many acupuncturists find that the addition of a low-level electrical current makes the treatment more powerful. Wires are attached to the acupuncture needles after the needles are inserted, and these wires are hooked up to a box that delivers an electrical current. Your acupuncturist adjusts this current by turning a dial. You should feel a light buzzing at your acupuncture points. If the buzz is annoying or uncomfortable, tell your acupuncturist, and they can turn down the 'juice' until it no longer bothers you.

✔ **Using heat and herbs (moxibustion):** To stimulate your acupuncture points, your acupuncturist may burn a small amount of a herb called *mugwort* (or *moxa* in Chinese) over your acupuncture points, taking care not to burn your skin.

✔ **Cupping:** Small glass cups are heated and placed over your acupuncture points to create a vacuum-like effect. As they cool, the cups invigorate these areas and leave interesting sucker-shaped marks afterwards, which slowly fade.

Discovering what acupuncture can do for you

Acupuncture treats ailments ranging from asthma to ulcers, but its primary use is for pain relief. Many people with osteoarthritis, rheumatoid arthritis, gout, fibromyalgia, and Raynaud's phenomenon swear by acupuncture, and some studies show that it can relieve the pain of osteoarthritis and/or fibromyalgia. Although no scientific explanation for its effectiveness exists, acupuncture does produce real responses in the body, including stimulation of your immune and circulatory systems and the release of endorphins, your body's natural painkillers.

You may need several acupuncture sessions (perhaps as many as six) before you begin to notice a difference, but once the beneficial effects set in, they often last for weeks, months, or even longer. Unfortunately, acupuncture doesn't work for everyone, so this therapy's a case of trying it and seeing how it works for you.

Finding a good acupuncturist

The British Acupuncture Council is the main regulatory body overseeing the practise of acupuncture in the UK. Members of the British Acupuncture Council have completed a thorough training of at least three years in traditional acupuncture and biomedical sciences. These members carry the letters MBAcC after their name and are covered by Medical Malpractice and Liability insurance. For a list of registered acupuncturists in your area, contact: The British Acupuncture Council, phone: 0208-7350400 – there is usually a small postal charge. Alternatively, visit www.acupuncture.org.uk and click on Find an Acupuncturist.

Some doctors are trained in acupuncture. To find a medically qualified acupuncturist in your area (usually a general practitioner (GP)) contact the British Medical Acupuncture Society, phone: 01925-730727; or visit www.medical-acupuncture.co.uk and click on Find a Practitioner. (See Appendix B for more information.)

Finally, ask the members of your health-care team for referrals, because more members of the traditional Western medical community are becoming aware of the benefits of acupuncture. (Who knows? Maybe some of these people see acupuncturists themselves!) Asking doesn't hurt, and your medical team members may be able to give you some good leads.

Pressing your buttons with acupressure (shiatsu)

Acupressure (which the Japanese call *shiatsu*) is a lot like acupuncture, but instead of using needles to unblock your energy flow and restore balance, the therapist presses on your acupuncture points using their fingers, hands, or special tools. Because acupressure involves hands-on manipulation, this therapy is often considered another form of massage instead of a version of acupuncture. Because acupressure is actually a combination of these two methods, both acupuncturists and massage therapists often use it.

Instead of lying on a padded table as you do during an acupuncture session, during acupressure you lie on a mat on the floor for better resistance against the pressure exerted during treatment. Using his or her thumbs, fingers, whole hand, elbows, or feet, the practitioner applies pressure and manipulates your body along meridians to improve your flow of *chi* (energy). They may also use tools, such as wooden rollers, balls, or pointers. As the practitioner works to unblock your chi, he or she also works to transmit some of their own energy into your body. Your acupressure session may include stretching or other kinds of massage, and some practitioners also give diet and lifestyle tips.

Discovering what acupressure can do for you

Acupressure is designed to produce the same pain-relieving and energising results as acupuncture – without the needles, of course! Like massage, acupressure has a calming and soothing effect, and that alone may help to ease some of your symptoms almost immediately. Although good studies demonstrating acupressure's effectiveness don't currently exist, it does work for some people, without side effects (when the therapy is properly done). At the very least, an acupressure session is usually a pleasant experience.

Finding a good acupressurist

Contact the Shiatsu Society, phone: 0845-1304560 or visit www.shiatsu.org to find an accredited acupressurist. (See Appendix B for more contact information.)

Many massage therapists also use acupressure techniques. To find such a therapist, check out the Massage Therapy UK Web site at www.massage therapy.co.uk and click on Practitioner Directory.

You may also find referrals for an acupressurist through your healthcare team, rehab centre, pain management centre, or chiropractor.

Restoring healing energy with Reiki

The word *Reiki* (pronounced 'ray-kee') is a combination of two Japanese words – *rei*, meaning a higher intelligence or spiritual consciousness, and *ki* (or *chi* in Chinese), meaning the life force or energy that animates all plants and animals. Therefore, *Reiki* is a healing energy guided by a higher intelligence or a spiritual power.

A Reiki practitioner administers the treatment by laying their hands on specific parts of your body and applying little or no pressure. (You remain fully clothed.) Some practitioners don't actually touch, but rather place their hands directly above the person's body. The practitioner then channels healing energy into you, which helps to relieve energy blockages and balance the life-force within your body. This technique is sometimes used along with some form of massage. The basic principle of Reiki is that the practitioner can channel universal life energy, which creates and maintains all forms of life, into someone else as a force for healing.

Discovering what Reiki can do for you

Enthusiasts say that Reiki can help to ease the pain and other symptoms of virtually every kind of illness and injury while increasing the effectiveness of all kinds of therapy. Although the practitioner may not actually touch you, those who have experienced Reiki say that they feel a glowing radiance flowing throughout their bodies after a 60- to 90-minute session. Stress reduction, relaxation, and an increased sense of wellbeing are typical benefits of a Reiki session.

Finding a good Reiki practitioner

Reiki is increasingly used in complementary therapy centres, GP surgeries, hospitals, hospices, and facilities that care for the elderly. Check out the Web sites for the UK Reiki Federation at www.reikifed.co.uk and the Reiki Association at www.reikiassociation.org.uk. Further contact details are in Appendix B.

Realigning and Releasing Tension: Western Hands-On Healing Methods

Although Eastern therapies are based on releasing energy blockages and restoring the chi, Western therapies contain a potpourri of approaches, ranging from manipulating the alignment of the spine to applying pressure to specific points on the sole of the foot. Each therapy is based on a different theory, and each takes a completely unique approach to pain relief.

Realigning the spine with chiropractic

First introduced to the Western world in the late 1800s by Daniel David Palmer, *chiropractic* is based on the belief that the body has the power to heal itself, and that this power is concentrated in the central nervous system, extending from the brain down through the end of the spine. According to Palmer, disease is the result of the spinal vertebrae causing undue pressure on nearby nerves. This pressure interferes with the healthy functioning of the tissues or organs served by those nerves, causing disease or damage. According to the chiropractic theory, manipulating the spine to relieve nerve pressure can eliminate illness and restore health.

Misalignments in the spine putting pressure on the nerves are called *subluxations* and are caused by injury, poor posture, stress, lack of exercise, or genetic problems, just to name a few. You don't necessarily feel that you have a subluxation (they're often very minor imbalances), and you probably don't realise that a misalignment in your back is causing the pain in your kidney – that's why you visit the chiropractor. They can tell by touch or other simple tests where your spine is out of alignment, and adjust it accordingly.

When you visit a chiropractor, he or she asks you about the location, duration, and intensity of your pain and how long you've had it. If the chiropractor feels it's appropriate, they may take an X-ray of the area.

After your X-ray, you lie face down on a padded table. The chiropractor feels along your spine looking for vertebrae that are out of line, tension in the muscles, swelling, or any other abnormalities. Then, they use a variety of methods to apply controlled, directed forces to your spine, including straight massage, acupressure, trigger point therapy, and myofascial release. All these methods fall into the category of *spinal manipulative therapy (SMT)* and aim to release stress, improve alignment, relieve pain, and improve function. Many chiropractors also use a tool called an *activator,* which resembles a tiny, rubber-tipped pogo stick. The activator delivers a precise, measurable force that, when applied to specific points on your body, helps adjust misalignments. The chiropractor may also 'crack' your back or neck to relieve pressure within a given area of your spine.

The term subluxation has different meanings in Western medicine and in chiropractic. In Western medicine, *subluxation* refers to the incomplete or partial dislocation of a joint, in which the bony surfaces no longer face each other. No such condition is correctable by chiropractic treatment. In chiropractic, a *subluxation* refers to subtle, minor imbalances in a joint, usually those involving the spinal vertebrae, which interfere with the spinal cord and/or spinal nerves, causing pain.

Discovering what chiropractic can do for you

Chiropractic is often a very effective treatment for acute lower-back pain, as well as a faster, better way to treat certain types of neck and back pain than standard Western medicine, massage, or acupuncture. Chiropractic is also a useful way to treat headaches, muscle spasms, knee pain, and shoulder pain. This therapy is used occasionally to relieve pain in the hip, knee, or shoulder, although it may not work as well in those areas as it does in the neck and spine.

Manipulating already-damaged joints can make them worse. Consult your doctor before trying chiropractic, and make sure that you let your chiropractor know that you have arthritis.

Finding a good chiropractor

Chiropractic is a fast-growing independent healthcare profession in the UK. Practitioners must be registered with the General Chiropractic Council (GCC) before they are allowed to see patients. Begin your search for a chiropractor through referrals from friends, especially if you know someone who has been treated by several chiropractors over the years and can compare their strengths and weaknesses. You can also check the General Chiropractic Council's Web site at www.gcc-uk.org (see Appendix B for more information), click on <u>Find a Chiropractor</u> and enter your town or postcode for a referral list. When narrowing down your choices, look for a chiropractor who:

- ✔ Has experience in treating patients with your type of arthritis.
- ✔ Spends at least 20 minutes with you each session, performing hands-on work.
- ✔ Doesn't pressure you to buy vitamins or supplements.
- ✔ Doesn't rely on gadgets, such as back massaging beds, infrared lamps, waterbeds, or vibrators.
- ✔ Takes few, if any, X-rays.
- ✔ Performs myofascial release or some other soft-tissue massage before adjusting your spine.

You may need several treatments before you see a noticeable improvement. However, if you aren't getting results after five or six treatments, chiropractic (or your current chiropractor) may not suit you.

Rubbing away muscle tension with massage

Massage is the manipulation of body tissues by rubbing, stroking, kneading, or tapping using the hands or other instruments, such as rollers, balls, or pointers. For most kinds of massage, you lie on a padded table, wearing little or no clothing, covered by a soft flannel sheet. Your body remains covered by the sheet throughout the massage, except for the area actually being treated.

If you're uncomfortable with the idea of disrobing in front of the therapist, remember that you only need to take off enough clothing to reveal the areas that you want massaged. Keeping your underwear on is definitely okay! Being massaged while sitting in a chair fully clothed is also possible (sometimes this is done in the workplace).

The therapist asks you what kind of massage you like (invigorating, relaxing, and so on), if and where you're experiencing any pain, and how firm or soft a touch you prefer. If you like, the therapist may darken the room and play soft music during the massage. Oil or lotion (usually pre-warmed) is used so that the therapist's hands glide over your skin without causing friction.

Speak up! Having a whole body massage is not necessary unless that's what you want. If you just want work done on your neck, feet, and hands, for example, say so. And don't be afraid to give your therapist feedback during the massage: Tell them what feels painful, what feels soothing, what you like more or less of, what kind of pressure feels best, and so on. The therapist adjusts the technique and pressure accordingly. The whole point of massage is for you to relax and feel comfortable, so state clearly what you need.

Many kinds of massage are available; following is a list of some of the most popular:

- ✔ **Swedish massage:** Also known as *effleurage*, Swedish massage involves the gentle kneading and stroking of muscles, connective tissue, and skin, using oils or lotions. Sometimes clapping or tapping movements are also used. Therapists can make this method of massage as gentle or as vigorous as you like. If you have fibromyalgia, rheumatoid arthritis, or another particularly painful form of arthritis, a gentle Swedish massage may be just what you need to help you relax.

- ✔ **Shiatsu:** Also known as *acupressure*. (See the 'Pressing your buttons with acupressure (shiatsu)' section earlier in this chapter.)

- ✔ **Deep tissue massage:** This method of massage involves the exertion of intense pressure to relieve chronic tension deep within the muscles. Using fingers, thumbs – and sometimes elbows – aching, knotted, or chronically tense muscles are slowly stroked across the grain to release tension and induce relaxation. Deep tissue massage is sometimes painful and may cause soreness during and after the session. But if favouring your painful joints causes chronic tension to develop in other parts of your body, deep tissue massage is a good way to release the tension.

Make sure you consult your doctor before trying deep tissue massage.

- ✔ **Rolfing:** *Rolfing* was developed in the 1950s by Ida P. Rolf, a biochemist who discovered therapeutic bodywork when an osteopath successfully treated her for a respiratory problem. Dr Rolf's treatment is based on the idea that both physical and psychological health is affected by the alignment of your body. If your body is out of line, poor physical, mental, and emotional health results.

To correct body misalignment, the Rolfing practitioner stretches and manipulates the thin membrane (called the *fascia*) that covers each bone, muscle, organ, nerve, and blood vessel. The fascia can tighten in response to stress, injury, or chronic misuse. To release this tightness, practitioners use their fingers, knuckles, or elbows to apply intense pressure. Administered in one-hour sessions once a week for ten weeks, Rolfing is uncomfortable at best; at worst, the therapy's quite painful. But proponents of this method claim that it can produce marked improvement in muscle function and reduced strain on the joints. Combined with special breathing techniques, Rolfing may also help to release the buried emotions that create chronic physical tension.

Rolfing is too painful for many arthritis patients. Make sure that you get your doctor's permission before trying out this kind of massage.

✔ **Myofascial release:** *Myofascial release* is a milder form of Rolfing, in which the practitioner applies gentle but steady pressure to the fascia to stretch it and release tension.

✔ **Sports massage:** This form of massage is intended to ease soreness; assist in healing sports injuries, such as sprains, strains, tendonitis, or muscle soreness; and prevent future injury. Like Swedish massage, sports massage involves kneading and stroking the muscles and connective tissue, with an emphasis on the areas of your body that the sport affects most (for example, the shoulder and arm of a bowler in cricket, or the knees and legs of a football player). If you have an injury or an inflamed joint, make sure that your massage therapist is a qualified expert in this type of massage.

✔ **Trigger-point therapy:** Using the fingers to apply prolonged, deep tissue pressure to specific points on knotted, painful muscles, *trigger-point therapy* relieves tension and helps muscles to relax. This therapy causes the pain sensors in the pinpointed area to 'overload', so they either send fewer pain messages or stop sending them altogether. In some cases, trigger-point therapy is a helpful treatment for fibromyalgia.

Trigger-point therapy is a treatment that feels so good – when it stops! For example, say that you have chronic tension in your neck, which you just can't seem to release. To perform trigger-point therapy, your massage therapist or chiropractor asks you to lie face down on a padded table, and then proceeds to apply intense thumb pressure to a specific point where your neck and shoulders meet. (Yes, it hurts!) Your therapist maintains this pressure for a good 30 to 45 seconds (or as long as you can stand it), but after the pressure is released, your chronic neck tension disappears (or at least, be greatly reduced).

As with deep tissue massage and Rolfing, check with your doctor before engaging in trigger point therapy.

Injured and/or inflamed joints are not massaged directly, as injured tissue can undergo further damage, and the increased circulation stimulated by massage may make swelling worse.

Discovering what massage can do for you

Like most kinds of hands-on therapy, massage can significantly affect your well-being – at least temporarily. A slower heart rate, increased endorphin levels, decreased pain levels, and improved relaxation are just a few of the positive results. Like a nice warm bath, a good massage can increase your circulation and then go two steps further. Massage helps your body to clear away by-products of metabolism that can irritate nerve endings, and it increases your level of *endorphins* – the body's natural morphine – to ease pain.

Some types of massage are not appropriate for all types of arthritis. Consult your doctor for guidelines before getting massage therapy, especially if you have rheumatoid arthritis, osteoarthritis, or ankylosing spondylitis. Also, avoid massage if you have a fever or infection, if you're experiencing an arthritis flare-up, or if you're coming down with an acute illness.

Drink plenty of water before and after a massage. Massage can release built-up toxins in the muscles, and keeping well-hydrated helps your body to flush them out.

Finding a good massage therapist

Locating a skilled massage therapist who is experienced in treating clients with arthritis is a top priority. Fortunately, your health-care team, rehab centre, pain management centre, chiropractor, or physiotherapist can often steer you to someone suitable.

For a therapist who specialises in a particular type of massage, consult the Web site of the Massage Therapy Institute of Great Britain at www. cmhmassage.co.uk and click on Find a Therapist. You can also visit www.massagetherapy.co.uk (see Appendix B for more information).

Just as important as technical qualifications is the chemistry between you and your therapist. The gender of the therapist, in fact, is an issue for many people. If you feel a little strange about accepting a massage from a male therapist, for example, you should automatically narrow your search to include women only. Remember, if you don't feel completely comfortable with the therapist you choose, you won't enjoy all the benefits of massage. So, shop around; you may want to try several therapists before deciding on one person. Keep in mind that many massage therapists come to your home with their massage tables and all the accoutrements in tow. All you have to do is pick up the phone!

Promoting energy balance with polarity therapy

Like traditional Eastern systems of healing, *polarity therapy* is based on the belief that the body contains energy systems that are balanced in good health, and that unbalanced or blocked energy leads to pain and disease. The aim of polarity therapy is to find these blockages and release them using the hands to touch specific points on the body, to help restore balance. After balance is achieved, the body returns to a healthy state.

During your first visit, the practitioner interviews you, observes your body and the way you move, and manually feels certain areas of your body to determine the location and degree of your energy blockages. The therapy itself involves touches that vary from light to firm, but you don't have to disrobe, and the touching involves your verbal feedback. A typical session lasts from an hour to an hour and a half.

Discovering what polarity therapy can do for you

Your polarity therapy practitioner works to help you increase your awareness of subtle energetic sensations. For example, you may feel mild waves of energy coursing through your body, tingling, warmth, or general relaxation. Your practitioner may also offer advice on diet and lifestyle. The aim of polarity therapy is to relieve your pain and to help your body heal itself, but currently no studies confirm that polarity therapy actually achieves these goals.

Finding a good polarity therapy practitioner

To find a practitioner of polarity therapy, see the Web site for the UK Polarity Therapy Association at www.ukpta.org.uk. Click on <u>Practitioners</u>, and then click on your county to get a list of referrals. Further contact details are in Appendix B.

Relieving pain and encouraging healing with reflexology

Reflexology involves applying pressure to specific points on the soles of your feet, the palms of your hands, or your ears, which are thought to correspond with various organs and other parts of the body. Reflexology theory maintains that your body is divided into ten zones, each running lengthwise from head to foot and down one arm through one of the ten fingers. Applying pressure on one part of the zone is believed to help relieve pain and encourage healing in another part of that zone.

The reflexologist manipulates a specific area – most commonly on the bottom of your foot, but sometimes on the palm of your hand or your ear – that corresponds to the diseased or painful area. They use a map of the foot, hand, or ear to indicate the points that can stimulate healing in the heart, stomach, lung, pancreas, kidney, colon, eyes, ears, throat, and even the tonsils. For example, your reflexologist may press an area just outside the middle of the ball of your foot to stimulate your lungs. Reflexologists use special thumb, finger, and hand techniques, without the addition of oils or lotions, to stimulate your body parts. For most people, reflexology is a relaxing and pleasant experience – as long as you're convinced that your feet are clean and sweet-smelling!

Discovering what reflexology can do for you

No studies exist that prove that reflexology is an effective treatment for arthritis. But, like most kinds of massage, reflexology is helpful in reducing the stiffness people with osteoarthritis and rheumatoid arthritis experience. Reflexology may also help to increase circulation, which is beneficial if you have Raynaud's phenomenon.

Finding a good reflexologist

Take a look at Web site for the British Reflexology Association at www. britreflex.co.uk (see Appendix B for complete contact information). Click on Practitioners, and then click on your county for a list of referrals.

Transmitting healing energy through touch therapy

In *touch therapy*, also known as *therapeutic touch*, energy is transmitted from the practitioner's hands to the patient's body in order to speed the healing process and ease pain. Like certain Eastern philosophies, therapeutic touch is based on the belief that the body possesses an energy field and that the energy within this field is ordered and balanced to maintain health. Disease occurs when the energy in this field becomes unbalanced.

Although the practitioner does not actually touch your body, he or she can discern where problems exist in your energy field by meditating while holding his or her hands over your body to feel the vibrations. The practitioner then channels energy into your body to help ease the pain and speed healing. One session of touch therapy usually takes about 30 minutes.

Discovering what touch therapy can do for you

Some studies find that therapeutic touch is effective, including one study performed on 25 patients with osteoarthritis. The study participants were divided into three groups: One received standard Western medical care, another received therapeutic touch, and a third received a simulated version of touch therapy. Those participants who actually received touch therapy experienced a significant decrease in pain along with an increase in mobility, which the other participants did not. However, other studies do show that touch therapy has little or no effect. In spite of this finding, therapeutic touch is widely practised, is used by many nurses and doctors, and is the subject of a great deal of scientific research. If you're in pain, you may want to give therapeutic touch a try.

Finding a good touch therapy practitioner

To find a good touch therapy practitioner, contact the British Complementary Medicine Association at www.bcma.co.uk, or the Institute for Complementary Medicine at www.icmedicine.co.uk.

Chapter 14

Other Complementary Approaches

● ●

In This Chapter

▶ Discovering the benefits of aromatherapy

▶ Understanding bee venom therapy

▶ Exploring electromagnetic therapy

▶ Finding out about food intolerances

▶ Looking into MSM

▶ Delving into hydrotherapy

▶ Peeking at prolotherapy

● ●

*Y*ou're probably familiar with herbs and homeopathy (and if not, check out Chapter 12), but many people use additional complementary methods to ease the symptoms of arthritis. This chapter looks at some of the more exotic therapies, how they're performed, and what they can do for you.

Even if you're lucky enough to find both a therapy that works and an excellent practitioner, you still need to work with your physician and other members of your healthcare team. Studies show that people with arthritis who completely ignore traditional medicine in favour of alternative methods can find their health deteriorating at an alarming rate. These therapies are used to *complement* traditional medicine, not act as a substitute for it.

Breathing In the Healing: Aromatherapy

Aromatherapy is one of the oldest healing arts, dating back over 4,000 years to the ancient Egyptians. Aromatherapy uses a wide variety of fragrant substances called *essential oils* to treat physical and emotional ills. Producing deliciously enticing smells, these oils are taken from the fruit, flowers, bark, stems, or roots of medicinal plants such as basil, bergamot, cedar wood, chamomile, jasmine, and rose.

The essential oils most often used for arthritis pain include benzoin, birch, black pepper, chamomile, eucalyptus, ginger, and juniper.

The unique aroma of each essential oil, when inhaled, is believed to trigger beneficial physiologic and emotional responses. Lavender, for example, is soothing and relaxing, which is why this oil is recommended for people who are stressed or anxious. Ginger, on the other hand, is energising and warming and is sometimes used as a mild aphrodisiac to spice up your love life.

One study shows that people with arthritis who use aromatherapy can reduce their intake of painkillers while maintaining their current level of comfort. Because aromatherapy acts on the central nervous system, it can also ease anxiety and depression, reduce stress, induce relaxation or sedation, give you a lift, or act as a mild stimulant.

Delivering good scents

Massage is perhaps the most effective delivery system for aromatherapy. A few drops of essential oil are mixed with a plain *carrier oil,* such as almond or corn oil, and massaged into the body. Some oils have a medicinal effect when absorbed into the skin, but most work through an effect on the smell-sensitive parts of the brain. Aromatic oils are also used in steam inhalations, and warmed in special heaters to scent the air.

With the exception of lavender oil, essential oils are rarely applied directly to the skin in their undiluted state because they are too strong and irritating.

When inhaling steam, remove the pot from the hob and allow it to cool. Inhaling the steam from a boiling pot can cause burns and swelling of the respiratory tract.

Sniffing out how to get aromatherapy

Many people perform aromatherapy on their own, but seeing a professional first to find out how to do it safely and effectively is a good idea. Many oils are not suitable for use during pregnancy or if you have high blood pressure, for example. You can find a certified aromatherapist by contacting one of the aromatherapy organisations listed in Appendix B.

Fighting Pain with Bee Venom Therapy

Bee venom therapy is quite popular in Asia and Eastern Europe, and many people swear it eases their symptoms of arthritis. Bee venom contains a potent mix of chemicals that, paradoxically, are used to relieve joint and muscle pain – especially in sports injuries, multiple sclerosis, and arthritic and rheumatic conditions. Although the traditional method involves the sting of a live bee, the venom is also given via injection in some countries. But there are a few drawbacks to these jabs, including their potential to cause dangerous allergic reactions. Therefore, receiving the venom in the form of a topical cream or as a homeopathic remedy is safer.

Homeopathic bee remedies are prepared from the whole honey bee, including its sting, and are known as *Apis mellifica*, *Apis mellifera*, or *Apis mel.* This remedy is used to treat inflammation accompanied by burning and stinging, including inflammation of joint linings – in other words, arthritis. Bee remedies are said to work best in restless people who resemble 'queen bees' in that they love to organise everyone else and have a sting in their tail for those upsetting them!

Being stung in a good cause

Traditionally, bee venom is administered either directly on or near the site of your pain or on specific acupuncture or trigger points. Applying the live sting of a bee is an interesting procedure. The bee, held in long tweezers, is placed on the designated spot and allowed to do its thing. Not surprisingly, the target area is often numbed with ice beforehand to help dull the pain. The procedure is usually repeated several times before you see any arthritis pain-relieving results. And, as you can imagine, this therapy hurts. Don't administer bee stings at home!

Bee-ing aware of the benefits

Surprisingly, bee venom has powerful pain-relieving and anti-inflammatory effects. There are no studies to document bee venom's prowess in humans, but it helped to prevent induced arthritis in rats!

This treatment is potentially fatal if you develop an allergic reaction to the bee venom. Before beginning bee venom therapy (assuming you can find a willing practitioner), ask your doctor to test you for an allergy to bee stings. If you are allergic, *do not* use this treatment! And even if you aren't allergic, having someone else present when you are stung, as well as an anaphylaxis emergency treatment kit in case you suddenly develop an allergic reaction, is imperative.

Applying bee balm

Bee venom cream, or bee balm, is available in many health-food shops. A 30 g tube contains venom equivalent to 300 bee stings, and is harvested using an electro-stimulant technique that does not harm these amazing insects. The balm is often mixed with other painkilling remedies, such as capsaicin (derived from chilli peppers).

You apply the bee balm twice a day and let it sink into tissues to stimulate release of cortisol – one of the body's most powerful anti-inflammatory hormones.

Use a tiny amount on a test area before using the full dose, in case of sensitivity. Do not use bee balm if you are allergic to bee stings, have high blood pressure, a serious heart condition, or muscle spasms such as those that can occur in fibromyalgia.

Mesmerising the Pain with Electromagnetic Therapy

Electromagnetic therapy is a way of accessing your body's own electric and magnetic fields through acupuncture points on the skin surface. Pain is considered to result from imbalances in these biological electric and magnetic fields.

Practitioners believe that electromagnetic therapy frees imbalances and build-ups of electromagnetic energy that irritate nerves and muscles. As a result, wearing electromagnetic patches can quickly reduce pain and relax spasms. The therapy also improves circulation and hastens healing.

Patching up the pain

Electromagnetic therapy involves the use of special patches that contain a rare earth magnet (an alloy of neodymium, iron, and boron) coated with purified zinc and surrounded with tiny copper spheres. These elements are pre-aligned and attached to adhesive tape to ensure the correct magnetic pole is in contact with the body.

Electromagnetic patches generate three different electromagnetic fields:

- **Magnetic** with the south pole of the magnet facing away from the skin.
- **Micro-electric** due to copper and zinc forming a battery bridged with moisture from the skin.
- **Induced electric current** due to the magnetic field acting on the copper microspheres.

These fields interact to produce pulsations of energy said to have a beneficial effect on the flow of electromagnetic energy through the body.

Going with the flow

The body's energy is thought to flow through channels known as *meridians*. These meridians are accessed through classic acupuncture points (*acupoints*) on the skin surface, and this practise forms the basis of ancient therapies such as acupuncture and acupressure.

When your body's electrical energy flow is abnormal, acupoints on the surrounding skin often become painful to touch. These tender acupoints are known as *tsubos*. In acupuncture, acupoints are stimulated with fine needles to generate electrical impulses and restore energy balance. In electromagnetic therapy, *tsubos* are stimulated with the tiny electromagnetic pulses released from the patches.

Electromagnetic patches are applied to clean, dry skin over acupuncture points (especially tender tsubos) near painful areas. For small areas, or mild-to-moderate pain, only one patch is necessary. If pain is more extensive or severe, several patches are used to treat a larger number of acupoints.

Patches are left on the skin, undisturbed, for five to seven days. You wear the patches during all your normal daily activities, including bathing and showering. After five to seven days, the patches are gently peeled away and discarded. New magnets are applied if necessary, though resting for a day or two before re-starting treatment is usually beneficial.

Do not use electromagnetic therapy if

- ✔ You have an infection at the site of the patch.
- ✔ You have an open wound at the site of the patch.
- ✔ You have a heart pace-maker.
- ✔ You're pregnant and want to put the patch on your abdomen
- ✔ The patch causes skin irritation.

Keep patches well away from computer disks and other magnetic media, as the magnetic field may wipe the stored information they contain.

The copper component of the magnet may cause slight discolouration on some skin types, but this is harmless and naturally wears off over a few days. Absorbing a little copper through your skin may even prove beneficial (see Chapter 21 for more about the benefits of copper in copper bracelets).

Picking up your electromagnetic patches

Electromagnetic patches are widely available in pharmacies, health-food shops, and even some supermarkets. Packets of patches are usually supplied with booklets that show acupuncture points and tell you where to position the patches depending on which area of your body is affected.

Finding Out about Food Intolerance

Increasing evidence suggests that inflammation in the body increases 'leakiness' in your gut so that partially digested food proteins enter your circulation. These particles can trigger reactions in your white blood cells, making them more active and aggressive. The over-activity of these immune cells may result in the symptoms associated with food intolerance. Eliminating the foods that trigger this reaction from your diet may improve your joint pain and stiffness.

Food intolerance is linked with a number of health problems, including irritable bowel syndrome, migraine, eczema, psoriasis, and joint pains.

Getting tested for intolerance

Food intolerance testing aims to identify the foods to which your white blood cells are over-reacting. Food intolerances are best identified through blood tests. These tests either measure levels of specific anti-food antibodies (of a protein class known as *immunoglobulin G* or *IgG*) or look at what happens when your white blood cells are incubated with different food extracts. If you have elevated levels of IgG antibodies against certain foods, or if your white blood cells develop changes in their shape and appearance on exposure to certain foods, you are advised to avoid these foods for a period of time.

Covering the controversy

Although controversial, ongoing clinical trials suggest that avoiding foods identified through food intolerance tests are effective in helping some people with non-specific joint pains and rheumatoid arthritis. The tests with the most evidence to support them either measure your levels of specific, anti-food IgG antibodies, or analyse changes occurring in your white blood cells

No scientific evidence suggests that hair analysis, muscle strength testing, or electrodermal testing for food intolerance are of any clinical use.

Fighting Arthritis with MSM

In some countries, including Russia, a drug called DMSO (dimethyl sulfoxide) is used to treat several different types of inflammation, including joint problems.

When DMSO is broken down within the body, about 15 per cent of it is converted into an organic compound called *methyl-sulphonyl-methane* or *MSM*. MSM has many of the same benefits of DMSO but fewer detriments; therefore, it's available as a food supplement that doesn't require a prescription. (In the UK, DMSO itself is licensed, on a named-patient basis, only for treating a bladder problem called interstitial cystitis.) MSM seems to help fight inflammation and may help to alleviate some of the symptoms of rheumatoid arthritis (RA).

When James Coburn won the Academy Award for Best Supporting Actor in 1999, he gave the marketing campaign for MSM a real shot in the arm by claiming that MSM made it possible for him to fight the pain and disability of rheumatoid arthritis and continue working. Since then, MSM has taken off as a 'natural' pain-relieving and inflammation-fighting treatment for osteoarthritis, rheumatoid arthritis, gout, and fibromyalgia. MSM is also said to help neutralise an acid stomach, fight allergies, and to ease constipation, among other things. Unfortunately, no real scientific proof exists for any of these claims. And much more research is needed before MSM is deemed safe.

Using MSM

MSM is available as tablets, capsules, powder, gel, cream, and lotion and is often combined with other substances that are beneficial for joint health, such as glucosamine, chondroitin, or vitamin C.

The recommended standard dose for tablets/capsules of MSM is 500 milligrams twice a day. You may start by taking 250 milligrams or less twice a day, and watch for side effects such as gastrointestinal problems. If all goes well, gradually increase the amount until you reach the standard dose. In some people, individual doses as low as 50 milligrams are effective, and most people can tolerate doses up to 1,500 milligrams, although for severe conditions, even higher doses are needed to achieve relief.

However, consult your doctor before taking MSM, and don't stop taking your other arthritis medication(s) unless he or she advises you to do so.

MSM may produce blood-thinning effects, and if used in conjunction with blood thinners such as heparin, aspirin, or certain herbs, can cause excessive bleeding or prolonged clotting time. Consult your doctor or a pharmacist about adverse interactions before taking MSM.

Getting MSM

MSM is widely available in pharmacies, health-food stores, and on the Internet. Before you buy, you may want to check out the content and quality of various brands of MSM at www.consumerlabs.com to get the most cost effective because it can work out expensive.

Whirling the Pain away with Hydrotherapy

Hydrotherapy is an ancient treatment using water (both hot and cold), steam, and ice to stimulate and soothe the body; thus, rearranging its energies and encouraging healing. The Romans gained fame for their public baths, where people 'took the waters' to ease the pain of arthritic joints. A modern hydrotherapist may recommend a variety of treatments, including colonics to rid the body of toxins, drinking plenty of distilled water to flush toxins away, taking short cold baths or showers to increase circulation, using warm baths, saunas, or steam rooms to increase circulation and sweat out toxins, and applying cold compresses to ease joint pain.

Although bathing in mineral waters (and sometimes drinking them) is touted as a health aid, evidence suggests that bathing in plain-old warm water works just as well!

Understanding hydrotherapy

Water is applied either to the entire body or to specific areas in the form of liquid, steam, or ice. This therapy is delivered via showers, baths, *sitz baths* (baths in which you're immersed only up to waist level), warm and cool compresses, wet-sheet wraps, hot blankets, saunas, and other techniques.

Hydrotherapy can also involve internal treatment through drinking water and/or having *colonic* irrigation (an enema that flushes out the colon).

No evidence exists that colonic irrigation is beneficial for arthritis. As this therapy flushes out healthy bacteria from the large bowel, it may result in future digestive problems. Many therapists advise taking lots of expensive supplements afterwards, too. If a therapist recommends colonic irrigation, question him or her very carefully about why he or she thinks it helps – and about the total cost implications.

Finding a good hydrotherapist

To find a specialist in hydrotherapy, contact one of the alternative medicine organisations listed in Appendix B. Look for someone experienced in treating arthritis, as some forms of hydrotherapy are detrimental to your condition (for example, cold water therapy for Raynaud's may further constrict blood vessels that are already overly constricted).

Peering into the Possibilities of Prolotherapy

Prolotherapy or *Ligament Sclerosant Therapy,* involves injecting an inflamed joint, or the area surrounding a joint, with dextrose (sugar) water. This therapy is a non-surgical way to treat several musculoskeletal conditions. '*Prolo*' is short for 'proliferation', and this therapy is believed to promote the proliferation (growth) of new ligament tissue surrounding joints where weakened and damaged tissue is causing joint instability and chronic pain.

Fighting inflammation with inflammation

Prolotherapy fights inflammation by creating even more inflammation – much like fighting fire with fire. When injured, *ligaments* – the structures that connect the bones within a joint and hold those bones in place – can have a hard time healing. Blood supply to the ligaments is limited, so the healing process is often slow and incomplete, leaving the ligaments loose, damaged, and weak. Unfortunately, the ligaments do have plenty of nerve endings, ensuring that you feel plenty of pain as a result. Injecting sugar water into the area surrounding a ligament, where it attaches to the bone, increases inflammation and brings extra blood, nutrients, and oxygen to the weakened tissue, which may help the healing process.

Getting your sugar-water fix

If you're interested in prolotherapy, ask your doctor if this treatment is appropriate for your condition and, if so, whether it's available on the NHS in your area. A number of pain clinics offer this treatment. Unfortunately, the waiting list for referral to an NHS pain clinic is often long.

Part IV
The Arthritis Lifestyle Strategy

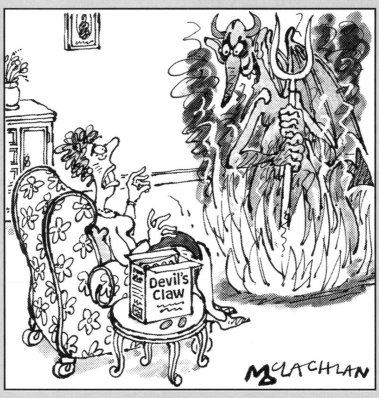

"This is just a courtesy call – How's
the arthritis?"

In this part . . .

Even though arthritis is a medical problem that continues to baffle doctors, you can do a great deal to lessen your pain, improve your ability to perform everyday tasks, increase your enjoyment of life and, in some cases, even slow the progression of the disease.

In this part, we tell you how to fight arthritis pain through diet and supplements; how to keep your joints as loose and mobile as possible through exercise; how to protect your joints by walking, sitting, moving, and lifting correctly; and how to deal effectively with stress, depression, and anger. Plus, you get loads of tips on how to make day-to-day living with arthritis easier.

Chapter 15

Fighting the Pain with Foods and Supplements

*T*he idea that food can cause or relieve arthritis isn't new. More than 200 years ago, English doctors prescribed cod-liver oil to treat gout and rheumatism. More recently, some health writers have insisted that people with arthritis should eat or not eat specific foods. The debate is in full swing. Do certain foods cause arthritis? Is there an 'Arthritis Begone' diet? All the evidence isn't yet in, but thanks to the studies currently available, more and more physicians are convinced that diet plays a valuable role in arthritis-treatment plans.

And what about supplements? Can food supplements eliminate arthritis pain, unlock 'frozen' joints, or prevent the immune system errors that lead to rheumatoid arthritis (RA)? Researchers have not yet come up with definitive answers, but more and more scientific evidence suggests that supplements are helpful in the battle against arthritis. So get ready to discover more about some of the foods, 'food parts,' and supplements that can help you manage your arthritis – and a few that are best avoided.

Reviewing in detail all the supplements that people take for various forms of arthritis is beyond the scope of this book, but this brief account gives you enough information to start a discussion with your doctor.

Discuss *everything* that you plan to take with your doctor. Subtle and sometimes hidden reactions can develop from the combination of body chemistry, supplements, medications, and disease processes that may make your condition worse.

Finding Foods That Heal

Researchers have long known that foods and the vitamins, minerals, and other substances they contain can aid in the battle against arthritis. Way back in the 1920s, researchers looked into treating osteoarthritis (OA) with the mineral sulphur. In 1963, a letter to the editor in the prestigious medical journal *The Lancet* described the use of a B vitamin called pantothenic acid in treating OA. What is new today is that researchers are finding out why certain foods are helpful – exactly *why* an apple a day keeps the doctor away.

Various studies link poor nutrition to rheumatoid arthritis, juvenile arthritis, and other forms of arthritis. However, the connection between nutrition and arthritis isn't yet fully understood. For example, researchers can't say that eating too few apples causes arthritis or that drinking too much beer *always* triggers gout. However, good nutrition *is* an important part of the battle against arthritis.

Which fruits, vegetables, meat, or fish should you eat? While no absolute rules exist, the results of studies and case histories suggest that the following foods are helpful:

- ✔ **Apples:** Not only can an apple a day keep the doctor away, but it also has the potential to hold arthritis at bay. Apples contain *boron*, a mineral that appears to reduce the risk of developing osteoarthritis. And boron also helps relieve pain in people with osteoarthritis.

- ✔ **Broccoli:** This vegetable contains a powerful antioxidant and detoxifying agent called *glutathione*. New studies show that people with low amounts of glutathione are more likely to develop arthritis. Other foods rich in glutathione include avocados, cabbage, cauliflower, grapefruit, oranges, potatoes, and tomatoes.

- ✔ **Cantaloupe:** This sweet fruit contains large amounts of vitamin C and *betacarotene,* the plant form of vitamin A. These powerful antioxidant vitamins help to control the oxidative and free radical damage contributing to arthritis. (For more on oxidative and free radical damage, see 'Saving Your Joints with Supplements' later in this chapter.)

- ✔ **Curry:** A combination of spices that often includes turmeric, garlic, cumin, cinnamon, and so on, curry contains powerful antioxidants that help to relieve inflammation and reduce pain.

- ✔ **Fish:** The omega-3 fatty acids in Norwegian sardines, Atlantic mackerel, sablefish, rainbow trout, striped bass, and other fish may help to reduce inflammation and pain. Just three-and-a-half ounces of anchovies, for example, contain almost a gram and a half of omega-3 fatty acids.

Omega-3 fatty acids help to regulate your *prostaglandins* – hormone-like substances that play a role in inflammation and pain. However, anchovies are extremely high in sodium, so if sodium-sensitivity or water retention is a problem for you, choose a different kind of fish. Because anchovies also are high in *purines* (nitrogen-containing compounds), they are best avoided if you have gout. (See 'Using omega-3s and omega-6s to fight arthritis pain and inflammation' later in this chapter.)

✔ **Garlic:** An ancient treatment for tuberculosis, lung problems, and other diseases, garlic also appears to relieve some forms of arthritis pain. Although not yet tested in large-scale, double-blind studies, garlic is helpful in many case reports. These helpful benefits are due to the sulphur in garlic, which has been known for many years to help relieve certain arthritis symptoms.

✔ **Grapefruit and other citrus fruits:** The skin, peel, and outer layers of citrus fruits are rich sources of *bioflavonoids* like quercetin, hesperidin, and rutin. Bioflavonoids help to increase capillary strength and permeability, fight inflammation, inhibit viruses, and strengthen the collagen that's so important to joint health.

✔ **Grapes:** These sweet, bite-sized fruits are a good source of the mineral boron, which is important for strong bones. Grape skins also contain *resveratrol*, a compound that can block the inflammation causing arthritis pain.

✔ **Mango:** A sweet treat, mangoes are packed with three powerful antioxidants. One medium mango provides 90 per cent of your daily requirement for vitamin C, 100 per cent of your betacarotene needs, and about 25 per cent of your vitamin E quota.

✔ **Nuts:** Almonds, peanuts, and hazelnuts are good sources of boron, a mineral that helps keep bones strong and certain arthritis symptoms at bay.

✔ **Oysters:** Oysters are an excellent source of zinc: Six medium-sized oysters offer about 125 milligrams of the mineral, which is well over the recommended daily amount (RDA). RA patients often have low blood levels of zinc, and depleted zinc supplies are associated with the joint pain and stiffness of arthritis.

Stay away from raw oysters, which are notorious for their high bacteria levels and are especially unhealthy for people with compromised immune systems or liver disease. Eat oysters either well-cooked or not at all.

✔ **Papaya:** Long used as a folk medicine for diarrhoea, hay fever, and other problems, a single papaya contains three times the RDA for vitamin C, an important antioxidant, plus more than half your daily allotment of betacarotene.

✔ **Spinach and other leafy greens:** Unfortunately, eating spinach won't dispatch arthritis as quickly as Popeye does Brutus, but the vitamin E found in this vegetable helps reduce the pain of RA, inhibits the prostaglandins that 'stir up' your inflammation, ease certain symptoms of fibromyalgia, and improve or stabilise lupus lesions.

✔ **Water:** Drinking eight glasses of water per day can help prevent kidney stones in some people with gout. Eight glasses is also the amount most health experts recommend to keep your body well-hydrated and healthy.

✔ **Whole-grains:** Whole-grains such as wheat, rye, and barley are good sources of B vitamins, which help to relieve some of the symptoms of arthritis. For example, vitamin B12 has reportedly helped reduce the pain of both chronic and acute bursitis. Niacin helps improve joint mobility in people with osteoarthritis, and may help lessen the skin lesions seen in lupus. Vitamin B6 reduces pain and improves performance according to a study of people with carpal tunnel syndrome. Because whole-grains are an excellent source of B vitamins, eating plenty of servings on a daily basis may help you battle arthritis.

Managing RA Mediterranean-style

Fat is considered a bogeyman because it is often linked with heart disease and is said to contribute to obesity, cancer, and a host of other ills. You're told to cut the fat off your meat and cut the fat out of your diet. But at least one diet that is high in fat, the *Mediterranean diet*, is actually good for you – and may help to ease rheumatoid arthritis (RA).

The Mediterranean diet was first studied over 50 years ago, when researchers noticed that people living on the Greek island of Crete had low rates of heart disease and certain types of cancer, plus a long life expectancy, even though they ate plenty of fat. Countless studies since that time have found the same results in other areas of the Mediterranean region – Greece itself, Italy, southern France and parts of Spain, Portugal, North Africa, and the Middle East. What are these people doing that the rest of us aren't? Part of the answer has to do with the kind of fat they eat.

Olive oil, which has long been linked to heart health, is the main fat used in the Mediterranean diet, replacing other oils, butter, and margarine. Olive oil can actually help lower levels of harmful cholesterol, and contains antioxidants that discourage artery clogging and chronic diseases, including cancer. But olive oil is only one part of this super-healthy style of eating. The bulk of the Mediterranean diet is made up of plenty of plant foods (vegetables, fruits, whole-grain breads, pasta and cereal, nuts, and legumes), eaten as fresh and as close to their natural state as possible. Cheese and yoghurt are eaten every day and small-to-moderate amounts of fish, poultry, and eggs are eaten a few times a week. Red meat is included just a few times a month, while a glass or two of red wine (which is loaded with antioxidants!) is taken just about every day, with meals. Sweets are limited, and fresh fruit is a favourite dessert. (See Figure 15-1 for the Mediterranean diet food pyramid.)

If you have RA and you love hummus, tabbouleh, and baba ghanouj (traditional Greek foods), or you just like the idea of a fresh, plant-based diet, you're in luck: The Mediterranean diet may help ease RA-related pain and swelling. When people with active RA were placed on either a Mediterranean diet or a standard Western diet for three months, those who ate like the Greeks had much less inflammation and much greater physical function and vitality. Researchers concluded that the Mediterranean diet seemed to suppress the activity of RA, at least for the short-term.

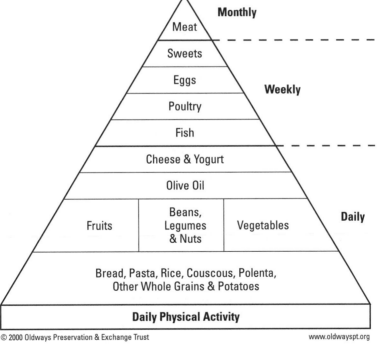

Figure 15-1: The Mediterranean diet provides a host of health benefits and helps ease the symptoms of RA.

© 2000 Oldways Preservation & Exchange Trust   www.oldwayspt.org

Daily beverage recommendations: Drink six glasses of water. If you drink wine, do so in moderation.

Using omega-3s and omega-6s to fight arthritis pain and inflammation

The benefits of olive oil come from its rich content of a type of fat called oleic acid, which is classed as a *monounsaturated fat.* Two other kinds of fat, the *omega-3* and *omega-6 fatty acids,* can also help fight arthritis. Omega-3s are converted to natural anti-inflammatory substances called *prostaglandins* that help decrease the inflammation and pain that plague so many arthritis sufferers. And a certain type of omega-6 fatty acid – *gammalinolenic acid,* or *GLA* – can help lessen pain by calling off the disease-related invasion of white blood cells that trigger the joint swelling and tenderness seen in rheumatoid arthritis.

Omega-3 fatty acids

Studies show that omega-3 fatty acids, which are found primarily in certain fish, can help to reduce the pain of osteoarthritis, as well as the joint stiffness and tenderness experienced with rheumatoid arthritis. The omega-3 fatty acids are believed to help fight arthritis by 'dampening' the inflammation response; thus, reducing joint pain and tenderness.

In one study, women with rheumatoid arthritis were compared to women of the same age who did not have the disease. The researchers found that women who ate more than one serving of grilled or baked fish (other than tuna) per week had less risk of developing rheumatoid arthritis than those who did not. Another study found that people who already had RA could ease pain and inflammation and reduce their use of non-steroidal anti-inflammatory drugs (NSAIDs), pain relievers such as aspirin and ibuprofen, just by eating a diet rich in antioxidants and omega-3s.

Omega-3s can undoubtedly help in the battle against arthritis, especially rheumatoid arthritis, and to some extent Raynaud's phenomenon and lupus. Good fish sources of omega-3 fatty acids include mackerel (Atlantic, Pacific, and Spanish), herring (Atlantic and Pacific), salmon (king, Chinook, and pink), and roe. Check out the sidebar 'Sources of omega-3 fatty acids' for more. Fish that come from cold water are generally the best sources of omega-3 fatty acids. Fish from warmer waters and those raised on fish farms have smaller amounts. Some non-fish foods, such as green soya beans, black walnuts, and flaxseed oil, also contain omega-3 fatty acids.

Omega-3 fatty acids have some long, complicated names such as *alpha-linoleic acid*, *DHA (docosahexaenoic acid)*, and *EPA (eicosapentaenoic acid).* But these fatty acids are often referred to simply as omega-3s or *fish oil* (because that's where you typically find them in their most concentrated form).

You can also get omega-3s through supplements. If you use a supplement, make sure that it clearly lists the amount of DHA and EPA per capsule. There is no RDA for fish oil: Some authorities suggest taking 3 grams of DHA and/or EPA per day.

What does 'omega' mean?

Fatty acids are built around a line of carbon atoms. There may be a few, 6, 10, 12, or more carbons lined up, one behind the other, like a line of school children. Each of the carbons has a 'left hand' and a 'right hand', and can 'hold' one hydrogen atom in each hand, off to either side. If each of the carbons in the line is holding two hydrogens, one in each hand, the fatty acid is saturated. Like a sponge that's full of water (saturated), the fatty acid can't possibly hold any more.

Often, however, some of the carbons in the line 'let go' of one of their hydrogens. When that

happens, the fatty acid is either monounsaturated or polyunsaturated depending on how many carbons have let go of a hydrogen.

If the first carbon holding only one hydrogen happens to be the third in line, the fatty acid is called an omega-3 fatty acid. If the first carbon holding only a single hydrogen is sixth in line, it's called an omega-6 fatty acid, and so on. The fatty acids are called 'omega' this or 'omega' that because the counting starts at the side of the fatty acid called the omega side.

Take supplements only after discussing them with your doctor. And make sure your doctor always knows what supplements you're taking, as some may interfere with certain aspects of your treatment.

Taking fish oil thins the blood, which is dangerous if pushed too far. Overly thin blood may not clot properly, which causes bleeding that can increase to dangerous levels. Consult a doctor before taking fish-oil supplements if you take blood-thinning medication, NSAIDs, supplements that contain ginger, or anything else that thins the blood.

Don't deep-fry your fish. Doing so destroys the omega-3s.

Supporting your joints with Cod-Liver Oil (CLO)

Whereas omega-3 fish oils are extracted from the flesh of oily fish, such as salmon, *cod-liver oil* (as its name suggests) is derived solely from the liver of cod. And if, as a kid, this was forced down your neck by a kindly carer (usually a granny) you'll recall just how yucky it is. CLO contains at least three times less omega-3s than standard fish-flesh oils. Clever manufacturers have worked out how to concentrate them during processing, however. The main advantage of cod-liver oil over standard fish oils is that it contains high amounts of vitamin A and vitamin D, which are both good for bones. Therefore, CLO is aimed at people with arthritis, while omega-3 fish oils are often just promoted for the heart and circulation (although they're excellent for joints, too).

Sources of omega-3 fatty acids

The best sources of omega-3 fatty acids are generally fish that come from cold water. Fish from warmer waters and those raised on fish farms have less omega-3. The following statistics are calculated on 3½-ounce servings of fish.

Fish	Grams of Omega-3
Roe	2.3
Atlantic mackerel	2.3
Pacific herring	1.6
Atlantic herring	1.5
Pacific mackerel	1.4
King salmon	1.3
Spanish mackerel	1.3
Pink salmon	1.0

You also find omega-3 fatty acids in other foods, including butternuts, black walnuts, and green soya beans.

Suggested doses range from 500 milligrams to 2 grams daily, but it's important to watch the vitamin A content. Vitamin A is best limited to less than 5,000 IU or international units (1,500 micrograms) per day although intakes of up to 10,000 IU (3,000 micrograms) are considered safe.

Fish-oil supplements can cause belching and mild nausea. Shaking fish oils together with milk or juice emulsifies them, breaking them down into tiny suspended globules that are more quickly absorbed; which helps to avoid 'fishy burps'. Emulsified fish-oil supplements are also available in shops

Do not take cod-liver oil during pregnancy as excess vitamin A is harmful to a developing baby.

Seek medical advice before taking fish-oil supplements if you have a blood-clotting disorder, are taking a blood-thinning drug such as warfarin, or have diabetes.

The good omega-6 fatty acid – GLA

Although most of the omega-6s are best avoided (see the section 'Avoiding Foods That May Be Trouble', later in this chapter), one of them gives hope to people with arthritis: *Gammalinoleic acid*, or *GLA* for short. Your body converts GLA from another omega-6 fatty acid, linoleic acid and, oddly enough, although linoleic acid *promotes* inflammation, GLA actually helps to *calm* it down. Some studies show that GLA helps to reduce the number of tender joints, pain, and inflammation in RA patients. In a study of 56 people with active RA, taking 2.8 grams of GLA for six months significantly improved joint pain, stiffness, and grip strength.

An often-suggested dose of GLA in supplement form is 1.8 to 2 grams per day. If you decide to take a supplement, make sure that it lists the GLA content on the label so you know exactly how many capsules or spoonfuls you need to take to get the desired dose. To get 1.8 grams of GLA, you need to take a lot of borage or blackcurrant oil, and even more evening primrose oil.

Getting a grip on arthritis with green tea

Green tea, that delicious drink sometimes referred to as a 'cup of steaming medicine', has been linked to prevention of heart disease, strokes, and certain kinds of cancer. Green tea also appears to protect against the cartilage breakdown seen in OA because unfermented green-tea leaves contain large amounts of some potent health promoters called *catechins*, which are powerful antioxidants and disease fighters. Two of the most potent catechins, EGCG and ECG, may actually block cartilage-destroying enzymes. So when you drink green tea, your precious cartilage is better able to stave off the breakdown process and stay intact. It may not work if your joints are already severely damaged, but if you start drinking green tea early enough, you may keep OA at least somewhat in check. (Tell your kids!)

Green tea's EGCG can also put a damper on the inflammation response. (See the nearby sidebar 'What oxidants and free radicals do' for more on the inflammation response.) And green tea may help boost bone density through certain compounds like fluoride, flavonoids, and phytoestrogens.

For best results, look for the higher grades of green tea, use flow-through tea bags, allow the tea to steep in just-boiled water for 3 minutes, and drink at least 3 cups of tea per day. Also, ensure that your tea bags are kept in an airtight container because exposure to air or dampness lessens both their antioxidant content and their flavour.

Avoiding Foods That May Be Trouble

No foods actually *cause* arthritis. At worst, a food may exacerbate a pre-existing condition. For example, alcohol can trigger gout, but only in certain people. However, some foods are known to give some people trouble, so you may want to consider cutting back or avoiding intake of the following:

- **Nightshades:** Peppers, potatoes, eggplant, and tomatoes are some of the members of the nightshade family of vegetables. Some people feel that eating nightshades aggravates their rheumatoid arthritis and other forms of the disease. Although it hasn't been proven, if you feel that eating nightshades worsens your symptoms, avoid them.

- **Organ meats:** Liver, kidney, sweetbread, and other offal contain the purines that can trigger gout. If you have gout, avoid offal and other foods high in purines, including sardines, anchovies, and meat gravies.

✔ **Processed meat:** Cold meats, hot dogs, bacon, and other processed meats contain various chemicals that may trigger allergic reactions, bringing about arthritis-like symptoms. Or, these processed meats may cause flare-ups of existing arthritis conditions. Whether these substances actually trigger arthritis and allergies, or whether they tend to replace the vegetables, fruits, and whole-grains that provide nutrients needed to hold arthritis at bay is not clear.

✔ **Foods containing linoleic/arachidonic acid:** The omega-3 fatty acids help reduce inflammation, but linoleic acid, an omega-6 fatty acid, does the opposite. Linoleic acid is found in oils such as corn, safflower, and sunflower. This oil is used to make many kinds of fast food, and large amounts of it are fed to the cattle that eventually end up on the meat counter at your local supermarket. Linoleic acid is converted into arachidonic acid, which the body uses to build substances that trigger inflammation and arthritic pain. Naturally, the less linoleic acid you consume, the better for your arthritis! To avoid linoleic acid, switch to olive, flaxseed, or canola oil for cooking, eat less meat and poultry, and avoid fast foods. At the same time, increase your consumption of fish and other foods that contain the helpful omega-3 fatty acids (see the 'Sources of omega-3 fatty acids' sidebar, earlier in this chapter).

Watch for food allergies

If you notice that a food tends to make your arthritis worse, try eliminating it from your diet for a while. Reports (including some published in prestigious medical journals) abound of arthritis cases seemingly cured when the sufferer stopped eating certain foods, including cheese, corn, milk, and various members of the nightshade vegetable family. Most likely, their arthritis-like symptoms were the result of simple food allergies or food intolerances. A food allergy/intolerance diagnosis may not apply to you, but it can't hurt to check it out.

To test for a food allergy/intolerance, eliminate all foods that contain the suspected culprit for at least two weeks and keep a diary so that you can write down everything you eat and drink, plus your symptoms – especially any reactions or changes in the way you feel. After the two-week period, if you notice no difference, gradually add the foods back into your diet, one at a time, in small amounts, once again recording your diet, symptoms, and any changes. Symptoms can occur one, two, or even more days after eating a food to which you are intolerant, as reactions are often delayed rather than immediate. Remember: This test is not a true, scientifically valid elimination diet. Only a health professional can conduct a scientifically valid elimination diet.

Another option is to have a blood test that measures your levels of specific anti-food immunoglobulin G (IgG) antibodies. Many people find that avoiding foods to which they have raised levels of IgG helps improve chronic symptoms, such as joint pains. You can get an IgG food-testing kit at most pharmacies. You take your own fingerprick sample of blood and send it to a laboratory for testing. For more information on food-allergy testing, visit www.york test.com.

Saving Your Joints with Supplements

Evidence suggests that careful use of supplements is very helpful in preserving and improving joint function. And not just the omega-3 and omega-6 fatty acids can help you out. Antioxidants, which are free radical scavengers, plus some regular vitamins and minerals, also have beneficial effects.

Take *all* supplements with care, because even helpful ones can interact with medicines or herbs that you're taking and cause trouble. Supplements can increase the effect of blood-thinning medications (which makes you more likely to bleed unnecessarily), counteract the effectiveness of some immune system suppressing drugs, increase the side effects of NSAIDs, make alcohol and sedatives more powerful, hinder the absorption of certain nutrients, and so on. Always let your doctor know about *all* the supplements, herbs, and other substances you're taking. Consult your doctor before beginning to take supplements, increasing or decreasing the dosage, or discontinuing their use.

What oxidants and free radicals do

The following is a short list of the damage that oxidants and/or free radicals can cause:

✔ They can attack the fatty membranes surrounding body cells. With repeated hits, the cell membrane may eventually become damaged and unable to ferry water, oxygen, and nutrients into the cells and carry waste products out. In short, the cell is unable to function properly.

✔ Sometimes they harm the outer wall of the cell, and parts of the cell leak out. In the wake of the spill, neighbouring cells are damaged.

✔ They can severely damage the DNA that makes up the genetic blueprint within your cells. When this happens, your cells are unable to grow, function, and/or repair themselves properly.

✔ They can increase the inflammation response. The inflammation response is the body's answer to foreign invaders, such as bacteria, and to injury. During the inflammation response, fluid rushes to the afflicted area, and the immune system is mobilised. Inflammation is a by-product of your immune system's attempt to destroy the foreign invader or repair the damage.

✔ They can hamper the immune system – the same internal defence system that goes awry in some forms of arthritis. (The immune system sometimes uses oxidants and free radicals to fight off certain germs. However, these same 'weapons' can harm the immune system, rather like a soldier getting shot with his own gun.)

What you need to know before taking supplements

Before you buy anything, see your doctor or pharmacist and bring a list of any medications, over-the-counter drugs, vitamins, minerals, herbs, and other supplements that you're currently taking. Be aware that some supplements can interact with medications, change the results of medical tests, and cause side effects. Ask your doctor or pharmacist if the supplement combinations and amounts you're taking are okay for your health and your body. Then, tell your doctor or pharmacist about any supplement you're planning to take and ask these questions:

- Can it interact with any medications I'm taking?
- Can it interact with any other supplements I'm taking?
- Can it have an effect on any of my medical conditions?
- Are there side effects I should watch for?
- Is there any good research that shows this supplement is safe?
- Is there any good research that shows this supplement is worth taking?
- What kind of results can I expect?
- How much do I take?
- How often do I take it?
- How long do I take it?
- How will I know when I should stop taking it?

Of course, your doctor or pharmacist may not know the answers to these questions and if that's the case, you may want to see a registered nutritional therapist, or just do the research yourself. You can contact the organisations listed in Appendix B for the latest nutrition and diet information. And you can find several excellent reference books in the library or at bookshops on the topic of dietary supplements. Don't turn yourself into a guinea pig: Get the facts before you take any supplements.

Fighting damaging oxidants and free radicals

Oxidants and free radicals are perfectly normal substances in the body; they're the result of normal metabolism. Unfortunately, if not properly controlled, oxidants and free radicals can cause damage to cells, tissues, and organs and have been linked to many ailments, including arthritis. Researchers can't absolutely say that they *cause* arthritis, but oxidants and free radicals are implicated in actions that lay the groundwork for trouble – or make current trouble worse.

Fortunately, many oxidant-quenching and free radical-corralling substances (called *antioxidants* and *free radical quenchers*) are found in foods and supplements. The following sections go over some of the substances that may help you fight the cellular damage contributing to your arthritis.

Vitamin C

This popular vitamin works together with vitamin E to scavenge free radicals or stabilise them so they're no longer dangerous. Vitamin C also reactivates used vitamin E so it can charge back into the fray. Researchers report that vitamin C may help to halt the progression of osteoarthritis as well as decrease OA pain.

Fresh fruits and vegetables, especially papaya, guava, Kiwi fruit, cantaloupe, berries, oranges, broccoli, cauliflower, and asparagus are good sources of vitamin C. An often-suggested dose is 500 to 1,000 milligrams of vitamin C per day in supplement form.

Vitamin E

Vitamin E, like NSAIDs, slows the action of prostaglandins, which play a major role in producing pain. This vitamin also helps control the free radicals that damage cells and tissues in and around your joints. A third way that vitamin E helps is to stabilise the *proteoglycans* (water-loving molecules in your cartilage). Individual reports have also suggested that vitamin E helps in the treatment of Raynaud's phenomenom.

Vitamin E is found in a variety of foods, including green leafy vegetables, broccoli, Brussels sprouts, seeds, nuts, green beans, and wheat-germ oil. An often-suggested dose of vitamin E is 400 to 800 IU (international units equivalent to 268–536 milligrams) per day in supplement form.

Selenium

Selenium, an essential mineral with antioxidant properties, works together with *glutathione peroxidase* (one of the body's internal defenders) to control free radicals. Selenium also makes vitamin E more effective.

You find selenium in whole-grains, Brazil nuts, fish, poultry, and meat; smaller amounts are present in fruits and vegetables. Selenium levels in food vary depending in part on how much is in the ground where the food is grown. An often-suggested dose is 100 to 200 micrograms per day in supplement form.

Warding off OA with boron

The vital mineral *boron* doesn't get much respect from anyone as most people – and doctors – are not familiar with it. But boron helps to regulate calcium (a mineral key to bone health), keeping it from leaving your bones and body. One way that boron is thought to work is by increasing oestrogen levels, helping the bones to hold on to more calcium and magnesium. Although boron's role in arthritis control isn't completely clear, it can help relieve inflammation and appears to help combat both osteoarthritis and rheumatoid arthritis. Studies of populations have shown that osteoarthritis is more common in areas where there are low levels of boron in the soil.

Boron is found in a variety of foods, including apples, peaches, peas, beans, lentils, peanuts, almonds, and grapes. An often-suggested dose is 3 to 9 milligrams per day in supplement form (as sodium tetrahydraborate).

Lowering homocysteine with folic acid, vitamin B6 and vitamin B12

The combination of vitamin B6, folic acid, and vitamin B12 helps lower blood levels of *homocysteine*, an amino acid linked to a higher risk of heart attack and stroke. Homocysteine levels are often high in people with lupus. Vitamin B6 may also help to relieve the pain and stiffness of carpal tunnel syndrome and, in some cases, can make surgery unnecessary.

You find vitamin B6 in brewer's yeast, sunflower seeds, and brown rice; folic acid in green leafy vegetables; and B12 in meat, fish, and dairy products. An often-suggested dose of these three for reducing elevated homocysteine levels is 5 milligrams of B6, 650 micrograms of folic acid, and 50 micrograms of B12 in supplement form.

Fighting OA and RA with vitamin D

Vitamin D helps you to build strong bones by aiding the absorption of calcium and is also vital for preventing bone loss and muscle weakness. But did you know that vitamin D may ward off both OA and RA, too? Studies find that getting too little vitamin D may actually triple the rate at which OA progresses! Those who get adequate amounts of vitamin D are less likely to develop OA of the hip. And, if these people do develop OA of the hip, the disease seems to progress at a slower rate.

A large-scale study begun in 1986 followed nearly 30,000 women (who did not have RA) over the course of 11 years. Those who consumed less than 200 IU (international units) of vitamin D each day had a 33 per cent greater risk of developing RA. Researchers aren't sure why vitamin D helps guard against RA – perhaps because it affects the immune system. Whatever the reason, getting ample amounts of vitamin D appears to protect.

Your body can manufacture an adequate supply of vitamin D from getting just 20 minutes of direct sun exposure per day on an area about as big as the back of your hand. But, 400 to 800 IU of vitamin D from dietary sources is still recommended. Good food sources include fortified milk (which has additional vitamins added), egg yolks, butter, cheese, fish oil, and fortified cereals.

Pumping up cartilage with collagen hydrolysate

Also known as hydrolysed collagen or gelatin, pharmaceutical-grade collagen hydrolysate (PCH) may help cartilage to absorb *collagen*, the 'netting' that holds your proteoglycans (water-loving molecules) in place. Collagen gives cartilage its elasticity and ability to absorb shock. When collagen fibres weaken and thin, your cartilage dries out, cracks, and is more likely to show signs of wear and tear. PCH, when taken with the hormone calcitonin, may help plump up your cartilage, inhibit the breakdown of bone collagen, and help bone to repair. The effectiveness of PCH is still controversial, with much of the research coming from Germany.

Made from the hides and bones of pigs, cattle, sheep, and chickens, collagen hydrolysate is available in powder, tablets, and capsules and is generally safe when taken in daily doses of up to 10 grams.

PCH that comes from chickens can cause allergies in those allergic to chicken or eggs. PCH that comes from cattle has a remote chance of contamination with mad cow disease. Some people taking PCH experience nausea and stomach upsets.

Combating Raynaud's with niacin

Niacin is a member of the vitamin B family. Niacin was first noted early in the 20th century during the battle against *pellagra*, the disease that causes blotchy skin rashes, confusion, weakness, memory loss, and other problems. Pellagra is rarely seen today, and doctors are primarily interested in niacin's ability to keep your skin, nerves, and intestines healthy; to lower cholesterol; and possibly to guard against cancer.

Niacin also has some antirheumatic properties that help damp down inflammation. For example, people with Raynaud's who are given a niacin preparation report fewer and shorter attacks of the disease compared with those given a placebo. And, people with OA experience significant improvements in joint mobility and overall severity of their disease after three months of taking niacin; they are also able to lower their NSAID dosage by an average of 13 per cent.

Nuts, liver, fortified grains and cereals, peanut butter, milk, cheese, and fish are all good sources of niacin. Although a typical daily dose of niacin for health maintenance is 15 to 20 milligrams, therapeutic doses are closer to 4 grams. Niacin is best taken in the form of niacinamide to minimise side effects (for example, severe facial flushing).

Niacin can produce liver damage when taken in 'therapeutic' doses. Don't take high doses of niacin except under a doctor's supervision.

Zapping RA and psoriatic arthritis with zinc

The mineral zinc is necessary for many aspects of good health. Although no one has shown that a lack of zinc causes arthritis, researchers know that the amount of zinc in the blood of at least some people with rheumatoid arthritis is lower than normal, which suggests that zinc supplements may help some people with the disease.

Unfortunately, the results of studies with zinc on arthritis are mixed. One study using zinc sulphate shows that it improves RA, while another found that it eases symptoms of psoriasis. But other studies have found that zinc has no significant benefit. These mixed results have led some researchers to suggest that zinc may not help everyone, but can greatly aid carefully selected people with arthritis who have low levels of this important mineral. And, side effects aren't an issue with zinc: Hundreds of thousands of people take it every day without a problem.

You can find zinc in oysters, seafood, eggs, meat, wheat germ, and plain yoghurt. An often-suggested dose is 50 milligrams per day in supplement form.

Relieving Arthritis Symptoms with Other Nutritional Substances

Omega-3 fatty acids, GLA (the 'good' omega-6 fatty acid), antioxidants, free-radical quenchers, vitamins, and minerals: The nutritional arsenal against arthritis is growing larger every year. And more substances are joining the battle. The sections here cover a few of the non-vitamin, non-mineral, non-antioxidant substances that are gaining recognition.

Alleviating inflammation with aloe vera

Made from the leaves of the aloe plant, aloe vera juice is an ancient beauty aid – one that reportedly kept Cleopatra's skin fresh and soft. Aloe vera is also an all-purpose balm that was carried by Alexander the Great's soldiers as they conquered much of the ancient world. Today, the popularity of aloe vera juice is partly due to its inflammation-relieving properties. Many people drink aloe juice as a laxative and health booster, and use aloe vera creams or gels to treat sunburn, cuts, burns, and abrasions. Aloe vera juice contains numerous vitamins, minerals, and amino acids, which may explain its many beneficial effects.

There are reports that drinking aloe juice can help to relieve symptoms of rheumatoid arthritis, as well as other inflammatory forms of arthritis. A few animal studies back up these claims, and many people with arthritis are eagerly awaiting human studies to show that aloe can help to knock down arthritis symptoms. Meanwhile, many people insist that moderate amounts of aloe juice relieve swelling.

You can find aloe vera in juice, cream, gel, and capsule forms. An often-suggested dose is 200 milligrams per day in capsule form.

Battling inflammation with bromelain

An enzyme found in pineapple, bromelain is often used as a digestive aid because it can help to break down protein. But bromelain also has anti-inflammatory properties that may help to reduce the swelling and pain of arthritis. In one study, 73 people with OA of the knee who were administered bromelain, combined with rutin (a citrus flavonoid) and trypsin (a pancreatic enzyme), found that this relieved pain and improved function as successfully as an NSAID. In another study, involving 80 people with acute knee pain of less than three months' duration, those taking bromelain for one month showed improvements in knee health, with a greater effect than those taking the higher dose.

Bromelain comes in capsule form, and an often-suggested dose is 80 to 320 milligrams per day, divided into two or three doses.

Bromelain can increase the effects of medications that thin the blood. Large doses of this enzyme can cause stomach upset or cramps. Avoid bromelain if you're allergic to pineapple.

Curtailing the pain with capsaicin

Chilli peppers have a long history of use to treat numerous ills, including (surprisingly enough) indigestion! Today, researchers know that *capsaicin,* the ingredient that gives chillies their bite, can help relieve pain. Applying cream that contains capsaicin stimulates the pain impulse (it feels hot!) and then blocks it. It works by depleting the nerves' supply of substance P, a messenger that carries the pain message to the brain. Substance P also revs up the inflammation process, so decreasing your substance P stores can translate to less pain *and* less swelling.

Creams containing small amounts of capsaicin are available in pharmacies without a prescription. Apply the cream to the painful area, following the instructions on the label. Stronger versions are also available as prescription-only treatments.

Some people find capsaicin irritating, so if you decide to try it, start with a very small trial dose and work your way up.

Guarding your joints with grapeseed extract

Medical researchers haven't yet discovered all the ins and outs of grapeseed extract, a potent antioxidant that appears to help vitamin C cross into certain body cells. With a good supply of vitamin C safely tucked inside, these cells are better able to prevent and/or repair oxidative damage. Grapeseed extract may also help combat the inflammation associated with many forms of arthritis by slowing the body's release of inflammation-producing enzymes. Some evidence suggests grapeseed extract can help strengthen connective tissues.

Grapeseed extract is available as a supplement. Typically recommended is a *loading dose* (a large dose to get things going) of 75 to 300 milligrams per day for three weeks, dropping down to 40 to 80 milligrams per day for maintenance.

Don't use grapeseed extract if you're currently taking blood-thinning medication, because it increases the risk of bleeding.

Fighting disease with flaxseed oil

Many people swear by flaxseed oil, which contains many 'building blocks' the body can turn into the helpful omega-3 fatty acids known as EPA and DHA. Although there aren't any good studies showing that flaxseed can actually ease the symptoms of RA and other inflammatory disorders like lupus, flaxseed does increase levels of EPA, while decreasing certain markers of inflammation in the blood – encouraging signs. One study found that flaxseed oil put the kibosh on autoimmune reactions just as effectively as EPA. And, taking flaxseed oil brings some hefty side benefits: It helps inhibit tumour growth, balance your hormones, ward off heart disease, and reduce high blood pressure.

Flaxseed comes in oil or capsule form, and as flour or meal. Grind whole seeds into meal, or your body just passes them right through without absorbing the helpful linolenic acid. The oil spoils easily and is not suitable for heating to high temperatures (as in frying), although you can cook with it and bake with the flour or meal. An often-suggested daily dose is 1 to 3 tablespoons of the oil, the equivalent in capsule form, or up to 40 grams of the flour or meal.

Giving OA pain the boot with ginger

Ginger has a long history of more than 2,000 years' use in China as a treatment for coughing, diarrhoea, vomiting, and fever. Today, we know ginger contains ingredients that can ease nausea, alleviate motion sickness, and prevent heart attacks by thinning the blood. But ginger also may help ease the hurt of osteoarthritis, thanks to its pain-relieving and anti-inflammatory properties. One double-blind study found that 225 milligrams of highly purified ginger extract, taken twice daily, reduces OA knee pain.

Don't take ginger if you have gallstones or are on medications for blood pressure, heart problems, blood thinning, or diabetes. Ginger can cause heartburn, diarrhoea, or stomach discomfort in sensitive people.

Treating OA with glucosamine sulphate and chondroitin sulphate

In early 1997, two supplements burst upon the arthritis scene: Glucosamine sulphate and chondroitin sulphate. Although touted as new, vets have used these supplements for years to relieve arthritis or arthritis-like symptoms in horses and other animals.

Unlike standard drugs for osteoarthritis designed to relieve symptoms, glucosamine and chondroitin (both components of human cartilage) appear to slow the progression of OA, reduce cartilage loss, and to improve pain, inflammation, and joint function. Glucosamine, which in supplement form comes from shrimp, crab, or lobster shells, provides the building blocks for cartilage growth, maintenance, and repair. Chondroitin, which comes from pork by-products or the tracheas of cattle, helps attract water to the cartilage (improving its shock-absorbing properties) and slows the action of certain enzymes that prematurely destroy cartilage.

When the results from the many studies that use either or both of these two supplements are pulled together, they give a promising picture. Here are some of the exciting results:

- People with osteoarthritis report significant and consistent improvement in joint function and pain – as much or more than they experience with traditional medications (NSAIDs).
- People who have difficulty walking are able to increase the rate at which they walk a measured distance by 30 per cent or more.
- Symptoms, such as pain, sometimes disappear altogether.
- Erosion of cartilage is sometimes slowed or halted.
- Study participants experience few or no side effects.
- People taking glucosamine and chondroitin sulphate can often reduce their NSAID dosage.
- The positive benefits do not fade with time, unlike the benefits reaped from many other medicines.
- The medicinal effect continues even after patients stop taking the supplements.
- The two supplements are as effective as ibuprofen, an often-prescribed NSAID, but are better tolerated because they lack the side effects typically seen with drugs.

Of course, not everyone experiences all the positive benefits of these two substances, and researchers don't yet know who is most likely to benefit. Glucosamine and chondroitin are not fast acting, like pain pills, so you can expect to wait anywhere from a few days to several weeks before you feel the difference. If you don't notice any improvement within a few months, the two supplements probably aren't for you.

Many different brands of glucosamine and chondroitin sulphate supplements are available. An often-suggested dose is 500 milligrams of glucosamine three times a day and 400 milligrams of chondroitin three times a day.

Several forms of glucosamine exist, including glucosamine sulphate, glucosamine hydrochloride, and n-acetyl glucosamine. Although most studies are carried out using the sulphate form, the hydrochloride form is believed to work as effectively. Some researchers feel the n-acetyl form is weaker than the other two forms.

If you're allergic to sulphates, avoid glucosamine sulphate and chondroitin sulphate. Also, glucosamine may cause a reaction in those allergic to shellfish, and chondroitin taken with medications that thin the blood (like NSAIDs) can increase the risk of bleeding.

Looking at a Possible Link between Lupus and Food

There are no easy nutritional answers for *lupus*, one of the more puzzling and complex forms of rheumatic disease. Studies with mice suggest that a low-calorie, low-fat diet may help to improve the symptoms, possibly by reducing abnormal immune-system responses. And, because more and more evidence suggests that lupus itself is a serious risk factor for heart disease, you can protect yourself by lowering elevated cholesterol levels, stopping smoking, and taking steps to prevent diabetes, which are especially important parts of lupus treatment.

Taking certain vitamins may also help in the management of lupus. For example:

- Intravenous injections of niacin improve (but do not eliminate) skin lesions in people with systemic lupus.
- Pantothenic acid given in large doses causes improvement in people with systemic and discoid lupus.
- Injecting vitamin B12 into three patients with systemic lupus cleared up their skin lesions within six weeks.
- Vitamin E eases the symptoms in 9 out of 12 people with systemic lupus.
- Within one-to-six months, many people taking daily doses of pantothenic acid plus vitamin E enjoy improvement in their symptoms.

Chapter 16

Oiling Your Joints with Exercise

*W*arning: Not Exercising Is Hazardous to Your Health!' This truth is doubly true for people with arthritis as lack of exercise affects your joints, making them stiffer, less mobile, and more likely to degenerate. The old saying, 'Use it or lose it!' is also appropriate when living with arthritis. This chapter explores the elements of a good fitness programme and gives tips on setting up a plan that can help to strengthen your joints without disrupting your lifestyle.

Before you start any kind of exercise programme, consult your physician to determine whether your body can accommodate the stresses of exercise. Checking with your doctor first is especially critical when you haven't exercised in a while, you're over 40, or if you have heart disease or high blood pressure.

Reaching Different Goals with Different Exercises

Every good fitness plan, no matter how simple or complex, includes three basic kinds of exercise: Cardiovascular endurance, strength training, and flexibility. Believe it or not, these three types of exercise can help you build a strong, toned, and healthy body, which, apart from boosting your oomph factor, is better able to withstand physical, mental, and emotional stresses. As an initial goal, aim to follow a short, easy fitness plan that includes these three kinds of exercise. Then, you can slowly increase the length and intensity of the exercises as your physical fitness grows.

Ensure that a physiotherapist or exercise physiologist who is experienced in working with people who have arthritis designs and supervises your fitness programme. Any kind of exercise, whether cardiovascular endurance, strength training, or flexibility manoeuvres, can cause injury if done improperly, especially over time.

Building cardiovascular endurance

People who do cardiovascular-endurance exercises regularly don't necessarily develop bulging muscles or a penchant for day-glo lycra. However, exercisers do have less heart disease, more energy, less body fat, and lower blood-pressure and cholesterol levels, as well as a faster metabolism, higher self-esteem, and a greater sense of wellbeing.

After you warm up with some moderately paced walking or calisthenics (the posh word for exercises that use your body's weight rather than barbells), you can safely move on to exercises that rev up your body's motor. However, don't use your mobile phone at the same time, as cardiovascular-endurance exercises done properly quickly turn you into a heavy breather, as they make your breath come faster and your heart beat more quickly.

You can choose from a host of invigorating activities: Walking, swimming, cycling, ballroom dancing, and so on. If you enjoy the outdoors, try a brisk walk or hike. If you prefer climate-controlled conditions, you can dance, or ride a stationary bike. You can also try a water-aerobics class held in a heated pool.

Take advantage of the great variety of fun and exciting cardiovascular-endurance exercises available, and mix them up in your individual fitness plan. For example, you may swim during one session, ride a bike in the next, and take a jitterbug class in the third.

Doing different kinds of exercise that work out different parts of your body is important so that you increase your overall fitness and don't put too much stress on any one area.

Most people with arthritis tend to gravitate toward three kinds of cardiovascular-endurance exercises – walking, cycling, and water exercises – because they're easy on the joints. You may want to start with these exercises, and then begin to investigate other activities as you get stronger and more adventurous.

Walking

Unless you have severe trouble with your feet, ankles, knees, or hips, walking is an ideal exercise. Walking is easy, inexpensive (all you really need is a good pair of supportive shoes and some absorbent socks), and can be done just about anywhere. A good walk also provides the weight-bearing exercise you need to keep your bones in shape without the heavy impact on your joints delivered by running or jogging.

In order to get cardio benefits, though, you need to work your way up to *brisk* walking. Strolling is certainly pleasant and beneficial, but you have to pick up the pace if you want walking to qualify as a true cardiovascular-endurance exercise – and that means walking fast enough to make you somewhat winded (but not gasping for breath!).

Cycling

Whether you race through the park on an autumn day or pump away in the comfort of your kitchen, cycling is a great way to get your heart racing without putting much strain on your joints. Start cycling on flat ground. Then, after several sessions (and if your joints permit it), raise the level of incline on your stationary bike or find a road that slopes upward slightly as you ride your outdoor bike. Take it easy, though – strenuous uphill cycling is not recommended for those with osteoarthritis of the knees or hips.

As with walking, you need to pick up your cycling pace. Coasting along is certainly pleasant but doesn't count for much if you're trying to give your heart and lungs a workout. If you're riding outdoors, look for a place free of traffic lights, pedestrians, and other impediments, because you'll have a hard time raising your heart rate and keeping it there if you're forced to swerve or stop every two minutes.

Exercising in water

Exercising in water is just what the doctor ordered for most arthritis sufferers: It offers overall physical conditioning and great cardiovascular-endurance with little or no pressure on your joints. With water to buoy you, you can say goodbye to gravity's woes and get your heart pumping without feeling that nagging pain in your knees or hips.

Swimming is one of the best exercises for increasing your head-to-toe fitness. When you swim, more than two-thirds of the muscles in your body go into action, giving you a good, total workout in a relatively short time. Swimming is an efficient and enjoyable way to increase your overall strength, endurance, and flexibility – and it improves your posture!

If you like the water but aren't keen on swimming, water aerobics is a good choice. Offered by many local swimming baths, these classes are held in warm-water pools. Participants are led by a qualified instructor through a series of gentle range-of-motion, cardio-endurance, and flexibility exercises. Many people find that not only is their pain reduced during the time they're in the water, but also both their mobility and relief from pain are increased for hours (or even days) after a workout.

Strength training

Strength-training exercises improve the ability of your muscles to do work in two ways: They increase the force your muscles can exert *(strength)* and the length of time they can exert that force *(endurance)*. If you have arthritis, strength training is particularly important because strong, well-toned (but not necessarily beefy) muscles and other supporting structures help to absorb and ease the stress and strain placed on your joints. In contrast, weak muscles do just the opposite, forcing your joints to bear the brunt of impact, and encouraging joint misalignment or slippage. You also need strong weight-bearing joints (those in your spine, hips, knees, and ankles) and sturdy supporting structures (tendons, ligaments, muscles, and so on) to take on the additional load as your body tries to protect the injured or diseased joints by shifting the weight elsewhere. Performed regularly, strength-training exercises can help fight weakness, frailty, falls, disability, and may even help you get selected for a mud-wrestling team.

You can do two kinds of strength-training exercises: *Isotonic* and *isometric*. When performing *isotonic* exercises, your muscles move against the resistance of gravity, water, light weights, or your own body weight, and your joints bend and straighten. Weight lifting and swimming are two examples. *Isometric exercises*, on the other hand, are done *without* moving your joints. Muscles are contracted and released, but the joint stays in a static position. Often, your body itself provides the resistance. For example, clasping your hands in front of you and pushing them together is an isometric exercise for your arms and pectoral muscles. These exercises are great for toning your muscles and supporting structures on days when your joints are just too painful to move.

Weight and repetition are the basis of strength training. You can build your strength by gradually increasing the amount of weight that your muscles must lift, which makes your muscles bigger, bulkier, and more awe-inspiring. But by increasing the number of times your muscles perform a certain movement (repetitions or reps), you can increase your endurance, which is even more important even if it doesn't increase the number of wolf-whistles you attract. Bulkier muscles are less flexible, more likely to be injured, and less likely to improve joint range of motion than muscles that have been conditioned for endurance.

You don't need a set of barbells to do strength training. When a dancer slowly lifts her leg and holds it in position, she is lifting weight – the weight of her leg as gravity pulls against it. When a swimmer pulls his arms through the water, he is working against the resistance of the water. With exercises like dancing and swimming, you don't need additional weights!

Positive side effects of exercise

If you don't already have enough reasons to exercise, here are a few more that don't directly relate to joint health but certainly boost your health in other ways. Getting regular exercise can:

✔ Reduce stress

✔ Improve your quality of sleep

✔ Increase your physical abilities

✔ Regain or maintain your independence

✔ Reduce body fat while increasing muscle mass

✔ Improve your balance

✔ Increase the activity of your immune system

✔ Promote relaxation

✔ Improve your sex life

✔ Keep your bowels regular

✔ Enhance your emotional health

Doing different strength-enhancing exercises varies your workouts and makes your exercise plan feel fresh and interesting, while toning different muscle groups. Strength-enhancing exercises include the following:

✔ Isometric exercises

✔ Sit-ups

✔ Push-ups

✔ Leg lifts

✔ Weight training

✔ Swimming

✔ Stair climbing

✔ Cross-country skiing

✔ Dance or yoga (sustained poses)

✔ Running

Increasing flexibility

Flexibility exercises – otherwise known as stretching – increase your ability to bend, reach, twist, and stretch. These exercises help you maintain or increase your *range of motion* – the amount of movement your joints allow in various directions. Flexibility exercises also improve the elasticity of your muscles, which makes them more resistant to injury. If you have arthritis, flexibility exercises are crucial, because pain, stiffness, and restricted range of motion tend to make you move your joints less, which only increases the pain, stiffness, and limited movement over time in a particularly unpleasant vicious circle.

You may think that you already bend and stretch enough while doing housework or gardening, and that you can just skip flexibility exercises. But everyday activities don't move your joints through their full range of motion, so you need to make flexibility exercises a regular part of your daily programme – do them every day if possible.

Easing Joint Pain with Exercise

Countless exercises can help to make you stronger, fitter, more flexible, and better able to fight arthritis. The exercises you choose depend upon what you and your physiotherapist feel are the best ones for your particular condition. The simple exercises outlined in this section are particularly good for stretching or strengthening the indicated areas.

As you do the stretching exercises in the following sections, keep these tips in mind:

- ✔ Always stretch slowly and carefully – don't bounce. Move your body to its maximum position, hold it in place for at least five seconds, and then ease into your stretch just a little more before releasing.

- ✔ Don't hold your breath while stretching – breathe slowly and deeply and try to relax into the stretch.

For some of the exercises in this section, you need an exercise mat to protect your weight-bearing joints from excessive pressure when they're in contact with the floor.

Stretching your neck

Use this exercise to stretch and relieve tension in your neck muscles:

1. **Sit cross-legged on your exercise mat, hands resting comfortably on your knees or thighs.**

2. **While facing to the front, drop your head to the right side, as if trying to touch your right ear to your right shoulder.**

   Don't scrunch up your shoulders!

3. **Put your right hand over the top of your head, and your left hand on top of your left shoulder.**

4. **Exert gentle pressure with each hand, stretching your neck.**

5. **Repeat on the other side.**

Stretching your hand and wrist

This exercise stretches and strengthens your fingers and wrists:

1. **Make a fist.**

2. **Fling your fingers out to their straightened position, fingers spread.**

3. **Return to the fist position.**

4. **Repeat five times for each hand.**

The following exercise increases finger and hand flexibility:

1. **Open your hand flat.**

2. **Touch the tip of your thumb to the tip of each of your fingers, one at a time.**

3. **Repeat ten times per hand.**

Extending your shoulder and arm

Use this exercise to strengthen your upper back and shoulder muscles:

1. **Get on your hands and knees on an exercise mat.**

   Make sure that your neck is straight and parallel to the floor.

2. **Slowly reach your right arm out in front of you, keeping your arm straight, parallel to the floor, and about the height of your ear.**

   Point your fingers at the wall on the opposite side of the room. (See Figure 16-1.)

3. **Hold for five seconds, if possible, and then slowly return your arm to its starting position.**

4. **Repeat with your other arm, and then alternate, doing as many reps as you can manage.**

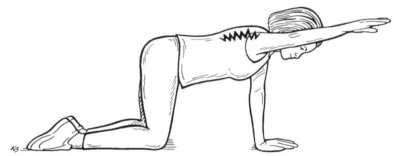

Figure 16-1:
Shoulder arm extension. This exercise strengthens your upper back and improves posture.

Stretching your side

This exercise tones your side and back muscles and helps prevent sudden back spasms that can result from turning or twisting the wrong way.

1. **Stand straight with your feet about 45 centimetres (18 inches) apart.**

2. **Bend your left elbow, placing your left hand at your waist.**

3. **Straighten your right arm above your head while trying to keep your right shoulder level with the left one.**

4. **Bend slowly toward the left (toward your bent elbow), keeping your right arm above your head, as shown in Figure 16-2.**

5. **Hold this position for a count of five.**

   You should feel a pull in your right side.

   Be careful not to push your right hip to the side as you bend – that's cheating, and it can put stress on your knees.

6. **Slowly return to an upright position.**

7. **Repeat on the other side.**

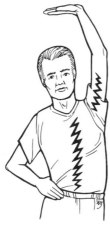

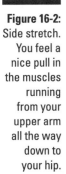

Figure 16-2:
Side stretch.
You feel a
nice pull in
the muscles
running
from your
upper arm
all the way
down to
your hip.

Lifting your lower back and pelvis

This exercise tightens your rear-end muscles and stretches your lower back:

1. **Lie on your back on your exercise mat, knees bent and a couple of inches apart, with the soles of your feet flat on the mat.**

   Your arms should be straight and about 7 centimetres (3 inches) away from your sides, with your palms flat against the mat.

2. **Tighten your buttock muscles and slowly raise your pelvis, supporting your weight with your feet and your lower arms.**

   Try to keep your spine straight – don't arch up – but don't let your rear-end sag, either. You need to have a nice straight line from your shoulders to your knees. (See Figure 16-3.)

3. **Hold this raised position for five seconds.**

4. **Slowly ease your back down, vertebrae by vertebrae, beginning with your upper back and ending with your tailbone.**

5. **Repeat slowly at least five times.**

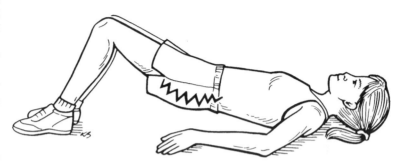

Figure 16-3:
Lower back and pelvis lift: A good exercise for tightening your buttocks and releasing tension in your lower back.

Stretching your hamstrings

Use this stretch to help you loosen up your lower back and the back of your thighs (hamstrings), as well as to improve your ability to bend over:

1. **Lie on your back on your exercise mat with your knees flexed and arms at your sides.**

2. **Bend your right knee and grab the back of your thigh with both hands.**

3. **Pull your knee toward your chest, keeping your foot pointed rather than flexed.** (Flexing stretches the sciatic nerve.)

4. **While holding onto your thigh, extend the lower part of your leg until your leg is completely straight, as shown in Figure 16-4.**

   If you can't straighten your leg in that position, lower your leg until you can straighten it. Hold for a count of five.

   To benefit from this exercise, you need to keep your working leg as straight as possible, your supporting leg bent, and your back flat on the ground.

5. **Bend your knee and move your leg back to the mat.**

6. **Repeat with the other leg.**

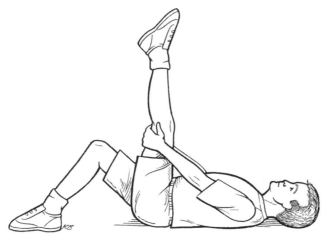

Figure 16-4:
Hamstring
stretch. This
manoeuvre
loosens up
your hip
joint and
stretches
the back of
your thigh.

If your arms aren't long enough to hold your leg while it's straightening, slide a towel or a belt around the back of your thigh and hold on to the ends of it.

Doing mini sit-ups

This exercise is great for tightening the abdominal muscles, which support your lower back. The mini sit-up causes your abdominals to contract and hold at the point of maximum resistance, without putting too much strain on your back and neck muscles.

1. **Lie flat on your back on your exercise mat, bend your knees, keeping your feet flat on the floor.**

   Keep your knees no more than an inch or two apart.

2. **Fold your arms across your chest and raise your head, neck, and shoulders off the floor, as shown in Figure 16-5.**

   Your head and neck curl forward, but not so far forward that your chin is on your chest.

3. **Hold this position for a count of five.**

   Try not to let your stomach muscles pop out; instead, suck them in.

4. **Slowly release and roll back down to your starting position.**

5. **Repeat this exercise five times, if possible.**

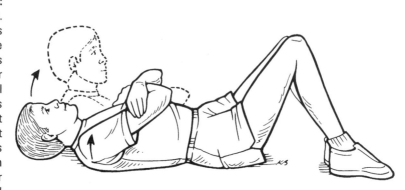

Figure 16-5:
Mini sit-up. This exercise tightens your abdominal muscles without putting a lot of stress and strain on your back and neck.

If you can't get your shoulders completely off the floor at first, don't worry. Do the best you can and work toward that goal in the long run.

Extending your hip and back leg

The buttock muscles are important in maintaining good posture. When the buttock muscles are contracted and 'tucked under', the stomach muscles automatically contract, too. This contraction helps you support your lower back, while avoiding the sway back, stomach out, knees locked position, which is so detrimental to your joints. Use this exercise to tighten up your rear-end muscles:

1. **Get on your hands and knees on an exercise mat.**

   Make sure your neck is parallel to the floor.

2. **When you feel comfortable and balanced, flex the toes of your right foot.**

3. **Slide your right leg out behind you until it's straight and supported only by your toes.**

4. **Slowly lift your right leg up until it's parallel with the floor, as shown in Figure 16-6.**

5. **Hold the position for five seconds.**

6. **Lower your leg slowly, bend it, and bring it back to its original position.**

7. **Repeat this exercise with your left leg.**

Figure 16-6:
Hip and back leg extension. This exercise helps support your lower back by strengthening the buttock muscles.

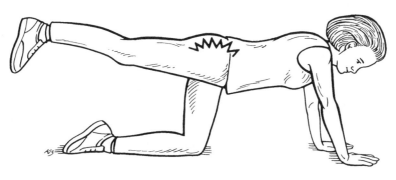

Rotating your ankle

This exercise is great for increasing the range of motion in your ankle:

1. **Lie on your back on your exercise mat, legs bent, and arms at your sides.**

2. **Raise your right leg into the air, keeping it bent, and hold onto your right thigh for support.**

3. **Rotate your foot slowly in a circle to the right, as if drawing a circle in the air with your big toe.**

4. **Rotate four times to the right and four times to the left.**

5. **Repeat the exercise with your left foot.**

Using Yoga to Ease Arthritis Pain

Yoga is an ancient way of bringing your physical, mental, and spiritual selves into balance and harmony; thus, achieving the highest form of good health. All of the many kinds of yoga involve assuming various sitting, standing, or lying-down postures called *asanas*. The postures are held for anywhere from seconds to minutes and are accompanied with deep breathing.

The benefits of yoga for arthritis sufferers are many, including relaxation, stress reduction, increased energy, improved flexibility, increased strength, and improved circulation. As an added bonus, many people find that regularly practising yoga helps to relieve depression, increase alertness, and improve overall wellbeing. Check out *Yoga For Dummies* by Georg Feuerstein and Larry Payne (Wiley), for more information on practising yoga.

The snake

Use this posture, or *asana*, to stretch your chest, stomach, and upper back muscles while strengthening your arms and upper body:

1. **On your exercise mat, lie face down on your stomach with your arms bent and hands palm down resting on either side of your neck, as shown in Figure 16-7a.**

2. **Pressing your hands and lower arms into the mat, slowly raise your head and upper chest until they're completely off the floor. See Figure 16-7b.**

3. **Gradually straighten your arms as you push your head, chest, and torso as far up as you can, as shown in Figure 16-7c.**

   Be sure to keep your pelvis flat on the floor and your legs extended.

4. **Hold the position for a count of five.**

5. **Slowly bend your arms as you ease your torso down to the mat.**

6. **Gradually return to the starting position with your face on the mat.**

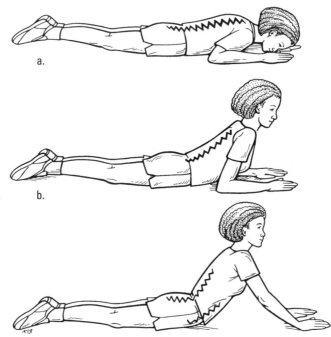

Figure 16-7:
The snake is a great stretch for your upper back, chest, and stomach muscles.

The cat

This exercise helps increase spinal flexibility:

1. **Get on your hands and knees on an exercise mat.**

   Make sure that your neck is parallel to the floor. Your knees need to be about 30 centimetres (12 inches) apart, with your arms straight down and your fingers pointing forward. (See Figure 16-8a.)

2. **Contract your stomach muscles and roll your head forward until your chin touches your chest as you round your back upward toward the ceiling.**

   Your entire torso should be contracted, forming a hollow. (See Figure 16-8b.)

3. **Gradually release the contraction and roll your head back to its original position.**

4. **Arch your back slightly, creating a curve going the opposite way.**

   Don't stick your rear-end out, let your stomach muscles relax, or sway your back to accomplish this position; these motions can put too much pressure on the disks between your vertebrae. (See Figure 16-8c.)

5. **Repeat, slowly forming the hump, and then ease into a slight arch.**

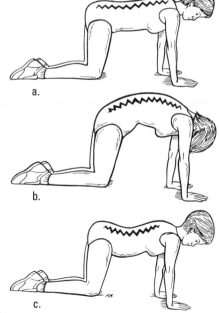

Figure 16-8: The cat. Contracting your stomach muscles then arching your back helps increase spinal flexibility.

The pretzel

Use this exercise to stretch your inner thigh and hip:

1. **Lie on your back on your exercise mat, legs bent and arms at your sides.**

2. **Cross your right leg over your left leg, with your right foot just clearing your left knee.**

3. **Grab your left thigh with both hands and pull it toward you while keeping your legs in the crossed position, as shown in Figure 16-9.**

4. **Hold this position for at least five seconds.**

5. **Slowly release, and then repeat with the opposite leg.**

Figure 16-9:
The pretzel. A nice, relaxing stretch that loosens your hip and increases the flexibility of your inner thigh.

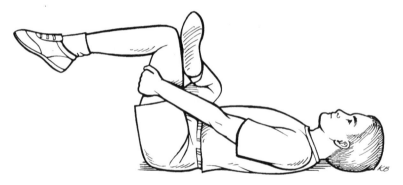

Knee-to-chest stretch

This exercise loosens up the hip joint while stretching your lower back and buttock muscles:

1. **Lie on your back on your exercise mat, legs extended and arms at your sides.**

2. **Bend your right leg, grab it with both hands just below the knee, and pull it gently toward your chest as far as you can, as shown in Figure 16-10.**

3. **Hold your leg at its maximum position for a count of five.**

   Make sure that your other leg is straight and on the floor.

4. **Slowly release, and repeat with your left leg.**

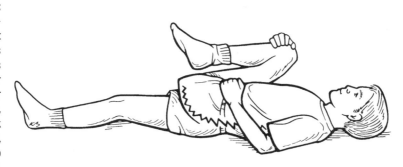

Figure 16-10:
Knee-to-chest stretch. This stretch is great for your lower back, buttock muscles, and hip joint.

The spinal twist

Exercises that twist the spine are good for maintaining the flexibility of the spine and the oblique muscles – muscles that run diagonally along your side and allow you to reach for something behind you without completely turning round.

1. **Lie on your back on your exercise mat, legs extended and arms at your sides.**

2. **Bend your right knee and bring it toward your chest, grabbing hold of it with both hands behind the thigh.**

3. **Extend your right arm straight out to the side, keeping it flat on the floor to make a 90-degree angle to your body.**

4. **Using your left hand, pull your right knee across your body, as if to touch it to the floor beside your left hip.**

    Your right foot stays in contact with your left knee, and your right shoulder stays flat on the floor. Your left leg stays straight.

5. **Turn your head to the right, as if looking at the right wall.**

6. **Hold this pose for a count of ten, and then slowly return to your original position.**

7. **Repeat, bending your left knee this time.**

    One time on each side is sufficient.

The child's pose

This posture stretches your entire back, your buttock muscles, and your upper arms, while putting you into a dreamy state of relaxation.

1. **Kneel on your mat with your legs tucked under you, heels directly under the buttocks.**

   Ensure that your knees are a comfortable distance apart.

2. **Roll your upper body head first toward the floor, until you can place your forehead as close to the floor in front of your knees as you can.**

   Place your palms on the floor on either side of your head.

3. **Slowly extend your arms in front of you as far as possible.**

   Your buttocks need to stay in contact with your heels, and keep your feet on the floor.

4. **Hold this position for a count of ten, and then slowly return to the kneeling position in Step 1.**

5. **Repeat five times.**

Doing Chair Exercises to Save Your Joints

If you like the idea of exercising without putting weight on your joints, consider these exercises, which you do while sitting in a straight-backed chair. The following subsections give details on some simple chair exercises you can use for warm-ups or, if performed more vigorously, as aerobic exercises.

Chair marching

This is a good exercise to do to music – try a brass-band march! Be careful not to slam your feet on the ground in your enthusiasm, though.

1. **Sit up tall in your chair with feet planted on the ground and pointing straight ahead.**

2. **March your feet in place, beginning slowly then gradually picking up the pace.**

   Lift your thighs as far off the chair seat as possible.

Chair running

With chair running, follow the directions for chair marching, but move at a much faster pace. Running on your toes is fine (it's too fast a pace to put your whole foot down), and you won't be able to lift your thigh off the chair as high as you do in chair marching. A couple of minutes of chair running are guaranteed to make you glow and start shedding layers.

Chair dancing

You can do the hora, the heel-toe polka, or the shuffle-off-to-Sheffield all while sitting in a chair. Not only does chair dancing warm you up, it's fun!

In addition to the following, many more dance steps can be performed from a chair; it only takes a little imagination. Try out some of your favourites; you may be surprised how enjoyable this kind of exercise can be.

Take small steps – you don't want to dance off your chair!

The hora

As with all dancing, the right music can make you forget that you're exercising and get you thinking that you're just kicking up your heels. Music for the hora can be found in the Jewish folk music section at your local music shop or library.

1. **Starting with your right foot, step to the side.**
2. **Cross behind your right foot with your left foot.**
3. **Step to the side with your right foot.**
4. **Do a small kick with your left foot.**
5. **Then kick with your right foot.**
6. **Reverse the movements: side- step with your left foot, back with your right foot, side with your left foot, kick right, kick left.**

Heel-toe polka

The count for this dance goes: heel, toe, step-together-step, or 1, 2, 1-2-3.

1. **Start with your right foot. Touch your right heel to the floor, and then touch your right toe to the floor.**
2. **Step to your right side with your right foot, then bring your left foot to meet it.**
3. **Step to the right again with your right foot.**
4. **Reverse: Left heel touches, then left toe, step side with your left foot, bring your right foot to meet it, step left.**

Shuffle-off-to-Sheffield

The sequence in this dance goes: hop-step, cross, step, cross, step, cross, step, with a count of 'and one and two and three and four'.

1. **Begin with both feet all the way to the left of your chair. Lift your right foot slightly off the floor and hop on your left foot.**

2. **Step to the side with your right foot.**

3. **Cross your left foot behind the right foot.**

4. **Step right again, cross left behind.**

5. **Step right again, cross left behind.**

6. **Step right.**

7. **Reverse, starting with your left foot.**

Chair fencing

Although real fencing is a strain on the knees – all that deep lunging! – chair fencing spares your knees while giving your arms a good workout.

1. **Sitting up straight, extend your right leg forward as far as you can while keeping your foot flat on the floor, toes pointing straight ahead.**

2. **Extend your right arm forward, in a thrusting position, with left arm against your side, elbow bent and fist curled against the front of your shoulder.**

3. **Reverse, extending your left leg and left arm. Continue to change positions, as if you were fencing.**

Maximising the Healing Effects of Exercise

Performing the proper exercises on a regular basis is a vital part of almost any arthritis treatment programme. But to gain maximum benefits, you also need to bone up on the proper exercise techniques, and always make sure that you're completely warmed up before exercising. Although a warm bath or shower can help, you can also do some light cardio or strengthening exercises until you break out in a sweat. If you have painful, inflamed joints, you may find that applying an ice pack before your warm-up helps keep pain to a minimum.

If you're in the midst of an arthritis flare-up, try a warm shower or bath, and then some gentle stretching to get a little circulation going. Take the stretching

What you may *not* know about exercise and arthritis

When you have arthritis, getting up and moving around is often the last thing on your mind, especially when you're full of pain. But studies show that exercise is actually your best friend because it can lessen pain perception, improve joint function, and even protect against the development of certain kinds of arthritis. Check out the following exercise facts to find out more:

✔ Those with osteoarthritis (OA) of the knee often experience less pain if they use free weights or machines with fixed weights to strengthen their knees before exercising.

✔ A team of Dutch researchers found that moderate-to-high intensity exercise (75 minutes, twice a week) performed over a two-year period helped increase functional ability in people with rheumatoid arthritis (RA), with no additional damage to the large joints. This finding was surprising because people with RA are often told that strenuous activity can increase joint inflammation.

✔ Kids who engage in vigorous physical activity may enjoy some protection against OA in later life, partly because exercise stimulates the production of cartilage. An Australian study found that inactive children had 22 to 25 per cent less cartilage than those who were just mildly active; but cartilage volume in the knee in children who were very active increased up to 15 per cent a year in boys and 10 per cent a year in girls. However, physical activities are not all good news, as too much high-impact exercise, or sports that contribute to joint injuries, can lead to premature OA.

✔ Both high-intensity *and* low-intensity aerobic exercise are equally effective in improving joint function, gait, pain, and aerobic capacity for people who have OA of the knee.

✔ T'ai chi, the ancient Chinese form of exercise that involves slow, fluid movements, helps improve physical functioning and ease the symptoms of OA. Those who participate in t'ai chi exercise programmes (one-hour sessions at least twice a week) can expect to see improved walking speed, bending ability, arm function, balance, management of arthritis symptoms, control of fatigue, and ability to do household tasks. One study found that this finding was true even for those people with severe limitations, such as those using a walking frame or oxygen tank, or who are obese.

easy, though. If stretching causes too much pain, stop; you can always try again later.

Warming up your muscles, through light exercise or a warm shower, is just one idea for making the most of your exercise sessions. Some other helpful tips include:

✔ Start slowly with a programme that you can do fairly easily.

✔ If you feel dizzy, nauseous, faint, or experience tightness in your chest, stop exercising and seek medical advice.

✔ Pick a cardiovascular-endurance activity that you can do continuously for ten minutes, if possible. (If not, try five minutes or even one minute, and gradually increase your time.)

✔ Make your cardiovascular-endurance exercises vigorous enough that you sweat, your heart beats faster, and your breath comes more rapidly. Find a pace at which you feel slightly short of breath but can maintain a conversation.

✔ Do your cardiovascular-endurance exercises three days a week (every other day, with one day off per week) for at least 10 minutes, working your way up to 30 minutes.

✔ Exercise at a slower pace to cool down after doing cardiovascular-endurance exercises. For example, you can walk slowly until your heart rate returns to normal.

✔ Do your strength-training exercises three days a week, on the days that you don't do cardiovascularendurance exercises. Leave one day a week free for rest.

✔ Do some flexibility exercises (stretching) before your strengthening routine, and then again afterwards. Thse exercises help decrease the likelihood of injuring your muscles.

✔ Ask your physiotherapist to supervise your stretching sessions, at least in the beginning. Incorrect stretching can cause more harm than good. Stretching sessions should last from 10 to 20 minutes, with each stretch held for at least five seconds. As you become more flexible, you can gradually increase the holding time to 10, 20, or even 30 seconds. Stretch every day, if possible.

You can help to make exercise a permanent part of your life by keeping a positive attitude toward yourself, your body, and your programme. Remember, the more you exercise, the easier it gets.

Although exercise may help to ease your current joint pain and lessen tomorrow's pain, don't go for a jog when your arthritic knees act up or do push-ups when your wrist aches. If an exercise or activity hurts, or inflames your joints, *stop immediately*. Pain is a message from your body telling you that tissue is experiencing damage. Respect the pain; try a different kind of exercise, or call it a day and try again tomorrow.

Designing Your Workout Programme

This section gives you the low-down on how to make sure that your exercise programme is the best possible to improve your health, keep you safe, and maximise the benefits for you as an individual.

What you discover by reading this book isn't a substitute for professional advice. Doing the wrong exercises, or even the right exercises in the wrong way, can make your condition worse. Enlist professionals to help you design your exercise programme so you do the right exercises in the right way.

Your doctor can advise which kinds of exercise are helpful for your condition, how much is too much, and when to stop. A physiotherapist can also help by suggesting appropriate exercises, teaching you correct techniques and positioning, and urging you on when it's time to increase the length and/or intensity of your workout. (An *exercise physiologist* can do much of what a physiotherapist does, but make sure that he or she has experience working with arthritis.) And an occupational therapist can teach you how to use your joints in the least stressful ways.

Considering the basic game plan

With the help of your health-care professionals, you can devise an exercise plan individually tailored for you. Ideally, you'll do some kind of exercise six days a week, taking one day off to rest. A good exercise session contains the following elements:

- **Warm-up:** A good warm-up lasts at least ten minutes and makes you break into a sweat. If your joints can handle it, calisthenics (jumping jacks, jogging in place, and so on) make ideal warm-up exercises. If calisthenics are too much, try doing the slow version of the activity you plan to do next — slow walking or relaxed cycling, for example – before beginning a brisk walk or bike trip.

  Don't begin your warm-up with big stretches (for example, the hamstring stretch). Stretching a cold muscle invites injury. Save your flexibility exercises until after the bulk of your exercise session is complete. (A small amount of gentle stretching is okay during the warm-up, but take care.)

- **Cardiovascular-endurance exercises:** Most experts recommend that you do at least 20 minutes worth of continuous cardiovascularendurance exercises at least three times a week. Try to get in 20 minutes of walking, cycling, or water exercises every other day. However, if you haven't exercised in a while or if you're experiencing a lot of joint pain, 20 minutes' activity may not be possible. The best idea is to start wherever you are right now. If you can do only five minutes worth of aerobic exercises, then so be it; perhaps by next week you can increase it to six minutes. Just get moving and gradually improve.

  If you find that you're doing great at your present level and aren't experiencing any physical problems, you can increase the length of your cardio workout and/or the number of sessions you do per week. Just make sure that you don't do so much exercise that you exhaust yourself or cause injuries. See the earlier section, 'Building cardiovascular endurance', to find out more.

✔ **Strength-training exercises:** On the days that you don't do cardio exercises, do about 20 minutes of strength training in the form of weight training, swimming, stair climbing, or other exercises that involve pitting your muscles against some form of weight. Check out the earlier section, 'Strength training', to find out more.

✔ **Flexibility exercises:** Do exercises that involve stretching, bending, twisting, and reaching six or seven days a week for at least ten minutes. To avoid muscle strains and sprains, do flexibility exercises only after your body is well warmed-up. The safest strategy is to stretch at the end of an exercise session.

✔ **Cool-down:** At the end of your exercise session, it's important to cool down for five to ten minutes to help your heart rate, breathing, and blood pressure return to normal. Begin by tapering off your activity; for example, slow your brisk walking down to an easy stroll. When your breathing has become easy again, you may want to do some gentle stretches, which doesn't only improve your flexibility, but reduces your risk of future injury, removes waste products from your muscle tissue, and helps lower the amount of muscle soreness you may feel later on.

Figuring out if you're working hard enough

First of all, as long as you're doing some form of exercise, congratulate yourself! A whopping 50 per cent of adults, many with no excuses for their idleness, get no exercise at all. If you're at least making an effort, especially on a daily basis, you're definitely on your way to better fitness and better health.

But to get the most out of your cardiovascular-endurance exercises without running the risk of exhaustion, you need to remember two things while exercising:

✔ Your breathing should feel faster and harder, but not to the point where you're panting.

✔ Your heart should beat faster, but not pound in your ears!

So how do you work out if you're doing enough exercise, but not too much? Try using the Target Heart Rate system.

1. **First, subtract your age from 220.** (Example: 220 – 60 = 160)

2. **Then, multiply the answer by 0.9 and by 0.6** (Example: $160 \times 0.9 = 144$; $160 \times 0.6 = 99$)

Your two answers indicate the upper and lower ends of your target heart rate zone. For maximum cardiovascular-endurance benefits, your heart rate falls somewhere between these two numbers while you're exercising – so a 60-year-old should be somewhere between 144 and 99 beats per minute.

To work out your current heart rate, all you need is a watch or clock with a second hand and your own fingers:

1. **Place your index and second fingers across the inside of your opposite wrist.**

   There's a little dip on the thumb-side of the tendon that runs up the middle of your wrist. Slide your two fingers over that tendon and into this dip, where it's easy to feel your pulse.

2. **With an eye on the second-hand of your watch or clock, count the number of pulse beats you feel in 15 seconds.**

3. **Multiply by four, and you have the number of times your heart beats in a minute.**

If you check your heart rate either during or immediately after your cardiovascular-endurance session, you can work out whether you're in 'the zone' or not.

Here's an easy way to find out if you're working hard enough (or too hard) while exercising. You should be breathing too heavily to be able to sing, but not so heavily that you can't talk. If you can sing while you're exercising, you may want to step up the intensity a bit. But if you find that you can't catch your breath enough to talk during exercise, you're probably overdoing it.

Taking it easy!

Whenever you start a new exercise programme, add a new activity, or increase the frequency or duration of your workout, the number one rule is this: Start slowly. Many would-be exercise enthusiasts are sidelined by doing too much too soon, winding up either injured or just plain burned out! Your exercise sessions should emphasise enjoyment; they require some effort but should never be gruelling. If you're more than just a little bit sore a day or two after the workout, you've done too much.

Finding a good class

After you do some initial training with a physiotherapist or exercise physiologist, you may feel ready to join a class. You can enjoy several advantages by working out in groups – it's a lot less expensive than private instruction, classes usually have more space and a greater variety of equipment, and the friendships formed among classmates can make exercise more fun. Classes are often advertised in the local press, libraries and sports' centres.

Chapter 17

Protecting Your Joints through Good Posture and Movement

. . . .

In This Chapter

▶ Looking into biomechanics

▶ Sitting comfortably

▶ Saving your joints with correct posture

▶ Walking correctly

▶ Sleeping to protect your joints

▶ Lifting with minimum strain and stress

▶ Looking at seven keys to joint health

. . . .

Surprisingly, how you sit and stand are just as important as how you walk when it comes to determining how healthy or hurtful your joints are today and how well they fare tomorrow.

You probably think that sitting in a chair, standing in a corner, or walking down the street are natural behaviours that you instinctively perform correctly. After all, you've been doing these activities all your life. But believe it or not, almost everybody misuses their joints by doing some of these behaviours incorrectly. And over time, repeated abuse of your joints can cause permanent tissue damage and a lot of unnecessary pain. Luckily, using certain joint-saving techniques can take undue pressure off your joints today, thereby helping to prevent tomorrow's problems, too. This chapter advises you how to take a load off your joints while doing everyday things that you probably don't realise are harmful.

Believing in Biomechanics

Biomechanics is the study of how your body handles the impact of its own weight against gravity. When your body is in a biomechanically correct position, the force of the impact created by movement is spread out over a large area. During correct walking, for example, when your heel strikes the ground, the impact travels up your entire leg and is absorbed along the way by your foot, ankle, knee, and hip, and all their supporting tissues. But during incorrect walking, the brunt of the impact may be taken by the ankle and knee alone. By distributing the load as widely as possible and positioning your joints for maximum impact absorption, joint stress and damage is significantly reduced.

Everybody can use correct biomechanical (joint-saving) techniques. But if you already have joint problems, observing correct biomechanics is absolutely essential. Unfortunately, most people have a hard time analysing their own posture or the way they move, which means they also have a hard time working out just how they are overstressing their joints. So you may want to have an evaluation with a practitioner who specialises in biomechanics.

In addition to a physiotherapist or a doctor trained in sports medicine or osteopathy, you may want to consider a practitioner trained in one of the following areas to assess your overall body alignment (Appendix B tells you where to find more information about each):

- ✔ **The Alexander Technique:** Developed by F. Mathias Alexander, an actor who couldn't shake a lengthy case of laryngitis, the basis of this technique is that faulty posture and poor-movement habits contribute to problems in both the physical and emotional realms. (Alexander found that his laryngitis was the result of tension and moving improperly.) Students are taught to stand, walk, and sit in ways that are less stressful to the body through the use of movement, touch, and awareness.

- ✔ **The Feldenkrais Method:** Moshe Feldenkrais, a physicist, martial arts expert, and engineer, devised this method to heal a sports-related knee injury without resorting to surgery. By changing unhealthy movement habits, breathing deeply, and improving their self-image, people begin to ease their pain. Classes are held in which people are taken through exercises that increase flexibility, range of motion, and body awareness.

- ✔ **Trager Approach:** Milton Trager, a medical doctor, believed that stress and pain originate in the mind and that bodywork can change the mental and physical habits that lead to them. Although the Trager Approach is more like massage (you lie on a table, and the practitioner manipulates your body), the gentle movement of your body (rocking, stretching, and so on) can help you relax and increase your body–mind awareness.

Although no scientific studies prove that any of these methods work for arthritis, many physiotherapists extol their benefits for rheumatoid arthritis, osteoarthritis, and fibromyalgia. Ultimately, you have to decide for yourself whether one of these methods is worthwhile. (Several sessions and a significant investment of time and money may be necessary before you can come to a decision.) But if one of these methods does make you feel better, great! Just make sure that you find a properly qualified therapist (see Appendix B), listen to your body, and don't do anything that causes you pain.

Waxing Ergonomic at Your Workstation

With so many people permanently welded to their computer, the incidence of neck, back, wrist, and hand problems has risen phenomenally, giving birth to a whole new field of study – ergonomics. *Ergonomics* involves the design of equipment that 'fits' the body and allows it to function in its least stressful positions. As a result, body stress, strain, fatigue, and repetitive-movement injuries are reduced.

When sitting at the computer, think 90-degree angles rather than stylistic curves. Your head and torso remain erect, as if a piece of string attached to the top of your head is pulling you toward the ceiling. Your chin, arms, thighs, and feet are at 90-degree angles to your body as you type. See Figure 17-1 for an example of this position.

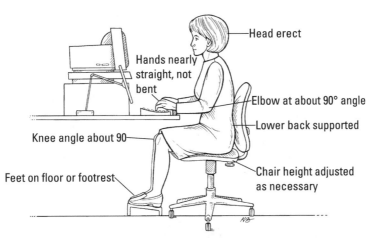

Head erect

Hands nearly straight, not bent

Elbow at about 90° angle

Lower back supported

Knee angle about 90

Feet on floor or footrest

Chair height adjusted as necessary

Figure 17-1: Sitting comfortably at your computer.

Remember – you are not an angle-poise lamp, and angling your head downward to read is stressful to your neck. A bookstand or a document holder that attaches to the side of your computer can help you maintain the proper position for your head and neck. When you're sitting at your desk and working at your computer, ensure that your body follows the alignment shown in Figure 17-1.

Take a look at your workstations (both at work and home) and see if they meet the following requirements – if not, start making some ergonomically correct changes today.

- Ensure that the top of your computer screen is just below eye level.
- Keep your eyes 45 to 70 centimetres (18 to 28 inches) away from the screen.

- ✔ Maintain your chin at a 90-degree angle to your neck when you look at the screen.

- ✔ Check that your shoulders are relaxed but not hunched over as you type, with your forearms making a 90-degree angle to your body, and your wrists and hands staying flat (not bent, flexed, or curled) on the keyboard.

- ✔ Make sure that your chair has adjustable armrests that support both your forearms and elbows at a 90-degree angle. This support eliminates neck strain and positions your wrists properly.

- ✔ Use a rolled-up towel or a cylinder-shaped pillow to support your lower back if your chair doesn't have a built-in lumbar support.

- ✔ Keep your knees bent, creating a 90-degree angle between your upper and lower legs.

- ✔ Place your feet flat on the floor or use an ergonomic footrest.

Save your own neck! Don't hold the phone receiver with your shoulder as you talk – either hold it with your hand or get a headset.

Even if your workstation is ergonomically perfect, sitting in one position for too long can wreak havoc on your body. Every 15 minutes or so, get up, stretch, and move around a little to get your circulation going and relieve muscular stress and strain. Do some head rolls, shoulder rolls, and neck stretches. Gently stretch your fingers toward the back of your wrist. Shake your arms and hands and let them dangle loose at your sides. Stop to make a cup of tea or fetch a glass of water at the slightest excuse. Your body will thank you for it!

Standing Tall: Body Alignment

You can start improving your posture right now, just by increasing your awareness of the general principles of good alignment. Correct posture doesn't just mean a straight back; holding yourself properly is a group effort involving many parts of your body.

Focusing on feet

As you may imagine, standing up straight starts at ground level. The way you position and use your feet not only determines your prowess as a dancer, it dictates how the rest of your body functions.

Aim to stand with your feet slightly apart and those twinkle toes pointing forward or just a little turned out. *Turnout* occurs when the toes point away from the centre of your body. Think of your feet as the hands of a clock, pointing at 12 when they're straight forward – a slight turnout puts your left foot at 11 o'clock and your right foot at 1 o'clock.

Distribute your weight evenly across your heel, along the inner edge of the outside of your foot, up to the ball of your foot. (Don't walk on the outside 'rim' of your foot, but don't transfer your weight in toward your arch, either.) Ensure that your weight is also spread over your big toe, second and third toes, and the ball of your foot directly under the big toe. Figure 17-2 shows an example of the proper distribution of weight on your foot. The black indicates where the majority of your weight rests, the stripped area bears the rest of your weight, and the white areas of your arch and first toe joints should be weight-free zones.

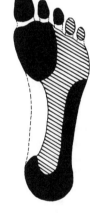

Figure 17-2:
Properly
distributing
your weight
on the sole
of your foot.

Many people carry their weight mainly on the inner edges of their feet, in a line that runs directly from the big toe down to the arch side of the heel. This position causes their arches to collapse and their ankles to roll inward or *pronate*. Because the feet and ankles make up the base of the body, pronation throws the alignment out of whack all the way up. (Can you imagine the result if the Eiffel Tower had pronated ankles?) Pronation is a major cause of poor posture and, if you pronate, simply trying to stand up straighter won't solve your posture problem. You need to correct the pronation first. (You may need to see a physiotherapist or request a referral to an orthotics department to help you correct the pronation.)

If you're a pronator, try rolling your weight more toward the outer edge of your feet, but not so far that your big toe is no longer bearing weight. See Figure 17-3 for the correct and incorrect position of your ankles.

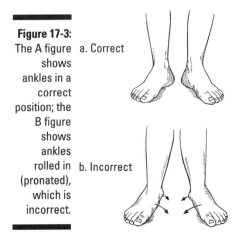

Figure 17-3:
The A figure shows ankles in a correct position; the B figure shows ankles rolled in (pronated), which is incorrect.

a. Correct

b. Incorrect

Bending your knees – just a bit!

Another cause of misalignment is *locked knees*, in which the front of the knee is completely straight (with no give in it at all) and the back of the knee is swayed back or *hyper-extended*.

Many people adopt the locked knees position because standing this way requires less muscular effort. Your leg and rear-end muscles aren't really holding you up as they should be; your leg bones are just locked into an unbending position. Your upper body is positioned as though perched on two stilts. The locked knee position is tough on knee joints because it forces them into misalignment, but the damage is even worse for the lower back, which automatically sways in response.

The locked-knees habit is a hard one to break because most people are completely unaware that they're doing it. If you have this habit, remind yourself to keep your knees slightly bent whenever you're standing, especially for long periods of time. Keep your knees slightly bent when you're queuing at the supermarket, the bank, or post office, and also when you're ironing, washing-up, waiting at a zebra crossing, or standing over your child while helping with homework. Standing this way takes a little more effort, but you build up your 'good posture muscles' and produce a healthier joint alignment if you do.

If you're queuing at the cinema, ease the pressure on your knees by shifting your weight subtly back and forth from foot to foot. Don't put all your weight on one foot; just transfer the bulk of the burden. If you find yourself standing for a long time (for instance, while ironing), you may try putting one foot up on a stool, which helps flatten your back and keeps you from slouching.

'Unswaying' your lower back

Your pelvic bones should face straight forward like headlights on the front of a car. If your pelvic bones point slightly downward, you may have a *sway back* – a lower back with an excessive curve. Swaying your back is often the result of locked knees and loose stomach muscles. A major cause of back pain, swaying puts extra pressure on the ligaments, muscles, and joints in your spine.

If you're wondering whether you have a sway back, try this test:

1. **Stand with your back to a wall and assume your typical relaxed posture.**

2. **Slide your hand behind your lower back into the space between your back and the wall, with your palm flat against the wall.**

3. **Your hand should almost be able to touch both your back and the wall at the same time.**

   If you have extra room between your hand and your back, you're probably swaying your back. Try contracting your buttock muscles and tucking them under in order to flatten your lower back. Contracting your stomach muscles helps, too.

One of the best ways to protect your lower back is to keep your stomach muscles firm and toned. If these muscles are weak, your centre of gravity is thrown off, your posture distorted, your back muscles and ligaments strained, and the discs in your lower back unduly stressed. Rather than just letting it all hang out when sitting or standing, contract your stomach muscles and tuck your rear-end under. Your posture improves automatically, the pressure on your lower back eases, and you give these muscles a mini-workout as well as displaying a more flattering silhouette.

Relaxing your shoulders

Your shoulders should line up with your ears – not hunched forward but not pinned back behind you, either. Rounding the shoulders is a common bad habit that lengthens upper back muscles and exaggerates the upper back curve while causing your chest cavity to cave in. Not only is this hard on your back and neck, rounding your shoulders is also a very low-energy position. Your lungs can't fill to capacity when your chest is sunken.

Pull your shoulders back to a midline position (pulling too far back throws off your alignment), and press down the area between your neck and shoulders, which helps to lengthen your neck. Raised shoulders are full of tension that eventually expresses itself as neck or back pain and can also trigger a stonking headache.

Holding your head high

Whether you're an Einstein or intellectually challenged, your head weighs anywhere from 4.5 to 5.5 kilograms (10 to 12 pounds); no wonder your neck sometimes bows under the strain of holding it up! Your neck has a gentle forward curve to it that's similar to the shape of a non-EU regulation banana. Many people jut their heads forward, though, distorting the natural shape of their neck and putting excessive pressure on their cervical vertebrae (the posh term for neck bones).

A jutting forward head is the natural result of the round-shoulders, caved-in-chest posture that so many people assume. To correct this posture, first pull your shoulders back until they line up with your ears, and open up your chest. Then gently pull your chin in toward your neck – not to the point of making a double chin, but a little more than what feels natural to you. Look straight ahead and keep your chin parallel to the floor as you do this.

Putting the posture points together

From stem-to-stern, here are the elements that make up the most efficient and least stressful ways to position your body:

- Head erect, with chin slightly pulled in
- Neck long
- Shoulders relaxed and slightly pulled back; they should line up with your ears
- Buttock muscles slightly tightened to counteract swayback
- Stomach muscles contracted
- Knees slightly bent
- Ankles directly over the feet (not pronated)
- Feet apart, weight evenly distributed across the heels, the first three toes, and the ball of the foot directly under the big toe

Now that you know how to stand correctly, you can do a lot to alleviate uneven wear and tear on your joints. But you don't just stand around all day – you keep moving, too! And, just as you can save your joints by standing correctly, you can also help your joints by moving in the right ways.

Reducing Joint Stress with the Right Stride

Walking is just putting one foot in front of the other to get from A to B, right? Wrong! A correct way to walk exists, and a surprising number of incorrect ways, too. And no matter how natural it may feel to you, walking incorrectly throws off your body's alignment. The end result of walking incorrectly is pain, uneven wear and tear on your joints, and (sometimes) permanent joint damage. Think of a car that's out of alignment: Eventually some areas of the tyres wear smooth, but others still have plenty of traction. If the misalignment goes on long enough, the tyres become worthless, and you have to buy a whole new set. Your joints wear out in exactly the same way – although buying a whole new set isn't usually an option. Figure 17-4 shows the correct position of the feet when walking, along with a couple of incorrect examples.

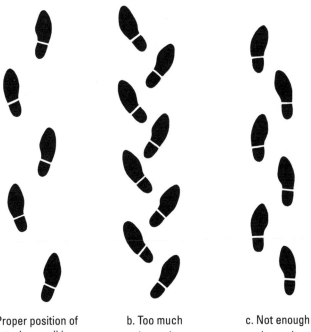

Figure 17-4:
Pointing the
way with
your toes.

a. Proper position of
feet when walking

b. Too much
turnout

c. Not enough
turnout

Correct walking is based on the principles of good posture with just a few additions:

✔ Turn your feet out slightly; just 15 or 20 degrees (see Figure 17-4). Feet that are turned out more than about 20 degrees (think ballet dancer), pointed straight ahead, or turned slightly inward (think pigeon-toed) throw off your body alignment.

✔ Make sure that your heel is angled downwards as it strikes the ground. (Remember: Avoid rocking in on your ankles.)

✔ Plant your feet about 20 to 25 centimetres (8 to 10 inches) apart as you walk. (Don't cross one foot over the other as you step.)

✔ Keep your knees in an ever-so-slightly flexed position at all times (no full straightening of the knee).

✔ Swing your arms naturally as you walk, moving them in a straight line forward and back, not around your body, keeping your palms facing your thighs.

✔ Keep your head erect, with eyes and chin just slightly lower than horizontal level.

✔ Tilt your body forward, almost as if you're falling toward the front, with your weight on the balls of your feet. This position brings your centre of gravity forward and helps stamp out the old locked-knees, swayback, stomach-out alignment. See Figure 17-5 for an example of proper and improper strides.

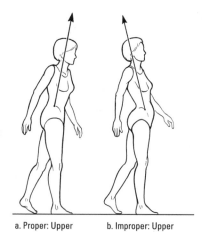

Figure 17-5:
Angling
your body
properly
when
walking.

a. Proper: Upper
body angled forward

b. Improper: Upper
body angled backward

Saving Your Joints When Hitting the Hay

Remember when you were a kid and loved flying through the air and belly flopping on your parents' bed? That approach is the exact opposite of the way you're to lie down today.

The best way to go from upright to lying flat is to follow these steps:

1. **Sit on the edge of the bed so that the edge of the mattress is just behind your bent knees.**

2. **Support your body weight by placing both hands flat on the mattress on the side nearest your pillow (unless you want to end up the wrong way round!)**

3. **Bend the elbow on the arm closer to your pillow and lean on it as you draw your legs up, knees bent, until you can lie on your side.**

4. **Adjust your arms, legs, and pillows until you are in your usual, most comfortable position.**

Although most people arise by sitting straight up in bed and then throwing their legs over the side, this action is much easier on your joints if you follow these steps:

1. **Scoot over to the edge of the bed while lying on your side facing the edge of the mattress.**

2. **Place your hands flat on the mattress and push yourself up while you simultaneously swing your legs down to the floor.**

   The weight of your legs counterbalances the weight of your upper body and helps pull you into a sitting position.

 If you're lying on the floor during an exercise session and you want to sit up, don't just throw your body up like you're doing a sit-up. Roll to your side and push off with your hands. Doing so helps to save your back and neck in the long run (although of course long runs don't really come into it – stick to long walks, instead).

Lifting without Losing It

Everybody knows that you don't just bend over to pick up a weighty load. This position puts great stress and strain on your back muscles, especially

Protecting your joints

Arthritis experts suggest the following seven tips to help you unload a great deal of joint stress and strain, and even prevent further bone and tissue damage:

☑ Respect pain.

☑ Avoid improper postures or positions.

☑ Avoid staying in one position for a long time.

☑ Use your strongest, largest joints and muscles for the job.

☑ Avoid sustained joint activities.

☑ Maintain your muscle strength and joint range of movement.

☑ Use assistive devices or splints, if necessary.

those in your lower back. But if you look at someone picking up a small child, you realise that improper lifting goes on all the time.

Always lift any size load (even baby-sized ones) in the following way:

1. **Make sure that the load is as close to your body as possible before lifting it.**

   The farther away an object is, the greater the strain on your lower back.

2. **Keeping your back straight and your neck in line with your spine, bend your knees until you can get your hands under the load.**

   Use two hands for lifting instead of one.

3. **After you have a good grasp, rise by straightening your legs, keeping your back straight at all times.**

Setting down a load is done in the same way; just reverse the process. And whenever possible, slide the load along the floor instead of lifting it. Or, even better, get someone else to shift it for you.

If you feel pain while lifting, you're overdoing it. Stop immediately and find another way to get the job done.

Chapter 18

Controlling Your Stress, Aggression, and Depression

*I*t's surprising how much your emotions affect the way you experience pain. When you feel happy and full of the joys of spring, discomfort from aching joints is much easier to tolerate than on days when you feel miserable, angry, or stressed.

This observation led to the development of the so-called *'Gate Theory of Pain'*, which suggest that 'gates' along your nerve pathways act like the portcullis of a castle; raising to let pain messages through, or lowering to block them out. And, the best part of this theory is that you can learn to shut the gates (before your pain horse bolts) so that not every discomfort automatically reaches your brain.

Several factors influence the opening and closing of your pain gates – including your feelings about pain and your experiences with it. Some of the things that get those gates swinging one way or the other are

✔ **The way you think about the pain.** Not only what, when, and where, but also your perception of its intensity, duration, and quality.

✔ **The way you feel about the pain.** Emotions that accompany your pain, such as fear, depression, anger, and despair.

✔ **Your tendency to take action in response to the pain.** For example, whether you tend to isolate yourself from others when you're hurt, immediately take painkillers, or take positive self-help measures.

✔ **Your prior experience with pain.** Memories, comparison of this pain to others, your perception of your own coping ability, and so on.

Thus, pain is more than the physical problem at the 'ouch point'. Your thoughts help determine whether the pain messages race through the gates to your brain, move at a more leisurely pace, or crawl slowly along taking a well-deserved break on the way.

Understanding Why You Hurt More Than You Have To

The bad news is that many people hurt more than they have to, because they're quick to think their unhappy thoughts that help beckon pain messages through the open gates. The good news is that positive thoughts and feelings can close those gates – a little or a lot – and make it harder for the pain messages to get through. Of course, pain is pain, and a brick dropped on your toe hurts. No amount of positive thinking can close the gate on that kind of pain message! But good thoughts can act as healing balms for a fair amount of the chronic pain that comes with arthritis.

Switching from one set of thoughts to another helps reduce your pain, but which thoughts are good and which are bad? The good thoughts are discussed later in this chapter. This section focuses on the thoughts and feelings you need to clear from your mind to help reduce pain, namely that trio of notorious gate openers: Stress, aggression, and depression.

Ratcheting up the pain with stress

Flare-ups of arthritis, especially rheumatoid arthritis are often associated with stress. In fact, any kind of pain, associated with just about any ailment, is usually worsened by stress. Therefore, reducing and managing stress is surprisingly helpful in managing pain.

Stress is your body's response to *stressors*, which are essentially anything that frightens, angers, annoys, scares, or challenges you. A stressor is therefore anything that forces you to change or respond to change. A car about to ram into you is a stressor, as is a nasty boss giving you a rough time, and a bank error not in your favour. Other stressors include illness, the loss of a loved one, and a failed relationship. Even good things, like getting married, having a baby, and going on holiday are stressors because they force you to respond to challenge or change.

But stressors and stress are two very different things. Nasty bosses, illness, and failed relationships are stressors, not stress. You may get tense, angry, or frustrated; you may feel helpless and hopeless when these stressors appear – now you're stressed. Or, you may simply ignore the stressors, laugh them off, or find a calm way to deal with them – the facts are the same, but you're not stressed.

Stress can make your pain gates swing wide open. If you respond to the stressors by getting stressed, a very good chance exists that whatever already hurts is going to hurt more.

Eliminating stress doesn't magically make all your pain disappear. (And, besides, eliminating stress probably isn't even possible or desirable.) But controlling your stress can help ensure that you don't hurt any more than you absolutely have to – and, let's face it, most people *do* hurt more than is necessary.

You're always going to face stressors, many of which you can't do anything about. But you *can* change your attitude toward these stressors. Reshaping your view of events and taking a more positive approach that calms your reaction to stressors (check out the section 'Discovering the Healing Power of Positive Thinking' later in this chapter) can help you reduce your stress and close the pain gates.

Increasing pain the 'A' way

People often equate the hectic pace of modern life with stress: You wake up early to get the kids ready for school, hurry to work, race through errands during lunch, drive the kids around to after-school activities, and then scramble to throw something together for dinner, with a mobile phone glued to your ear all the while. No wonder so many of us are stressed out by all this running around – or are we? Several studies suggest that feeling harassed and under pressure aren't to blame for stress; instead, anger and hostility are the culprits.

You may have heard about the *Type A personality* – the often angry, hostile, hard-driving, competition-loving person who seems to relish going into battle. Unfortunately, anger, hostility, and aggression can trigger stress and open the pain gates wide.

Are you a Type A personality? Do you

- ✔ Hate to waste any time?
- ✔ Feel compelled to accomplish something every second of the day?
- ✔ Love to compete with others, just for the fun of winning?
- ✔ Often think about your life and accomplishments in terms of money earned, cases won, opponents defeated?
- ✔ Feel somewhat unsatisfied after each success and immediately start working for the next?
- ✔ Jump to anger easily?
- ✔ Always feel you're behind or racing against the clock?

✔ Leave little time for hobbies and relaxation, often taking work with you on holiday?

✔ Generally dominate conversations, finding it boring listening to other people talk about themselves or their interests?

✔ Make snap decisions that you 'know' are right?

✔ Often feel like other people are in your way?

✔ Often find yourself locking horns with others?

✔ Feel threatened when someone questions your achievements?

If you answered yes to more than a few of the questions, you may be a Type A personality, and this may increase your pain.

If you're a Type A, the odds are that you can't simply stop acting that way. You can, however, do quite a bit toward reducing your hostility and calming both yourself and your body chemistry. Try integrating the following behaviours into your busy lifestyle:

✔ Slow down!

✔ Make a point to find someone or something to admire every day.

✔ Take time each day to relax – really relax, not just move your work to a nicer, seemingly more-relaxed environment.

✔ Make loved ones and friends a top-of-the-list priority.

✔ Go easy on others.

✔ Go easy on yourself.

✔ Have some fun!

✔ Accept things you can't change.

Heightening pain when you're feeling low

Depression, a common companion to lingering and painful arthritis conditions, also makes your pain feel worse because it affects both your body and your mind.

On the physical front, depression leads to inactivity – at times you may not even want to get out of bed; inactivity, in turn, leads to a general de-conditioning of your body, joint stiffness, decreased flexibility, and weak muscles – all of which increase arthritis pain, too. Depression also raises your sensitivity to pain because it causes insomnia, fatigue, irritability, stress, and anxiety.

On the emotional front, depression is associated with low levels of endorphins, your body's natural painkillers. Too few endorphins can mean increased pain.

Your perception of pain also increases when you focus on it. Depressed people typically withdraw from life and become inactive, which increases their self-awareness and focuses their attention on their pain. In short, although depression can result from pain, it undoubtedly causes pain, as well.

Understandably, as many as 80 per cent of people with chronic arthritis pain become depressed about it from time to time. That depression is hardly surprising, given that doctors are unable to cure the disease. The good news is that when depression is recognised and properly treated, pain tends to lessen as well. A study reported in the *Journal of the American Medical Association* in 2003 found that when 1,001 older adults with arthritis received normal or enhanced depression care, more than half of them enjoyed a 50 per cent drop in pain intensity, along with significant improvements in quality of life and their ability to function.

Identifying the symptoms of depression

Many people don't realise that they're depressed, because the signs of depression aren't always obvious. Besides sadness and feeling low, other possible emotional symptoms of depression include

- Anxiety
- Brooding
- Difficulty concentrating
- Disturbed sleep patterns
- Excessive or inappropriate crying
- Fatigue
- Feelings of worthlessness or hopelessness
- Irritability
- Loss of interest in formerly pleasurable activities
- Loss of sexual desire or pleasure
- Not laughing as much as usual
- Thinking and speaking slowly
- Withdrawal
- Weight gain or loss

And in some people, depression can show up as physical symptoms that can lead to expensive and unnecessary testing and treatment. These symptoms include

- Abdominal pain
- Back pain

✔ Headaches

✔ Worsening of joint pain

Any of these emotional or physical symptoms can and do strike from time to time; everyone gets the blues. But when several of these symptoms linger day after day for a couple of weeks or more, they are considered indicative of depression. If you're diagnosed with depression, see your doctor to help you get through this difficult period; full-blown depression is not something you should even think about coping with on your own.

Seeking medical treatment for depression

Always take depression seriously. If you recognise the symptoms of depression in yourself, feel unable to help yourself, or find yourself feeling suicidal, see your doctor immediately. Although many of the milder forms of depression respond well to the self-help approaches discussed in this chapter, more severe depression can require medication, face-to-face psychotherapy, and careful monitoring by a mental health professional.

Think about taking St John's wort, a herbal remedy that is as effective for treating mild-to-moderate depression as many prescribed antidepressant drugs. Check with a doctor or pharmacist for potential interactions if you are taking any prescribed medications, however.

Lifting your mood to ease your pain

If you have arthritis or any other painful condition, you need to guard against depression and look for ways to take control of your situation and your life. Thinking good thoughts is like a medicine for the body – it increases your body's production of natural painkillers, helps boost your immune system, and speeds healing.

Depression, on the other hand, increases the sensation of pain, weakens your immune system, and interferes with your ability to participate in treatment and rehabilitation.

Although no instant cure for depression exists, several approaches can help to lift your mood:

✔ **Express your feelings.** Don't pretend everything is alright just to please your doctor. If you're frustrated or angry because you're stuck with arthritis and its resultant pain, say so. This doesn't mean that you should throw a temper tantrum, although it can help to go somewhere private to scream and shout as loudly as you can. In public, however, look for the middle ground between bottling up your feelings and blowing your top. Express yourself in an assertive, yet moderate and positive way. Tell your doctor what hurts and ask for help. If a certain pill or procedure doesn't help, say so and ask for another approach. Tell your family if your pain is preventing you from performing your normal activities and ask for help and understanding. Joining a support group and expressing your feelings there can also be helpful. (See Appendix B for more information about support groups.)

✔ **Don't get caught in the 'Love Me Because I Hurt Syndrome'.** Some depressed people start to subconsciously enjoy what they consider the good parts of being depressed (for example, you get lots of sympathy, you're excused from certain chores, you're allowed to act up, you're given extra treats, and so on). Don't get attached to these secondary gains from depression. Remember, depression can breed more depression, so you need to break the cycle as soon as possible.

✔ **Exercise regularly, even when you don't feel like it.** Take brisk walks, ride a bike, or otherwise rev up your body chemistry to increase the production of *endorphins*, which are your own natural feel-good hormones. As they're chemically related to morphine, endorphins help damp down your pain, too.

✔ **Avoid seeing yourself as a victim.** Some forms of arthritis are still mysterious, but they're physical diseases, not the results of curses or black magic. New breakthroughs are constantly happening and new therapies and drugs are constantly under development. At the very least, you can manage your disease. And you can always hope that someone discovers a cure in the near future (more positive thinking).

✔ **Walk, talk, and act positively!** Even if you don't feel good, try to approach life with a positive attitude. If possible, don't shuffle; instead, walk tall and with vigour. Don't mumble; speak clearly and enthusiastically. Don't look down at your feet; look up. Don't avoid other people's gazes; look them straight in the eye. Even if you're only pretending, always walk, talk, and act positively. You may be surprised to find that soon you're not acting any more – you really are feeling better.

Discovering the Healing Power of Positive Thinking

Stress, aggression, and depression can change your perception of pain, pushing the pain gates wide open and making you hurt more than you have to. Your perception is one of the reasons why doctors have trouble treating your pain: They can tell how much cartilage is worn away and guess how much it hurts, but they can't gauge whether your attitude is making the pain better or worse.

Just thinking positively may help you close the pain gates, a little or a lot. For example, researchers found that people with positive expectations before going into hip replacement surgery are more satisfied with the results than those who doubt the benefits. And those people who imagine that the op means they can enjoy complete relief of pain actually *do* experience significantly less pain and better physical function than those who aren't so optimistic. So you really can make good things happen just by expecting them. Shame it doesn't work with Lottery numbers!

Thinking positively doesn't mean that you have to love everyone you meet and love everything that happens to you. Even positive thinkers still get upset now and then, and avoid people or situations they don't like. Letting off a little steam once in a while or staying away from annoying people is actually an excellent idea.

The next sections present a few of the many techniques you can use to make yourself better equipped, emotionally, to deal with physical pain, and to keep from making that pain worse than necessary. Which approach is best for you? The approach that works. Everyone responds differently. Give all the techniques a try; the ones that help you to control your stress and your pain most effectively are the ones for you to use.

Relaxing the pain away through biofeedback

Although your body usually runs things as it sees fit, you *can* override some of its instructions. Biofeedback operates on the premise that 'seeing' what's happening inside your body helps you control it. During biofeedback sessions, you're hooked up to sensitive, electrical equipment that monitors your blood pressure, heart rate, muscle tension, body temperature, and so on. The machine(s) may beep or flash a light every time your heart beats. A continuous display may show fluctuations in your body temperature or blood pressure, and lights may change colours in response to changes in your skin temperature.

These numbers, displays, lights, and beeps give you something tangible to work with as you try to control what's happening inside your body. After working out these relaxation and visualisation techniques, you can often alter your bodily functions for the better – and see the results on the monitors. For example, with practise, many people can lower their heart rates and otherwise calm themselves, even in the midst of stress.

Biofeedback is a wonderful teaching tool that gives immediate reinforcement as you practise relaxation techniques. Eventually, you can apply these techniques in your daily life without the equipment. Many Physiotherapy and Occupational Therapy departments offer biofeedback for reducing problems such as muscle tension.

Quieting your mind with meditation and programmed relaxation

Practised in many different forms, meditation helps you quiet both your body and your mind. Some forms of meditation are exotic, using chants, incense, and foreign terms, but others are plain and simple. However, all forms of meditation have one thing in common: A strong, deliberate focus on something outside of the self. Meditation reduces stress by giving you a break from your thoughts, problems, and the stressors in your life.

In basic meditation, you focus strongly on a *mantra*, a special word that is believed to have mystical powers. Repeating your mantra over and over again in your mind is a way of keeping your mind still. As thoughts and images drift into your mind, you simply ignore them and concentrate on your mantra, and soon, they just drift right out again.

Programmed relaxation, also known as the *relaxation response*, is another form of meditation. But instead of focusing on a mantra, you tune in to your muscles, feeling them tighten and relax in a programmed manner. Programmed relaxation can help relieve the stress that accompanies chronic pain, reduce your overall pain load, and help you sleep better.

You can find out more about meditation and programmed relaxation from many sources, including meditation centres. You can also find a meditation or programmed relaxation practitioner by contacting the organisations listed in Appendix B.

Moving to a stress-free place through guided imagery and hypnosis

Although no hard scientific data proves that guided imagery can dramatically change body chemistry and conditions, many people have benefited from finding out how to put themselves in a better place by imagining happy scenarios. For example, you may imagine yourself relaxing on a beautiful tropical beach when you're actually stuck in rush-hour traffic. You manage to remain calm, at ease, and even happy while those around you are ready to scream with road rage.

Hypnotherapy can produce the same effects as guided imagery. Hypnosis doesn't cure arthritis, but it can help you handle emotional upsets caused by pain, which can help ease the sensation of pain. Hypnosis can help you relax in the face of pain and stress, reduce your stress and anxiety, and make you feel as if you're no longer a prisoner to your pain.

You can find a hypnotherapist through the organisations listed in Appendix B.

Controlling your breathing

Think about your breathing when you're stressed: You probably take short, shallow breaths. But when you breathe in the opposite manner, with long, deep breaths, your body naturally moves toward a relaxed state. Making it a point to breathe slowly and deeply when you feel stressed can help short-circuit the stress cycle. And by focusing on your breath rather than your fear, frustration, anger, or pain, you can also help derail negative feelings.

Using cognitive behavioural therapy

Cognitive behavioural therapy (CBT) is a form of psychotherapy that helps you discover how certain thinking patterns can exacerbate your problems, and it guides you through how to change your habitual reactions to these problems.

A study of 53 people with rheumatoid arthritis (reported in the journal *Rheumatology* in 2003) found that CBT not only helped them deal with their anxiety and depression, but also decreased their disability and significantly improved their joint function. CBT fostered more positive attitudes toward the illness and challenged erroneous beliefs that tended to drag these people down (for example, 'I'm going to end up in a wheelchair, so why should I make things worse by exercising?'). The study participants found out how to couple optimism with realism and to manage their conditions more effectively.

Many (but not all) psychologists use cognitive behavioural therapy in their practices. To find a psychologist using CBT in your area, access the following Web site: http://www.babcp.org.uk and click on Find a therapist.

Laughing your way to relaxation

Laughter is undoubtedly the most enjoyable stress reliever. A good, hard laugh is believed to lower the levels of cortisol, one of the stress hormones. Laughter also helps you to relax all over. Laughing takes your thoughts away from whatever is going wrong in your life, so you can't stew in your own negativity. Many health experts actually believe that a good sense of humour is like a vitamin for the body and soul. And laughter heightens the activity of the body's natural defences. So the more time you spend laughing, the better your health!

Take steps to create opportunities for laughter. Spend more time with the friends who make you laugh and, most importantly, look for the funny side of whatever life throws you. If you can laugh at your problems, they can't control you. Almost every situation has a funny side – if you look hard enough.

Forgetting all about it

Even something as simple as distracting yourself from your problems is helpful. Instead of focusing on your pain, which only increases your stress, try going for a walk with a friend, doing an arts and crafts project, volunteering for a charity, going to a sing-along, watching an interesting film or television show, reading an engrossing book, or listening to some great music. Distraction doesn't cure arthritis, but it does help prevent the stress caused by focusing on pain.

Easing Depression and Anxiety with Prayer and Spirituality

Several studies show that people who belong to religious groups and regularly attend services are less depressed and anxious than those who don't. Studies with hospitalised patients support the notion that religion is an antidepressant. No one knows why depression and anxiety are affected by religious belief, but it is probably because following a religion makes you feel that:

✔ Someone very important (a higher power) is looking out for you.

✔ You belong to something large and wonderful.

✔ You have a role to play in life.

✔ You're loved.

✔ You belong to a community of people who can help support you.

You can also find plenty of opportunities to help others through your church, temple, or mosque; there's nothing like reaching out to others to help you forget about your own pain and feel better about yourself.

Dealing with 'helpful' loved ones

As if you didn't have enough in your life to make your blood pressure rise, well-meaning friends and relatives are likely to make you crazy by 'helping' you deal with your arthritis. Mary Dunkin (writing in *Arthritis Today*) describes the types of helpful loved ones who can drive you crazy with their advice. Beware of the following types:

✔ **The caretaker:** This person hates to see you suffering and tries desperately to get you to try one treatment after another. That's because *he or she* needs to see you well again; what *you* want takes second place in their mind.

✔ **The blamer:** This person insists that things can get much better if you just stop doing things a certain way, or thinking certain 'silly' thoughts. This is his or her way of getting out of helping you. After all, if you'd just shape up, everything becomes fine (according to them).

✔ **The evangelist:** This exceedingly 'helpful' person absolutely, irrevocably, and unshakably knows exactly what you need for a cure – and insists you try it. Maybe this thing cured him or her or someone they know, perhaps it helps them make money from the therapy they're pushing, or they just believes in it wholeheartedly. And he or she never lets up about it. This is the helpful loved one that's most likely to make you run and hide when you see then.

✔ **The minimiser:** This person has a very simple cure, even though you have a very complex problem. But no sweat – they know exactly how to set things right in one fell swoop. Of course, this cure doesn't wipe out your arthritis, but they continue to insist that it will, if you'll just give it a fair try. (He or she also thinks the answer to the nation's drug problem is 'just say no'.)

What do you say to the caretaker, blamer, evangelist, or minimiser and everyone else who offers unwanted advice? Just say *no!* Gently, but firmly, tell these people that you appreciate their concern, but you're following your doctor's advice.

Hand-in-hand with religion goes prayer, which itself is often an antidote to stress. The simple act of praying can relieve stress, and the thoughts expressed in many prayers can also have a calming effect. A favourite of many people is the Serenity Prayer:

> God grant me the serenity to accept the things I cannot change, the courage to change the things I can, and the wisdom to know the difference.

Of course, you don't have to have a religion to feel spiritual. Spirituality is the quest for a connection with a higher power, however you define that. You can also think of spirituality as a search for meaning in life and as an attempt to understand the world and your place in it. You can express your spirituality through religion, or you can find your own path. Some people approach spirituality through meditation or yoga. Other people commune with nature, write poetry, or do charitable deeds. The road to spirituality that you take is yours to choose. However you approach spirituality, you may find it a helpful balm for your pain.

Chapter 19

Living with Arthritis Day-to-Day

*A*rthritis or not, you need a life! Like everyone else, you probably have a lot on your plate – a job, family responsibilities, household and gardening chores, a social life, romantic interests, pets, hobbies, and maybe more. But some days, the twin demons of pain and fatigue may make you wonder if you can even hobble to the next room. On these days, you need to find the most efficient, least stressful ways of accomplishing your goals. But don't wait until you're having a rough day before starting to simplify your life. Start today by making a list of the things that you typically need to accomplish each day. Then, read this chapter to find ways to take on those tasks with greater ease and efficiency. Jot down ideas as you look through and start to make a plan.

Studies show that people who take an active part in managing their arthritis and finding new ways to cope with physical disabilities do better and feel less pain and fatigue. Don't marginalise yourself! In this chapter, we show you how to wrest control of your life away from arthritis by applying these three watchwords to your daily activities: *Organising*, *planning*, and *prioritising*. You may be surprised at how much you can accomplish as a result of applying these three tools, and how good you can feel about yourself, even on a bad day.

Taking Care of You

When you have arthritis, everyday stresses and activities become twice as hard to handle. But, you can help yourself by seeing an occupational therapist to learn the easiest, most efficient ways to get through the day, working out how to make the best use of your precious energy, and getting a good night's sleep. Another important part of taking care of yourself is taking care of your sex life, which can still form a happy, healthy, and fulfilling part of your life.

Working with an occupational therapist

The *occupational therapist (OT)* is a vital part of your treatment team, helping you get through your everyday activities despite your arthritis. Typically, an OT interviews and examines you to determine how your arthritis affects the things you do on a daily basis, such as getting into and out of bed, dressing, grooming, eating, drinking, cooking, getting around, shopping, doing housework, and working.

After the OT gets a sense of where and when you're having trouble, he or she comes up with ideas and recommendations. An OT can design splints or supports that conform to affected body parts, recommend and locate a wealth of assistive devices, and come up with plans to help you get through the day with greater ease and efficiency. An OT can also show you joint-protection techniques that reduce joint strain and help prevent further damage.

Many people are tempted to skip occupational therapy, thinking it's just about weaving baskets – it's not. And those who miss out on OT skills cheat themselves of a great opportunity to attack the practical problems posed by arthritis. Even though medical attention and physiotherapy are vital parts of the treatment programme, they don't help you work out how you're going to change a light bulb in the ceiling when you can't raise your arm, or how to get yourself a decent meal when you can barely shuffle around the kitchen. Occupational therapy exists to help you discover easier, more efficient ways of getting through the day. But possibly the most important thing that occupational therapy can show you, is how to conserve your energy.

Conserving your energy

Even if you're the most organised person in the world and follow absolutely every principle of arthritis management, you only have so much energy. After that energy runs out, you're like a car that's out of petrol – you have to pull over and stop. Don't waste your precious energy; conserve it so you have the fuel to get through the day's most important tasks.

Experts suggest the following ideas for conserving your energy:

  ✔ **Balance activity with rest.** Don't try to do everything at once; work in some breaks between activities. When you're tackling chores, don't do two difficult ones in a row: Alternate heavy chores with light ones. In the long run, pacing yourself lets you accomplish more tasks and experience less fatigue.

✔ **Plan ahead.** Find short cuts, combine activities that you can do simultaneously, work out what you can skip, and organise your job list for maximum efficiency.

✔ **Do the most important things first.** If you absolutely must do something today, do it first so it doesn't fall by the wayside as your energy wanes.

Getting a good night's sleep

The best fatigue fighter in the world is a good night's sleep. If you sleep well, you are better able to handle pain, less stressed and less depressed, and more energetic. Unfortunately, many people develop trouble sleeping as they grow older, especially if they're suffering from pain. To give your body the best possible chance of a good night's sleep, follow these sleeping guidelines:

✔ **Go to bed and get up at the same time every day (even on weekends).** Getting up at 7:00 a.m. Monday to Friday and then at 10:00 a.m. on Saturday and Sunday confuses your body's internal clock.

✔ **Keep your sleeping area as dark and as quiet as possible.** Block the light with heavy curtains or blackout blinds. Get a white noise machine or turn on a fan to cover up noises that may disturb your sleep.

✔ **Make sure that your mattress and pillow are comfortable.** A mattress that is either too hard or too soft and a pillow that doesn't support your head and neck comfortably can interfere with your sleep more than you realise. You have loads of options for mattresses and pillows – ask your OT for recommendations. (See Chapter 21 for more on choosing the right mattress.)

✔ **Use your bed for sleep and sex only.** Some people use their beds as the Piccadilly Circus of their lives – they eat, watch TV and DVDs, pay bills, read, play with the kids, do office work, and perform beauty routines while firmly ensconced between the sheets. Then, they wonder why they can't fall asleep there, too. Your mind should associate bed with just two activities – sex and sleeping. Bed is the place you go to relax, not to get on with the business of living.

✔ **Get some exercise every day, but not in the latter part of the evening.** Exercising after dinner tends to rev up your body, making it harder for you to fall asleep. Finish your heavy exercise by about 6:00 p.m. (Light exercise, like a stroll or some yoga before bedtime, is fine.)

✔ **Relax for about an hour before bedtime.** Doing yoga, meditating, reading, taking a warm bath, or listening to soft music or a relaxation tape are all good, relaxing activities to help you wind down before going to sleep. Don't try to do 101 chores before falling into bed. Even if you're physically exhausted, your mind is going to race and find it impossible to relax.

✔ **Stay away from caffeine in the evening (this includes coffee, tea, soft drinks, and cocoa).** Caffeine is a stimulant and can keep you awake, even if you ingested it hours earlier. A good rule of thumb is to avoid caffeine after 6:00 p.m.

Holding on to your sex life

Having arthritis doesn't mean that you can't have a romantic relationship. Nonetheless, you may find that sex takes a back seat when you're trying to manage pain, medication, emotional issues, and physical limitations. You may depend more on your partner during the day, which can change the nature of your relationship. Perhaps physical limitations and/or deformities due to arthritis mean that your self-image is altered. Some medications can also put a damper on sexual desire or performance.

Worrying if physical lovemaking is going to hurt your joints is also normal. Fear of pain alone can cause a lack of lubrication and/or orgasm in women, and problems getting and maintaining an erection in men. If both partners are acutely aware of the pain factor, then even when everything is going along okay, as soon as one partner winces, the other immediately gets concerned rather than desirous. Lubrication stops, erections disappear, and the thought of intimate relations goes out of the window.

Fortunately, satisfying and pleasurable sex is still on the menu. In fact, research suggests that some people with arthritis feel less pain for up to six hours after sex. Focus on the intimacy and closeness that sexual relations bring, rather than concentrating on some pre-ordained standard of performance, such as penetration. Gentle stroking, kissing, caressing, and massage are wonderful ways of expressing sexuality and nurturing one another at the same time. In most cases, intercourse is also possible, although it may require careful positioning and gentle technique.

To make sex easier and more pleasurable, try the following suggestions:

✔ Take a warm bath beforehand to relax your joints and muscles and ease pain. This can also help increase circulation to your fingers and toes, which is particularly important for those with Raynaud's. (Light exercise and stretching may help, too.)

✔ Take your pain medication so that it kicks in before your session.

✔ Talk to your partner about what feels good and what doesn't. Explore various methods of achieving mutual satisfaction. Good communication is an important part of any sexual relationship, and it's vital when difficulties exist.

Coping with arthritis when you're pregnant

Pregnancy can affect your body in several ways when you have arthritis. You may find that your joints are less stable and looser. The additional weight may increase symptoms of osteoarthritis in the knee. As your back tends to sway in response to the additional weight of the baby, then back pain, muscle spasms, or numbness and tingling in your legs can occur. An increase in water weight can also increase stiffness in your hips, knees, and ankles (the weight-bearing joints) and can worsen carpal tunnel syndrome.

On the bright side, some forms of arthritis seem to improve during pregnancy. Rheumatoid arthritis, for example, often improves before the beginning of the fifth month, with a decrease in joint swelling. Sometimes lupus and scleroderma improve during pregnancy as well. However, you may experience a flare-up soon after the birth of the baby.

See both an obstetrician and a rheumatologist during the course of your pregnancy. You can also continue to take your arthritis medicines (if advised to do so by your doctors); exercise to keep your weight under control, your joints flexible, and your muscles strong; follow a nutritious eating plan; observe the rules of joint protection; and use stress-management techniques to control mood swings and encourage relaxation.

 If you have sexual problems that you and your partner can't seem to resolve yourselves, seek help from a counsellor, doctor, or nurse experienced in dealing with the problems of living with arthritis.

Finding an Easier Way to Get through the Day

For many people, one of the most frustrating things about arthritis is that it gets in the way of their daily activities, making it hard or even impossible to do certain things that used to come easily. When arthritis pain strikes, it takes a big effort to get something off a high shelf or to bend over to make the bed, and just getting dressed is often very tiring. For this reason, learning how to simplify everyday tasks is important so that, like the best conservationists, you can save your energy expenditure.

Simplifying your household

You can make elements of your jobs around the house easier to manipulate and deal with on a daily basis. Try the following:

✔ If you have trouble closing the door behind you, install two cup hooks – one in the door, near the doorknob, and one in the door frame, just outside the hinge area. (Position the cup hooks so they're level with each other.) Run a string or elastic cord between the cup hooks. You now have a cord that's easy to grab and pulls the door shut behind you.

✔ Wrap rubber bands around a doorknob that's difficult to turn. Doing so gives you a better grip.

✔ Invest in a beaded seat cover on your car seats. They're not just for aging hippies – the beads roll and make it easier for you to get in and out of your car and to adjust yourself after you settle in.

✔ Instead of the traditional lace-up style of shoes, try the kind with Velcro fastenings.

You can also make your kitchen more functional for you. Personalising your kitchen makes your daily tasks easier and helps you to cope. A few ideas include:

✔ Screwing a cup hook underneath one of your cupboards and using it to pry open ring-pull cans. (In order to get the ring-pull started before the hook can grab it, slide a dinner knife or spoon under the tab and push it up slightly.)

✔ Putting lazy Susans (turntables) on your fridge shelves, in your cupboards, and in any other storage areas. Doing so eliminates reaching, straining, and shuffling things around as you try to get an item that's at the back.

✔ If dialling a phone is difficult, get a phone with an extra-large keypad or use a pencil to push the buttons. Most phones offer an automatic dial feature so you can call frequently dialled numbers with the touch of a button.

✔ Single-arm taps (the kind often found in kitchens that let you control the temperature and the amount of water with just one lever) are easiest to use and don't require two hands. Consider getting your kitchen and bathroom taps converted to this style. If you want to keep your double-arm taps, try getting wing-type handles that you can operate with your hand, wrist, or forearm.

✔ Use the pointed tip of a tin opener to open boxes with a 'press here' type of opening.

✔ Buy kitchen utensils (carrot peelers, tin-openers, and so on) with extra large, rubber-covered handles for easier gripping.

Making household cleaning easier

Back in the 1960s, a popular household cleaner claimed it was so fast and versatile that it whipped through your house like a 'white tornado', cleaning everything in sight in no time at all. Although the tips that follow won't exactly make a white tornado out of you, they may reduce the time and effort you spend on household chores. Remember to spread your chores out; don't try to get the whole house clean in one day!

If bending over while doing chores is difficult for you, use these tips to make cleaning easier:

- ✔ If you find it easier to sit while sweeping, cut down the length of your broom handle or use a child's broom. The broom does a better job of collecting dust and dirt if the bristles are sprayed with water or furniture polish first – or use the latest magic-duster style products that work using static electricity.

- ✔ For cleaning a dirty bath, mix together 125 grams (4.5 ounces) of automatic dishwashing powder and 500 millilitres (one pint) of hot water. Plug the bath, add the mixture, and swirl it around with a long-handled mop. Let the mixture stand for 20 minutes, then rinse thoroughly with cold water from the shower.

- ✔ Stop bending over to plug and unplug your vacuum cleaner as you move from area to area. Add a 30-foot extension cord instead.

If you have arthritis in your hands, eliminate chores that involve scrubbing with elbow grease or using intricate movements. Here are a few things to try:

- ✔ Cleaning the fireplace is a dirty, unpleasant job, but you can make it easier if you line the fireplace with aluminium foil before you put in the grate and add the wood. After the ashes have cooled, spray them with water (to keep ashes from flying), remove the grate, carefully pull the foil toward you, and put the whole mess in the dustbin.

- ✔ Instead of scrubbing a pot that has burned-on food, use one of the new spray-on products that promise to remove it in a matter of minutes.

- ✔ If clutching a duster hurts your hands, try putting old socks on both hands, spraying with a small amount of furniture polish, and then wiping off tabletops and counters.

- ✔ Foam pipe insulation is great for covering the handles of tools to make them easier to grasp and you can find it in DIY shops in several sizes. Slip the insulation on the handles of your knives, carrot peelers, screwdrivers, mops, or anything else that has a tendency to slip out of your hands.

Using assistive devices

One of the best ways to conserve your energy and keep from putting undue stress and strain on your joints is to use assistive devices – equipment that makes performing a task easier, safer, and more comfortable.

Assistive devices run the gamut from long-handled shoehorns to hydraulic seat lifts that boost you out of a chair, and from bath benches to computerised wheelchairs. Some of these devices may require professional installation; others are ready to use upon purchase. You can find many assistive devices in medical-supply shops, pharmacists, and mail-order catalogues, or your occupational therapist can steer you to reputable sources. Deciding which assistive devices are right for you is probably the hardest part – your OT also can help with that task. Here's a partial list of what's currently available:

- **Bathing and grooming:** Bath and shower grab bars, toilet safety frames, bath benches, foam tubing for handles (for example, toothbrush, hairbrush, and so on), raised toilet seats, toothpaste tube squeezers, long-handled bath sponges, and make-up and razor holders are just a few items that can make bathing and grooming easier to accomplish.

- **Dressing:** Button hooks, zip pulls, sock aids, long-handled shoe horns, shoe removers, cuff extenders, stretch shoe laces, and watch winders can help simplify dressing.

- **Food preparation and eating:** Large grip utensils (knives, carrot peelers, cutlery, and so on), jar-openers, tin-openers, ring-pull can openers, plastic bag openers, non-slip grips for plates and cups, easy-hold cups, and glass holders (with two handles) can aid in meal preparation and eating.

- **General household:** Doorknob turners, key turners, car-door openers, tap turners, voice-activated or speaker phones, telephone headsets, voice-activated computer programs (for correspondence), grabbers (long-handled devices that grab items), grips for phone receivers, and long-handled sponges and dusters for cleaning can make the handling of household tasks much easier.

- **Cleaning the house:** Use tools with long handles whenever possible. A long-handled mop can clean the bath or shower, and a long-handled feather duster can get those cobwebs out of the corner.

- **Getting around:** Walking-sticks, crutches, stair walkers, chairlifts, walking frames, portable stools, scooters, and wheelchairs can help you become more mobile.

For details of the Disability Information Services Web site which provides links to a number of organisations supplying assistive devices, see Appendix B.

Getting help from other people

If you live alone and don't have the luxury of assistance from family and friends, you can handle personal care, household, gardening, and transportation chores in several ways – without trying to do everything yourself. Home careworkers can come to your home and help you dress, bathe, do housework, prepare meals, get to the doctor's surgery, or do just about anything else you can imagine. Housekeepers and gardeners can take care of cleaning, laundry, and weeding. But if that kind of help is too pricey, look to the less expensive sources of assistance:

- ✔ Teenagers (either your own or your neighbour's) are often willing to do outdoor work or other chores for a small fee.

- ✔ A stay-at-home parent in your neighbourhood may appreciate making some extra money preparing meals for you, or taking you to the doctor.

- ✔ Your church, temple, synagogue, or mosque may have volunteers willing to help you out for free.

- ✔ Your doctor, social worker, or other healthcare workers may know of various non-profit organisations that can offer either inexpensive or free services. There's no harm in asking!

Joining an Arthritis Support Group

Support groups are as individual as the people who join them. Some support groups are quite structured, emphasising education, but others stress emotional support and the sharing of experiences. Some groups are designed for those with a particular kind of arthritis, such as osteoarthritis or rheumatoid arthritis, but most are all-inclusive.

Support groups generally have a leader, who is either a medical professional (for example, a doctor, nurse, psychologist, or social worker) or simply a member of the group. Member-run groups are often called self-help or peer groups.

If you think you'd like to try a support or self-help group, keep in mind that it may take some detective work and a sizable investment of time before you find the one you really like. Visit several groups and go to each one at least twice. The one-time meeting you observe may represent an off-night for an otherwise dynamic and helpful group (or a good night for an otherwise disorganised and not-very-helpful group).

One of the great things about support groups is they remind you that you're not alone. You needn't try to master all the arthritis terms and treatments yourself, because thousands of experts who've experienced something similar themselves are waiting to help you.

Finding help and hope through the group

Joining an arthritis or pain support group is often both educational and comforting. Within these groups, you can find the following:

- A chance to talk about your feelings
- A good reason to get out of the house, interact with people, and make new friends
- Encouragement
- Information
- People who can tell you what to expect from a certain test or treatment, because they've already experienced it
- People who understand exactly what you're feeling
- Role models – people who are much more advanced in their arthritis than you are, but who are living happy and productive lives
- Sympathy

Locating a support or self-help group

To find a support or self-help group (or a pool of groups from which to choose), ask the members of your healthcare team for referrals. You can also contact any of the arthritis organisations listed in Appendix B.

And, for those of you who don't want to leave the comfort of your desk, you can even find support groups on the Internet, such as www.arthritiscare.org.uk.

Dealing with Arthritis in the Workplace

When you have arthritis, you have some days when you just don't feel like going to work. But you may not have the luxury of staying home every time you have a flare-up, especially if they happen often. For this reason, simplifying your tasks at work, just like you did at home, to make them as easy on your joints and as energy-efficient as possible is important.

If your pain seriously interferes with your ability to do your job and you've done all you can to control it, you may want to consider leaving work behind and applying for disability benefits.

Easing the pain when you work

Many people spend their working hours sitting down in an office. While sitting down sounds easy, working on a computer, handling correspondence, and doing other paperwork is difficult if your hands hurt or you can't sit comfortably in a chair. Look into these ideas for streamlining paperwork and making desk duties easier:

- ✔ Large scissors with well-padded handles can make cutting easier.
- ✔ A rubber grip that fits around the barrel of a pen or pencil makes it easier to hold and less likely to slip.
- ✔ Rubber fingers (they look like a thimble made of rubber) can help you turn pages or thumb through a sheaf of papers without fumbling. Or, you can twist a rubber band around the end of your finger for the same effect.
- ✔ Seam rippers that quickly cut through stitches are a nice substitute if you have trouble handling scissors.
- ✔ Tape dispensers with weighted and rubberised bottoms make it easier to pull off a piece of tape using just one hand, because they won't move.

If you have internet access and your employer doesn't object to your handling some office tasks with online business transactions, you can cut down on the time you spend standing in long queues (putting strain on your joints) by doing the following:

- ✔ Banking by computer or through the post. Most banks now offer these services.
- ✔ Buying books, vitamins, presents, travel tickets, holidays – even cars – online. The days of pounding the pavement to do your shopping are gone!

Applying for disability benefits

People with long-term disabilities are often entitled to a variety of benefits. Your general practitioner (GP), social worker, hospital, Citizens' Advice Bureau, and the Internet – try www.disabilitybenefits.co.uk and www.dwp.gov.uk/lifeevent/benefits – can all provide information. But getting disability benefits doesn't necessarily mean that you can't still work. If you don't relish the idea of sitting at home, your local Social Security office can provide you with more details of the options available to you.

Part V
The Part of Tens

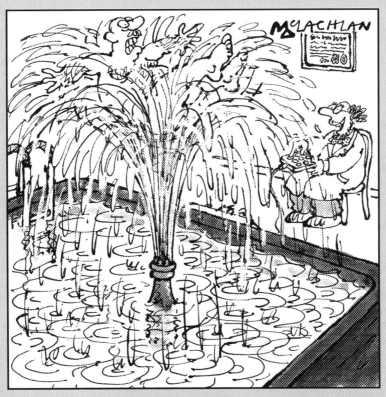

"It's a new type of hydrotherapy
- Let me know when you've had
enough, Mr Maybrick."

In this part . . .

This part of the book is a kind of "distilled" way of pre-senting some key information about managing your arthritis. We include tips for traveling with arthritis, ways to save prescription dollars, health professionals who can help you fight arthritis, new treatments that you might not have heard about yet, and myths about arthritis.

Chapter 20

Ten Tips for Travelling with Arthritis

*F*ew things are more exciting and invigorating than packing your bags and hitting the road, bound for some exotic destination or just getting out of your home town for a while to clear your head. But travelling with arthritis is not always easy, what with the additional strain on your joints, skyrocketing stress levels, change in routine, long hours sitting in cramped seats, jet lag, and having to haul loads of luggage and other travel paraphernalia. But don't give up – you *can* still travel when you've got arthritis, and you can even have a good time! You just need to plan a little more carefully than in the past. Consider this chapter the Ten Commandments of Travelling with Arthritis.

Talking to Your Doctor

Consider telling your doctor about your travel plans: Where you're going, for how long, what you plan to do, the kind of climate to which you're travelling, and the kinds of foods that you plan to eat. Then ask your doctor if he or she has any cautions for you. Do you have to limit yourself to certain kinds of activities? How much time do you have to spend resting every day? Do you have to carry your own luggage or ask others to carry it for you? How do you arrange for a wheelchair at the airport? Is pain the best gauge of when to stop an activity? Or do you stop before the pain sets in?

Ask your doctor about the possibility of carrying along a prescription for any medicines you may need in case you run out, and, if you think it's necessary, get a letter from him or her describing your condition (just in case) – although there may be a charge for this 'private' service.

You also need to arrange travel insurance, and understand exactly how it works in the country you are visiting. If, for example, you have an arthritis flare-up on holiday, how do you pay for a visit to the doctor, and how do you obtain reimbursement?

If you are planning to travel to the European Economic Area (EEA, which is basically the European Union (EU) plus Iceland, Liechtenstein, and Norway) or Switzerland after 1 January, 2006, you need the new European Health Insurance Card. Seek information about applying for the card from either the Department of Health Web site or your local post office. This card gives you access to free or reduced-cost emergency healthcare. You still need insurance to cover repatriation in the event of serious illness, however.

If travelling to a developing country, ensure that your insurance covers repatriation to fly you home if you need medical treatment.

Always carry your insurance and identity papers with you; don't leave them in your hotel as you never know when you may need them!

Reviewing Your Medications and Supplements

Make a list of every medicine, vitamin, mineral, herb, supplement, potion, cream, and liniment you use. Then bring all of them! Try to follow your normal routine as closely as possible; don't start flinging out what seems superfluous just before you go on a trip. That 'superfluous' item is often the very thing helping you avoid or clear a flare-up. Bring along familiar over-the-counter aids for pain, so you don't have to start experimenting with strange brands when you're in unfamiliar territory. If you're flying, pack your medications in a carry-on bag so you have them with you even if your luggage gets lost.

After you have every medicine and supplement assembled, count the number of days you're away, and make sure that you take enough of everything to last the entire trip. Then pack a little extra – they may not have what you need where you're going!

Before travelling to another country, find out which drugs it considers illegal. For example, Japan frowns on stimulants, while Greece and Turkey are strict about opiates like codeine. Carry all your medicines (prescription, over-the-counter, and even vitamins) in their original containers. If you're taking syringes or narcotic drugs, get a letter from your doctor explaining why you need them. Don't undergo endless delays and interrogations because you're carrying the 'wrong' medication!

If you're allergic to any medicines, keep a note of this information with your identity papers. If you're involved in an accident or have a serious illness, you may not be in a position to give any details.

Preplanning to Reduce Stress

Think through your trip and try to anticipate and solve any problems before you leave, so that you can travel without worry. For example, if you have trouble walking, request a wheelchair or motorised cart in advance. Keep your carry-on bag light and easy to manage, and make sure that all of your luggage has wheels and is well balanced. Make a daily plan that includes periods of activity, periods of rest, and plenty of time to sleep. Schedule some time to exercise and some time to soak in a hot bath, if you find these activities helpful. Build in an extra day to give yourself time to recover from jet lag. Don't just rush headlong into the unknown (your trip) without a plan, or your body may complain via an arthritis flare-up.

Finally, plan an emergency-exit procedure in case you need to cut your trip short. Purchase holiday insurance, or get open-ended plane tickets. You won't enjoy getting stuck far away and being unable to go home if you're not feeling well.

Eating Wisely and Well

Eating a healthy, balanced diet is always important, but especially when your body is stressed by an ongoing condition (arthritis) compounded with the strain of travelling. People with arthritis benefit from taking special care with what they eat as some foods can make their condition worse. Luckily, other foods can help to relieve some of these people's symptoms. In general, no matter where your destination, try to:

- Eat a wide variety of foods, focusing on whole-grains, fresh fruit and vegetables, with smaller amounts of meat, fish, poultry (110 to 170 grams or 4 to 6 ounces per day, maximum), and dairy products.
- Limit your intake of cholesterol, fat, sugar, and salt (sodium).
- Take it easy on the alcohol.
- Use olive oil, rapeseed oil, flaxseed oil, and others high in the 'good' fatty acid (linoleic acid), which can help lessen inflammation.
- Watch your intake of foods that contain the 'bad' fatty acid (arachidonic acid) such as meat, poultry, egg yolks, and full-fat dairy products.
- Eat fish that contain omega-3 fatty acids (mackerel, herring, salmon, and so on) a couple of times weekly.

Exercising, Even though You're on Holiday!

Regular physical activity strengthens your joint super-support structures, helping them take some of the load, while nourishing and moisturising your cartilage. Aerobic activity can tone you all over, strengthen your heart, increase bone density, and help you keep your weight under control (very important, especially for those with arthritis of the knee). Flexibility (stretching) exercises increase and maintain your range of motion, loosen up your muscles, and make your tendons and ligaments more resilient. At the same time, these exercises help to release tension and promote relaxation – translating into less pain and stiffness, greater ease of movement, and an improved mental attitude. In addition, exercise can increase your physical abilities, help prevent joint deformities, boost your immune system, improve your balance, and helps you maintain your independence.

Get plenty of exercise before you leave, to help carry you through a short trip. If you're travelling by car, get out and stretch every 90 minutes or so. If travelling by plane, get out of your seat and walk up and down the aisle every so often to ease joint stiffness and prevent *deep vein thrombosis* (a potentially life-threatening condition in which a blood clot forms in one of the deep veins of the body, usually in the leg). If you can find room, try a few stretches and some range-of-motion exercises. Set aside some time each day to stretch and do relaxation exercises in your hotel room (or wherever you're staying). And if your trip doesn't include plenty of walking, start each day with a brisk 20- to 30-minute walk. Walking is a great way to start the day, especially as the scenery is brand new to you!

Using Joint-protection Techniques

When travelling, the way you use (or abuse) your joints becomes crucial. Remember (and apply) these joint-protection techniques:

- Respect pain and, if something hurts, stop doing it and rest.
- Avoid joint-stressing postures or positions.
- Avoid staying in one position for a long time.
- Use the strongest and largest joints and muscles for the job.
- Avoid sustained joint activities.
- Maintain muscle strength and joint range of motion.
- Use assistive devices or splints, if necessary. (See the next section.)

Using Assistive Devices

Splints, supports, walking-sticks, pillows, motorised carts, wheelchairs, and anything else that takes a load off your joints are invaluable when you're travelling. Take advantage of the many little helpers designed to make your life easier and more comfortable:

- Use a horseshoe-shaped pillow to support your head and relieve neck pain while travelling in the car or flying.

- Support your back with a lumbar pillow wedged between the back of your waist and the seat.

- A small pillow atop the armrest in a plane or a car can make it easier and more comfortable to prop up your upper body.

- Wear your knee supports, or wrap your affected joints in elastic tape for greater stability.

- If you're planning on visiting museums but your knees hurt when you stand for long periods of time, bring along a small camping stool so you can pull up a chair whenever you want.

- Use walking-sticks, walking frames, motorised carts, and wheelchairs as needed.

Renting an Arthritis-friendly Car

The right car can minimise physical exertion, ease joint stress and strain, and make a driving trip much more comfortable. Contact the hire-car company at least six weeks before your trip to request a car that has as many of these arthritis-friendly features as possible:

- Automatic seat belts
- Cruise control
- Easy-access gear-stick and ignition
- Four doors
- Hand controls
- Lightweight doors
- Plenty of leg room
- Central locking
- Power seats (which adjust at the flick of a switch rather than you having to force them into position)

- Electric windows
- A steering wheel that tilts to provide different position options so you can find the one most comfortable for you.

Flying with Finesse

Flying is sometimes uncomfortable even for those who don't have arthritis, but it is torture for those with chronically stiff, achy joints. To make your flight as tolerable as possible, try the following:

- If your budget allows it, flying first-class or even club class is a lot more comfortable – from the seats and the amount of space you have, to the service. But flying first-class or club class is very costly.
- If you're flying coach, make your reservations early and request a seat in the first row or in an exit row, to ensure more leg room.
- Spend the extra few pounds and get a porter to handle your luggage – although this option is common abroad it's not always available in the UK, however.
- Request a wheelchair or motorised cart in advance if walking is a problem for you.
- Ask to pre-board so you can take your time to get settled. The airlines are usually happy to accommodate you.
- Arrange for a non-stop flight when possible, to avoid the hassle of getting on and off planes.
- Get up and move as much as possible during the flight to ease joint stiffness.
- Drink plenty of water during the flight, because the atmosphere inside the plane is extremely dehydrating.
- Travel during the less busy times (mid-week or midday, evening, and late at night) to avoid the crush of a crowd.

Taking a Test Run

If you're concerned about taking a long trip, try a smaller one first. Think of the little trip as a test run. You find out what works for you and what you need to work on to make a bigger trip more successful. Make a detailed list of what you brought and what you were lacking. When you get home, revise your list so you know exactly what to take next time. Each time you travel, make a note of what was missing and revise your list when you get home. Then refer to the list the next time you pack. You can become a seasoned traveller in no time. Happy wandering!

Chapter 21

Ten Drug-Free Ways to Reduce Pain and Stiffness

*E*ven though you have arthritis, you can live an active and comfortable life without drugging yourself up to the eyeballs. The following drug-free suggestions can help relieve pain and stiffness and may also help cut back on the number of prescription pills you pop each day.

Mastering Your Mattress

Sleeping on a comfortable mattress can reduce pain and stiffness, but sleeping on a mattress that's too hard or too soft can make your joint pain worse.

Signs that you may need a new mattress, or even a new bed (an adjustable one, for example) include:

- ✔ Tossing and turning at night, trying to get comfortable
- ✔ Waking with neck or backache
- ✔ Developing tenderness over bony prominences (especially hip or heel) from the pressure of sleeping on these areas

To solve the problem of sleeping (or, more likely, *not* sleeping) with arthritis pain, many people opt for one labelled as an *orthopaedic bed*. However, in reality there's no such thing; orthopaedic beds are just a manufacturer's name for one that is harder than normal, and this does not suit everyone. Although a firm mattress that evenly supports your weight is a good choice, there is no evidence that the harder the bed, the better – especially as you get older, when it's important to avoid excess pressure on the bits of you in contact with your mattress during sleep.

Lots of different types of mattress are now available and, when selecting a new mattress or bed, try lying on as many different surfaces as possible, to see which you find most comfortable. Don't feel embarrassed about asking the salesperson to leave you for 15 minutes to see how the surface suits you – they understand that beds are a very individual thing (and if they don't they need another job!) And if you sleep with someone, try out the bed together with your partner. If he or she moves, does it disturb you? Is there a tendency for one person to roll towards the other?

Although sleeping surfaces are an individual thing, I believe a *memory foam mattress* is best for anyone with back pain or osteoarthritis, as it gets you as close to weightless sleeping as possible. The term 'memory foam' doesn't mean the mattress remembers the contours of your body, although you can see your dent in the mattress for a few seconds after getting up; it refers to the fact that the foam material remembers its original shape and bounces back into it as soon as you get up. Memory foam is one of the many benefits to come out of the space program. NASA scientists originally developed the material to help astronauts withstand massive G-forces during space flights! These scientists soon realised that the visco-elastic polymer, which is heat and pressure sensitive, forms a perfect sleeping surface that naturally moulds to your body shape.

Unfortunately, memory foam mattresses are relatively expensive, although when you work out the nightly cost of sleeping on one over at least ten years, it doesn't seem so bad. If your own mattress is serviceable, but uncomfortable, an alternative is a memory foam overlay which goes on top to give firm support as your body sinks into the material. A visco-elastic polymer mattress overlay helps support the natural curves of your back, reduces the load on your pressure points, and helps your muscles and ligaments recover during sleep. Research shows that reducing the strain on your joints also reduces the number of times you toss and turn from the usual average of 80 to 100 times to less than 20 times a night. Improved restlessness means less pain; thus, reducing your need for both sleeping tablets and painkillers. Pillows, seat wedges, and back supports in the same material are also available. Buyers beware – these mattresses are so comfortable you won't want to get up in the morning!

Taking Regular Exercise

While getting enough rest is important, don't go overboard and rest all the time! Being inactive makes your muscles weak and increases joint stiffness, while regular exercise helps maintain your joint mobility and muscle strength.

Many people worry that physical activity damages their joints further. Far from it! Do go gently and avoid weight-bearing activities, such as jogging, that place extra strain on your lower limbs. Simple exercises such as walking, cycling, and swimming are best, though do avoid walking on rough ground. Ideally, you can ask a physiotherapist to suggest a regime tailored to your individual needs.

Chapter 16 has exercises and tips.

Eating Well

Like your heart, your joints thrive best on a healthy diet. Eat plenty of fresh fruit and vegetables – at least five servings per day. Fruit and veg contain antioxidant vitamins such as vitamins A and C, as well as carotenoids and the mineral selenium, which can reduce the rate at which your cartilage breaks down.

Antioxidants help to damp down inflammation and are remarkably effective in slowing the progression of osteoarthritis. In one study of 640 men and women, those with moderate-to-high intakes of vitamin C (two or more times the recommended daily amount) were three times less likely to develop knee pain or to see their knee osteoarthritis worsen than those with low intakes of vitamin C (up to about twice the recommended daily amount). An apple a day really does keep the doctor away – they are rich sources of protective antioxidants called flavonoids. In fact, following a full-blown vegetarian diet appears to have particular benefits for people with rheumatoid arthritis.

If you follow a vegetarian diet, maintaining good intakes of vitamins and minerals, especially of iron, zinc, and vitamin B12, is important as levels of these are often low in non-meat diets.

Eating oily fish such as salmon, trout, sardines, herrings, and mackerel also helps keep your joints healthy by damping down inflammation. Many people choose to take an omega-3 fish oil or cod liver oil supplement.

And if you're prone to gout, help lower uric acid levels by reducing your intake of purine-rich foods such as offal, shellfish, oily fish, game, meats, yeast-extracts, asparagus, and spinach.

For more dietary info, turn to Chapter 15.

Considering Hydrotherapy

For helping ease pain and stiffness, there's nothing like a warm bath. That's why hydrotherapy, in which exercise is performed in a warm, deep pool, gives such excellent results. Ask your doctor if a hydrotherapy pool is available in your area – many physiotherapy departments now have them. Chapter 14 has more information on hydro and other therapies.

Losing Excess Weight

If the pounds mount over the years, not only your silhouette suffers. Did you know that when you walk, the load on your lower limbs reaches up to five times your body weight? So, if you're just 4.5 kilograms (10 pounds) overweight, your legs bear the brunt of an extra 22 kilograms (50 pounds)! Sounds scary, but turn it round the other way and you realise that losing just half a kilogram (or 1 pound) in weight can reduce the strain on your legs to the tune of just over 2 kilograms (5 pounds) per step.

Switch to more fruit, vegetables, and salad stuff, and ditch those pies, pastries, cakes, biscuits and chocolates, which from now on are no more than occasional treats. Sob.

Keeping Warm

Cold is one of the worst culprits for encouraging stiff, aching joints. Get out those woolly jumpers, vests, and long-johns once Jack Frost starts making an appearance. Avoid cold draughts and keep as warm as possible in winter, especially when going out. Wrap up in multiple layers, wear hat, gloves, scarf, and thick socks, and don't worry about looking unfashionable.

If you have rheumatoid arthritis, try exercising your hands in hot, soapy water first thing in the morning and throughout the day. Frequent hot baths/showers are also soothing. Applying hot compresses or packs that you warm in the microwave (widely available from chemists) are worth trying too. And don't forget your hot water bottle or electric blanket when it's time for bed.

If using an electric over- or underblanket, check that it's in good repair and only use according to instructions.

Wielding a Stick

Using a walking-stick can more than halve the load on weight-bearing joints, and increase your stability and balance – as long as you wield it properly. Think of your stick as a third limb. Use your stick on the opposite side to your worst leg, so if your left hip joint is worse, hold the stick in your right hand, regardless of which hand is dominant. (If both legs are 'bad', you may need to use two sticks, crutches, or a walking frame.) First, put all your weight on your 'good' leg, then step forward a comfortable distance with your 'bad' leg and the stick at the same time. Once your weight is supported on both your stick and your bad leg, step through with your good leg. Sounds simple? You may need practise to overcome the urge to use the walking-stick on the same side as your bad leg.

Select a walking-stick at a height that leaves your elbow slightly bent during use, and try to maintain an upright posture when walking.

If you're experiencing difficulties with walking, ask for a review with an occupational or physiotherapist to select additional aids for you. Tips for walking correctly can be found in Chapter 17.

Wearing a Copper Bracelet

How copper helps reduce joint pain remains unclear, but is likely to centre on its involvement in the function of a number of antioxidant enzymes, including powerful *superoxide dismutase (SOD)*. Lack of copper reduces activity of SOD and may contribute to the development of inflammatory diseases. Copper is also involved in vitamin C metabolism and the synthesis of collagen – a major structural protein in bones and joints. Another theory is that copper bracelets work through a process known as iontophoresis, in which copper leaches excess sulphates from the body where they are deposited as a blue-green discolouration on the skin. Trace amounts of copper are absorbed through the skin, and in one study of 240 people with rheumatoid arthritis, those wearing copper bracelets had a statistically significant improvement compared to those wearing an inactive, placebo bracelet. Each copper bracelet lost an average of 13 milligrams of copper during the trial. The efficacy of copper bracelets is thought to depend on the level of copper in your body. If you are copper deficient, you may benefit from a bracelet, but if your level is already adequate, it may not help.

Cheaper copper bracelets may contain nickel, to which many people are allergic. If you are sensitive to nickel, only buy a bracelet guaranteed to be nickel free.

Using Magnetic Patches

Applying magnetic patches on tender spots around arthritic joints can ease pain and stiffness quite quickly. A double-blind study in Japan found that magnetic patches were 80 per cent effective in relieving painful, stiff shoulders compared with just 6 per cent for non-magnetised placebo patches. In another double-blind study involving 222 patients with acute and chronic muscle and joint pain, 90 per cent of those using magnetic patches reported significant improvement within five days, compared with only 14 per cent in the placebo group. Chapter 14 discusses patches in more depth.

Selecting Supplements

Lots of food supplements have proven anti-inflammatory actions that are at least as effective as those of non-steroidal drugs, but with significantly less risk of serious side effects. Combining these food supplements with physio-therapy and regular exercise can help to reduce pain and improve your mobility if you are unable, or unwilling, to take prescribed treatments. In some studies, supplements given together with prescribed painkillers helped to reduce the dose of drugs needed.

In general, each supplement tends to help around two-out-of-three people, but predicting in advance which supplement suits an individual is difficult. Use trial and error to find those supplements that are best for you. Information on the different supplements you can try is available in Chapters 11 and 15.

A common starting point is to take:

- ✔ Glucosamine sulphate (with or without chondroitin)
- ✔ Omega-3 fish oils
- ✔ A multivitamin and mineral, perhaps with extra vitamin C

If you have very inflamed joints, you can also add in anti-inflammatory turmeric, bromelain, Devil's claw, green-lipped mussel extracts, or MSM sulphur.

Always tell your doctor or pharmacist if you intend to combine supplements with prescribed medication, and check there are no known interactions.

Chapter 22

Ten Professionals Who Can Help You Fight Arthritis

*A*s you know, taking charge of your arthritis isn't just a matter of seeing your doctor once in a while and popping a few pills. Because arthritis is a multi-faceted disease, your war against it is fought on many fronts, involving the physical, the mental, the emotional, and the practical day-to-day business of living. For optimal effectiveness, you need to assemble a team of health-care professionals (think of them as generals) to help you attack arthritis in several ways.

The most important members of the team (after you) are your general practitioner (GP) and *rheumatologist*, a doctor who specialises in arthritis and other diseases of the joints, muscles, and soft tissues. But other members of the team, including the pharmacist, physiotherapist, occupational therapist, social worker, massage therapist, and others also play vital roles. Assembling a team is up to you, so research all you can about what each professional does and find the best to help you win your battles against arthritis pain and joint destruction.

Primary Care Physician

Having a great relationship with your GP is vital; he or she remains responsible for your overall health and wellbeing, even though they may refer you to a rheumatologist or other specialists. The role of your GP – or primary care physician – is crucial as hospital or clinic-based rheumatologists and other specialists don't provide regular health maintenance, which is essential for people with arthritis.

Important health-maintenance checks include cancer screenings such as cervical smears, breast examinations, and mammograms, which are especially important as some of the drugs used to treat arthritis and related conditions may increase your risk of cancer (although the benefits of treatment obviously outweigh the slight increased risk or your doctor won't suggest them). Paying attention to preventing and treating heart disease is also vital, as more and more research suggests that people with inflammatory arthritis of any kind are at increased risk of heart problems – especially if you regularly use non-steroidal anti-inflammatory drugs (NSAIDs – refer to Chapter 8). Your GP can also treat any co-existing diseases (keeping tight control of blood pressure in people with lupus who have kidney disease, for example, helps the kidneys to function properly for longer). Your GP can also provide vaccinations such as a yearly flu jab.

People receiving the best care often have close communication between their rheumatologist and their primary care physician. If your relationship with your GP has broken down, or if you have moved area, useful information on finding a new doctor is available from the British Medical Association Web site at www.bma.org.uk/ap.nsf/Content/registernhssurgery, the NHS in England site at www.nhs.uk/England/Doctors/Default.aspx, and from the NHS Direct site at www.nhsdirect.nhs.uk, phone 0845-4647.

Rheumatologist

A *rheumatologist* is a doctor who specialises in rheumatic diseases and has additional training and experience in the diagnosis and treatment of problems affecting the joints, muscles, and soft tissues. A rheumatologist treats rheumatoid arthritis (RA) and related diseases such as fibromyalgia, lupus, scleroderma, and Sjögren's syndrome. A rheumatologist's goal is to alleviate pain, ease inflammation and other symptoms and, as much as possible, ward off further damage to your joints.

Treatment from a rheumatologist is particularly crucial for those with rheumatoid arthritis. Taking DMARDs (disease-modifying antirheumatic drugs; refer to Chapter 8 for more details) is considered a first-line treatment for people with newly diagnosed RA. Studies show that those treated with DMARDs have less joint damage and better joint function, and they tend to live longer than those who aren't treated with these medications.

However, RA patients who receive care solely from a GP are less likely to receive these important medications than those consulting a rheumatologist. According to a Canadian study that followed nearly 30,000 RA patients over a five-year period, 80 per cent of those under the care of a rheumatologist had used a DMARD, compared to only 53 per cent of those seen by a general physician, and 14 per cent of those seeing just a GP. So seeing a rheumatologist may mean better treatment for many arthritis sufferers, particularly those with RA.

And for the biologic response modifiers (BRMs, refer to Chapter 8 for more information), official advice is to only use them under specialist supervision. For referrals to a rheumatologist in your area, contact your GP. Everyone has the right to request a second opinion on how their condition is treated!

Pharmacist

A pharmacist can do a lot more than just fill your prescriptions. This highly educated professional is a walking encyclopaedia when it comes to information on interactions between drugs, and between drugs and foods, herbs, or supplements. A pharmacist can give you suggestions for maximising drug effectiveness and minimising or avoiding side effects. They automatically keep track of all medications you're taking (assuming you get all of your drugs from the same pharmacy), and they can look for potential problems or overdoses. Some pharmacists can even check your blood pressure and screen you for high cholesterol. Bring your medication-related questions to your pharmacist, who is a gold mine of free, accurate, and trustworthy information.

Physiotherapist

A physiotherapist can help you put together a programme of exercises to strengthen muscles supporting your painful joints. They can also show you how to do these exercises correctly, without inflicting more joint damage. A physiotherapist can also help you increase joint and muscle flexibility, restore range of motion, and pump up your endurance without putting undue strain on your joints.

Although you won't need the services of a physiotherapist forever, it does take several weeks to get you on track with a good exercise programme and to supervise exercising and stretching to make sure that you're not doing more harm than good. A physiotherapist can also show you techniques using heat, cold, or water therapy to help manage your pain and improve your mobility. Ask your GP about referrals to a physiotherapist in your area. Some physiotherapists may also work privately – check the *Yellow Pages* or phone the physiotherapy department of your local hospital (NHS or private) for information about who's available. A search facility to find privately practising physiotherapists is also available on the Web site of the Chartered Society of Physiotherapy at www.csp.org.uk.

Occupational Therapist

An *occupational therapist (OT)* shows you how to overcome arthritis-related movement limitations through the use of special techniques or assistive devices that can ease the performance of daily activities. The OT interviews you and watches you in action, and then comes up with recommendations that can make it easier for you to get dressed, groom yourself, get around, shop, do housework, drive, or work. They may also design special splints or supports and show you techniques to reduce joint stress and help prevent further joint damage.

For referrals to OTs in your area, contact your GP. You can also search the directory of the Web site for Occupational Therapists in Independent Practice at www.otip.co.uk.

Registered Dietitian or Nutritionist

If you have osteoarthritis (OA) and are overweight, nutritional therapy is an important component in your recovery. OA of the knee is often a direct result of carrying too much weight, and losing as little as 5 pounds (or just over 2 kilograms) can do much to prevent arthritis of the weight-bearing joints or, at least, dramatically reduce the symptoms. But losing weight, as we all know, is a lot easier said than done, and getting the help of a professional is well worth the cost. A good dietitian or nutritionist can help you work out how to eat regular, well-balanced meals consisting of standard-size portions; distinguish between eating/food-related behaviours and feelings/psychological problems; and help you gradually lose weight and keep it off.

For referrals to dietitians in your area, contact your GP. For a list of nutritionists who offer private consultations, visit www.nutsoc.org.uk.

Many people can benefit from seeing a nutritional therapist who can advise on the best food supplements to take. Nutritional therapists with recognised experience, and who have professional indemnity insurance, are registered with the British Association of Nutritional Therapists. You can obtain a list of those registered by sending £2 plus a large (A4) self-addressed envelope to BANT, 27 Old Gloucester Street, London WC1N 3XX. A list of members of the Institute for Optimum Nutrition, who obtain the DipION qualification, is available at www.ion.ac.uk or you can find a therapist in your area by phoning ION on 0208-8779993.

Social Worker

A *social worker* can help you solve personal and family problems, locate community resources, recommend support groups or other special services, and help you deal with serious illness or disability. He or she can also help you apply for any benefits to which you are entitled and help you access after-hospital services such as meals-on-wheels.

For referrals to a social worker in your area, contact your GP surgery or Social Services department.

Chiropractor

A *chiropractor* manipulates the spine to relieve nerve pressure caused by poor posture, stress injury, disease, or lack of exercise. A chiropractor can help to relieve pain, release stress, improve joint alignment, and increase joint function using a variety of techniques. These techniques include applying controlled and directed forces to your spine using massage, acupressure, trigger-point therapy, and myofascial release. They can also apply a precise, measurable force to specific points on your body with a tool called an activator. A chiropractor may also manipulate your joints to increase your range of movement. (Refer to Chapter 13 for more on chiropractic treatment.)

To find a chiropractor in your area, contact the General Chiropractic Council by phone on 0207-7135155 or search at www.gcc-uk.org.

Mental Health Professional

A mental health professional can help you cope with the depression, anger, anxiety, relationship problems, or other emotional fallout that you may experience due to chronic illness. He or she can help you understand the origins of your emotional troubles, find new ways of handling these problems, and address co-existing conditions, such as alcoholism, drug abuse, or prescription-drug dependence. (More information is given in Chapter 18 for dealing with emotions and coping with depression.)

Anyone can call themselves a 'therapist' and set up a practice, so make sure that you consult a properly qualified mental health professional (a psychologist, counsellor, or psychiatrist). Psychiatrists are physicians and are therefore the only mental health professionals who can prescribe medication. But most mental health professionals can refer you to a psychiatrist if medication is needed.

For referrals to mental health professionals in your area, contact your GP, or phone the British Association for Counselling and Psychotherapy on 0870-4435252 or perform a search at www.bacp.co.uk.

Massage Therapist

If you have arthritis, your muscles often work overtime to favour the joints that hurt. A good massage therapist can help to ease the pain that settles into muscles doing double duty. Massage can also relieve some of your arthritis pain as it eases tension in the muscles surrounding painful joints and improves joint range of movement. In general, massage increases circulation, helps your body release the metabolic by-products that can irritate nerve endings, pumps up endorphin levels (your brain's own natural painkillers), and relieves tension. Massage also feels great, making it an effective way of helping you let go of pain, stress, and the extra tension in locked-up muscles. Check out Chapter 13 for more on the various forms of massage.

But don't turn your body over to just anybody. Find a massage therapist who's skilled in treating people with arthritis. Some kinds of massage are too rough or painful for certain kinds of arthritis, so consult your doctor first. But if you're having an arthritis flare-up, you have an infection or a fever, or you're coming down with an illness, avoid a massage as increasing circulation can sometimes increase inflammation.

To find referrals for a massage therapist in your area, search the Massage Therapy UK Web site at www.massagetherapy.co.uk.

Chapter 23

Ten Crackerjack New Treatments

*I*n the not-too-distant future, physicians may diagnose arthritis by looking at a map of your genes and treating the ailment through subtle genetic manipulation. Examining small variations in your genetic code can also pin-point which drugs work best for you and at what dose. Rather than the hit-and-miss approach of today, your doctor will individually tailor your prescriptions for you. Although this idea may sound far-fetched, much of the technology is already in place, and this rapidly evolving new branch of science even has a name – *pharmacogenomics*.

In fact, doctors may even prevent arthritis by studying a baby's genetic code and tweaking it to ensure that the young one's joints never begin the process of deterioration.

The medical profession is not there yet, but medical researchers are developing a host of new treatments. Some treatments are modern twists on older therapies; others, are entirely new ideas.

Anti-TNF Drugs for Rheumatoid Arthritis

If you have rheumatoid arthritis (RA), your immune system turns on your body, which is one reason doctors use drugs that suppress the immune system (disease-modifying antirheumatic drugs, or DMARDs) to control this disease. But this approach is a rather broad one, interfering with the immune system's helpful actions as well as its harmful ones. A new family of drugs, called *biologic response modifiers* or BRMs, address this problem by focusing on very specific parts of the immune system, trying to spare the 'good' parts of the immune response while stifling the 'bad' ones.

When overproduced, one of the 'bad' parts of the immune system, called *tumour necrosis factor (TNF),* can cause severe inflammation and tissue damage. Large amounts of TNF often go hand-in-hand with autoimmune diseases like RA, and a special subgroup of the BRMs called the 'anti-TNF' drugs can help to calm inflammation and ward off tissue damage.

Three of these anti-TNF drugs – etanercept, infliximab, and adalimumab – have made new strides in relieving RA symptoms and controlling the disease. Designed for those with moderate-to-severe RA who aren't helped by the standard disease-modifying medicines, these drugs calm down the body's immune system and decrease the effects of TNF, slowing the progression of RA. Although these drugs are covered more fully in Chapter 8, here's some extra low-down on each:

✔ **Etanercept** is injected just beneath the skin twice weekly to help the body regulate TNF and slow disease progression. In studies of etanercept, a little more than 60 per cent of patients enjoy a 20 per cent or greater improvement in joint pain, joint swelling, and other symptoms. The medicine works fairly quickly, so many people can handle daily chores with greater ease within two weeks.

✔ **Infliximab,** when combined with methotrexate (a standard medication for RA), produces dramatic improvements in RA symptoms compared with using methotrexate alone. Fifty-two per cent of those getting the combination of drugs enjoy significant reductions in swollen and tender joints, compared to 17 per cent on methotrexate alone. The improvement in symptoms occurs within two-to-six weeks (as opposed to months with methotrexate) and still remains after one year. Infliximab also significantly reduces long-term damage. The drug is given intravenously once every eight weeks, although the dose is occasionally increased to once every four-to-six weeks.

✔ **Adalimumab,** like infliximab, rapidly reduces the pain, tenderness, and swelling of joints seen in RA, and sustains those results over the long term. This drug also helps to slow or prevent progressive joint destruction. Clinical trials involving more than 2,400 patients show that treatment with adalimumab significantly improves physical function and health-related quality of life, and surveys of nearly 2,500 patients have also shown that the drug is generally safe and well tolerated. Adalimumab is currently approved as a treatment for RA.

The anti-TNF medications can bring dramatic results, but they are also costly and produce some serious side effects. A very small percentage of patients who are prone to infections develop deadly diseases, such as tuberculosis, while taking these medications. Because of the possibility of developing tuberculosis, every single person considering them must have a TB skin test and, in some cases, a chest X-ray before beginning treatment with anti-TNFs. Other side effects caused by these drugs include reactions at the injection site and headaches.

Rituximab for Rheumatoid Arthritis

Rituximab is an anti-cancer drug administered by infusion that is licensed for the treatment of a form of lymph cancer called non-Hodgkin's lymphoma. Recently, rituximab was shown to have excellent potential as a treatment for RA and lupus as well.

Rituximab belongs to a class of drugs called the *monoclonal antibodies*, which act like little 'smart bombs'. These drugs zero in on a targeted protein on the surface of certain cells and then attack and kill that cell, while sparing the healthy cells that surround it. Rituximab goes after immune cells called *B cells,* which are the most likely driving force behind the autoimmune reaction that causes RA. Treatment with rituximab kills about 90 per cent of these errant B cells and preserves the stem cells that produce new, healthy B cells.

A study of 161 RA patients, published in the *New England Journal of Medicine* in 2004, shows rituximab's exciting potential as a treatment for arthritis. Just two infusions of rituximab, taken either alone or combined with a standard RA drug, relieved RA symptoms for as long as six months in up to 40 per cent of patients. Only 13 per cent of those taking methotrexate (the most widely used RA drug) enjoyed similar results.

Rituximab is not yet approved for use as a treatment for RA or lupus, as much more study is needed. This drug may, however, prove the forerunner of a new wave of focused treatments that zero in on the causes of arthritis and other joint diseases.

The 'Mini-Open' Surgical Technique for Carpal Tunnel Syndrome

A new ten-minute surgical procedure, done on an out-patient basis, may provide excellent relief from the pain of advanced carpal tunnel syndrome (compression of the nerve and tendons that pass through the carpal tunnel, a corridor between the ligaments and bones in the wrist). Carpal tunnel syndrome causes pain, numbness, and tingling in the thumb, index, and middle fingers that can move all the way up to the arm and shoulder.

Splints, medications to reduce pain and inflammation, and steroid injections into the afflicted nerve are standard treatments. But those who don't respond to these treatments may opt for surgery. In the past, a longer, more complex operation was used, but today a new operation called the *mini-open technique* is becoming more popular. This technique allows better access to important structures in the wrist and sidesteps the pain and complications that come from making incisions in the more painful area of the palm of the hand. A tiny 2-centimetre incision (just less than 1 inch) is made in the palm, through which specially designed surgical instruments are inserted, allowing the surgeon to 'open up' the carpal tunnel and relieve nerve compression. Most people can use the affected hand the same day for regular activities such as brushing teeth, and physiotherapy is almost never needed. In most cases, the mini-open surgery cures the problem of carpel tunnel permanently.

Etoricoxib for RA, OA, and Gout

Etoricoxib is a relatively new medication used to treat osteoarthritis, rheumatoid arthritis, and acute gouty arthritis. As described in Chapter 8, etoricoxib is an NSAID that interferes with an enzyme called COX (cyclo-oxygenase) to relieve inflammation. There are *two* of these COX enzymes: COX-1, which helps keep your stomach healthy (among many other things); and COX-2, which plays a role in the inflammation process. Standard NSAIDs inhibit both COX enzymes, the good and the bad and as a result, your joints may feel better, but your stomach feels worse.

In contrast, COX-2 inhibitors are designed to spare the COX-1 'healthy stomach' enzymes while going after the 'inflammatory' COX-2 enzymes. So, like standard NSAIDs, COX-2 inhibitors relieve pain and inflammation, but are less likely to leave you with a raw, burning stomach or stomach ulcers (although some people do develop gastrointestinal bleeding and ulcerations while taking them). Etoricoxib, which is a more selective COX-2 inhibitor, goes even further than other 'coxibs', targeting the COX-2 enzymes 100 times more often than the COX-1 enzymes. In theory, this targeting should make etoricoxib even easier on your stomach.

Studies of RA patients show that etoricoxib reduces joint tenderness, swelling, and RA disease activity, working just as well as or better than a standard RA treatment: The NSAID naproxen. Also, in a quality-of-life study, etoricoxib significantly improved pain relief, physical functioning, social functioning, and the patients' general perception of health when compared to patients who were using naproxen. And the risk of developing kidney complications (a possibility with certain OA and RA drugs) was low. Etoricoxib also causes significantly less gastrointestinal blood loss than ibuprofen does.

When etoricoxib was compared to the commonly used OA medication diclofenac, it provided an equal amount of pain relief but worked faster, providing much greater relief within the first four hours. As an added bonus, etoricoxib is taken only once a day, compared with diclofenac's three times a day.

In patients with acute gouty arthritis, etoricoxib relieves joint pain, inflammation, and tenderness as quickly and effectively as the standard gout medication, indomethacin, but with fewer side effects.

Although a COX-2 inhibitor is a great idea for people with a history of stomach ulcers or who suffer from gastrointestinal side effects when taking traditional NSAIDs, it's important to remember that many people do well with traditional NSAIDS, which are quite a bit cheaper.

Bosentan for Scleroderma

Scleroderma, a disease that causes the body to produce too much collagen and store it in body tissues in harmful ways, has no cure. Thick, hardened, and rough skin with lumpy calcium deposits, joint swelling and locking, problems swallowing, and organ impairment are just a few of the devastating effects of this disease. One serious complication of scleroderma is a lung disorder called *pulmonary arterial hypertension (PAH),* in which abnormally high blood pressure develops in the arteries between the heart and the lungs. PAH causes shortness of breath and significantly reduces your ability to exercise or exert yourself. PAH is linked with changes in the lining of the blood vessels that service the lungs making it harder for them to deliver nutrients and take away waste from these vital organs. Scleroderma is a rare disease, but it's also fatal.

In the past, scientists thought that these unhealthy changes in the blood vessels were permanent. But in July 2003, a report of the long-term results of a medication called *bosentan* showed these blood vessel changes were actually reversible, as bosentan blocks a hormone that constricts blood vessels. Bosentan improves blood-vessel health, allowing many (but not all) people affected to walk farther and function better overall. This improvement in walking distance continues for as long as seven months after treatment is stopped. Bosentan also prevents the painful, debilitating hand ulcers often seen in those with scleroderma and significantly improves their hand function.

Another reason that bosentan is considered a breakthrough in the treatment of PAH is that it's taken orally. In the past, most PAH patients had to use a medication that was continuously infused through a central-venous line, so they were forced to carry around an infusion pump.

Bosentan does have two significant risks: It can cause birth defects and liver toxicity. Anyone who is pregnant, who may become pregnant, or who has liver disease should not take this medication.

MMF for Lupus-Related Kidney Problems

Mycophenolate mofetil (MMF) is an immunosuppressive drug used to help prevent the rejection of organ transplants. Several recent studies show that MMF is also a promising treatment for kidney inflammation in people with lupus. Lupus is sometimes treated with a very toxic chemotherapy drug, cyclophosphamide, which has serious side effects, including irreversible sterility, bone marrow suppression, and an increased risk of cancer. But MMF, which has far fewer side effects (there is often some bone marrow suppression), appears to reduce kidney inflammation and send it into remission in some cases. MMF is also effective as a maintenance therapy for those treated with cyclophosphamide who are already in remission. This effect is great news for people with lupus and kidney disease – at last, a treatment that is generally well tolerated and safe!

MMF is also helpful for treating lupus-related skin lesions, psoriatic arthritis, inflammatory arthritis, rheumatoid arthritis, and scleroderma, although it's not yet licensed for any of these uses. Remember that MMF *does* weaken your immune system, although it is generally safer than other immunosuppressive drugs. MMF is usually taken twice a day in capsule or liquid form, and common side effects include nausea, vomiting, loss of appetite, abdominal pain, diarrhoea, anaemia, and low white-blood cell count.

Cartilage Self-Transplants and Tissue Engineering

Simply popping in a new 'slab' of cartilage every time a joint went bad would be nice. Although doing so isn't yet possible, doctors have figured out how to use cartilage from a healthy joint to buff up a joint whose cartilage has seen better days.

The concept is simple: Use an arthroscope to take a small sample of cartilage from a healthy joint, 'wash' this cartilage clean, then let it grow and multiply in the laboratory. At the appropriate time, open up the damaged joint with an arthroscope and 'plant' the cultured cartilage into the bad joint. If all goes well, the new, healthy cartilage grows and multiplies in the new location, replacing the diseased cartilage and restoring the damaged joint to health. And you don't have to worry about tissue rejection, because it's your very own cells.

Cartilage self-transplantation is primarily performed on the knee. So far, results are promising, with up to 80 per cent of people reporting improved joint function several months or years later.

Researchers from Johns Hopkins University in the US are currently working on a new approach to the problem of old or worn-out cartilage. The approach involves harvesting cartilage stem cells (cells that have the ability to multiply) from adult goats, adding them to a nutrient-rich fluid, and injecting this fluid under the goat's skin. When an ultraviolet light or a visible laser is shone through the skin, the liquid hardens into a solid material called a *hydrogel*. In theory, this gel is suitable for injection into the joint, where the stem cells regenerate and eventually replace the damaged cartilage. Bone stem cells could work the same way to replace damaged bone tissue.

Although studies involving humans are years away, researchers hope that replacing joint parts with living tissue instead of metal or plastic parts can provide better, more long-lasting results.

Glass Therapy to Repair Bone and Treat RA

Although still in developmental stages, crushed-glass particles and tiny glass spheres form the basis of two new treatments for diseased bones and joints. Researchers at the University of Missouri-Rolla are crushing particles of glass and mixing them with a polymer in an attempt to create a solution suitable for injection into broken or diseased bones. Just as caulk fills cracks in your windowsill, this solution is designed to fill gaps in the broken or diseased bones, making them stronger.

Another development in the pipeline is tiny biodegradable glass beads made of radioactive material, which are injected into a joint to irradiate the diseased synovial tissue seen in RA. Delivering the radiation only to the diseased tissue means healthy tissues remain unaffected. The glass beads (which have a diameter of ⅕ to ¹⁄₁₀ the size of a human hair) eventually dissolve. This procedure was used in many studies to perform a non-surgical *synovectomy* (removal of a diseased joint lining). However, now that better medications for prevention and treatment of joint lining disease exist, (specifically the disease-modifying antirheumatic drugs – see Chapter 8), the need for synovectomies is less and less. The niche for glass therapy is probably as a way to handle stubborn cases of RA, rather than as a first-line treatment.

Therapeutic Tape for Osteoarthritis Pain

Researchers in Australia recently found that using special therapeutic taping techniques on osteoarthritic knees significantly reduced knee pain and disability, and the benefits lasted as long as three weeks after removal of the tape! The study involved randomly dividing 87 people with OA of the knee into one of three groups. The therapeutic tape knees were taped in a special way with hypoallergenic tape topped with rigid strapping tape. The control knees were taped in the same fashion, using hypoallergenic tape only, and the third group of knees remained untaped.

After three weeks, 73 per cent of those in the therapeutic tape group enjoyed less knee pain compared with 49 per cent of those in the control group and only 10 per cent who weren't taped. The therapeutic tape group also showed significant improvements in pain, disability, and quality of life compared with the no-tape group.

Although no one is quite sure why therapeutic taping works, researchers suggest that it helps improve joint alignment by 'taking a load off' the inflamed tissues.

The therapeutic taping technique is an easy-to-learn, inexpensive way of self-managing OA of the knee. If you're interested in finding out more about therapeutic tape, contact a physiotherapist. (See Appendix B.)

Improvements in Hip Replacement Materials and Techniques

Every year, approximately 43,000 people have a hip replacement in the UK. Joint replacement surgery gives a new lease of life to people with severe arthritis. But even though this surgery improves joint function, increases range of motion, and reduces pain dramatically, many doctors are reluctant to perform the operation too early, because the joint replacements themselves tend to wear out or come loose over time. Until recently, hip replacement implants were made of metal and plastic, and the plastic wore down over time, sometimes even causing joint infection. Revision surgery to install a new replacement is often required after as little as ten years. So in order to reduce the number of operations needed over a lifetime, young people and those who are particularly active often waited as long as possible before going under the knife. Yet delaying joint replacement surgery is often a bad idea. Studies show that those who delay joint replacement surgery until their decline in joint function is severe have the worst surgical outcomes.

Luckily, recent improvements in the quality and durability of the materials used in hip replacements mean that these delays are less necessary. New implants made completely of metal can increase the life of joint replacements substantially and reduce the risk of joint infection. So, scores of young people, baby boomers, and active adults previously considered unsuitable for joint replacement surgery can now enjoy the benefits of an artificial hip much sooner.

And even more good news exists: Hip surgery itself has become less damaging to the surrounding tissues and requires less time for recovery, thanks to a new, minimally invasive form of hip surgery that was pioneered in 2001. The incision is only 8 to 15 centimetres long (or 3 to 6 inches) – a far cry from the standard 30 centimetres! – which means that fewer muscles and other body tissues are cut. The smaller incision is possible because the ball-and-stem portion of the artificial joint is folded before insertion, so it fits into a much smaller opening. The stem is also shorter and narrower than the older varieties of artificial joint, so less drilling is required to make the shaft in the bone, which translates to less bone and tissue damage and a much faster recovery time.

Yet another new technique is also available – the minimally invasive '2-Incision' cementless procedure developed by Zimmer, a manufacturer of orthopaedic products and instruments famous for its walking frames. Rather than one large incision down the side of the hip and upper leg, two small cuts of just 4 to 5 centimetres (just under 2 inches) in length are made on either side of the hip joint. Then, rather than extensive cutting of leg and hip muscles to get at the joint, the muscles are simply moved to one side. Doing so reduces blood loss, allows you to get moving much more quickly after the operation, and promotes faster, less painful rehabilitation so you return to normal daily life more quickly. The only down side to this procedure is that it takes between one and two hours, which is longer than the traditional operation lasting 45 to 60 minutes.

In another advance, having a hip replacement using a prosthesis specially designed to your individual measurements is now possible. Your hip is scanned using computerised tomography (CT scanning) and a computer builds a three-dimensional image of the required prosthesis. The new hip is then custom-made using a computerised-milling machine that fashions the new hip from titanium. A special coating is then added. Your custom prosthesis fits snugly in all the right places – without the need for cement. The two surfaces of the artificial joint are covered with a hard-wearing ceramic liner. After the artificial joint is inserted, your own bone grows into the prosthesis to hold it in place. Where necessary, a hybrid operation is possible, in which just one of the components – either the ball or socket – is cemented in place while the other part remains cementless.

Part VI

Appendixes

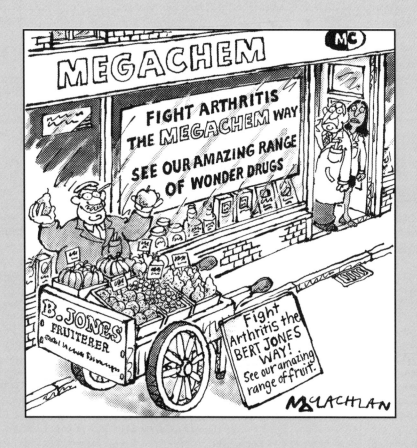

In this part . . .

*I*n Appendix A, we give you a glossary that defines the most frequently used terms relating to arthritis. You'll probably encounter these terms as you read and talk to others about arthritis.

Appendix B is a list of resources — associations where you can find a practitioner, get more information, find support groups, and more. A lot of good, free information can be found on the Internet as well, so we've listed Web sites whenever possible.

And in Appendix C, we tell you how to take stress off your joints by reaching and maintaining a healthy weight.

Appendix A

Glossary

Acupressure (shiatsu): A Japanese form of massage that aims to restore health by normalising the flow of energy in the body.

Acupuncture: A part of traditional Chinese medicine that uses the insertion of very fine needles to help balance the flow of energy in the body.

Acute pain: Pain that typically strikes severely and suddenly, builds, and then fades away. It occurs in response to injury, inflammation, surgery, and so on, and usually doesn't last long.

Alternative medicine: Healing techniques that fall outside of the realm of conventional, Western medicine.

Analgesics: Drugs that fight pain but don't interfere with the inflammation process (in cases where pain is experienced but without heat, redness and swelling as with osteoarthritis or fibromyalgia). A common painkiller is paracetamol.

Ankylosing spondylitis (AS): A disease that causes inflammation and stiffness of the spine and its joints, also resulting in the fusing or 'locking' of those joints.

Antibiotics: A class of drugs that either kills bacteria outright, or which disables them so your immune system can finish them off. The symptoms of Lyme disease and gonorrhoea are commonly treated with these drugs.

Antioxidants: Substances manufactured in the body and found in foods and supplements that help control the oxidation and free-radical activity that can damage body tissue and cause or worsen certain disease states.

Aromatherapy: A complementary healing system based on the belief that inhaling certain aromas or scents can help the body to heal itself.

Arthritis: A group of diseases (formerly called rheumatism) that strikes the joints and/or nearby tissues. The word arthritis means *joint inflammation*, although not all forms of arthritis cause inflammation.

Arthrodesis: Surgically immobilising a joint so that the bones grow together and 'lock' into position. This procedure is sometimes performed in cases of rheumatoid arthritis.

Arthroplasty: Surgical reconstruction of a joint using a combination of natural tissues and artificial parts; most commonly performed on the hip and knee.

Arthroscopy: Visual examination of the inside of a joint performed using a special scope that is passed through a small incision. Arthroscopy is used to diagnose certain types of joint disease and, in some cases, make repairs surgically.

Autologous chondrocyte implantation: The transplantation of healthy cartilage cells from a normal joint to a damaged one, so they can grow and supplement or replace ailing cartilage.

Ayurvedic healing: An ancient Indian healing art that uses diet, exercise, internal cleansing, herbs, massage, crystals, aromatherapy, colour therapy, gems, and other modalities to eliminate illness and restore balance to the body.

Bee venom therapy: The use of bee venom to relieve pain and inflammation. Although the venom is traditionally delivered via the sting of a live bee, or through an injection, it is now more commonly used in the form of a cream.

Biofeedback: A method for mastering how to exert some control over certain physiological functions, such as muscle tension or blood pressure. During a biofeedback session, you're hooked up to a machine that provides audio and visual feedback as, for example, muscle tension increases or decreases. Feedback from the machines shows you how certain body functions change as you relax.

Biologic response modifiers (BRMs): Also referred to as *cytokine inhibitors,* this new class of drugs is effective in reducing stubborn inflammation in rheumatoid arthritis, ankylosing spondylitis, and psoriatic arthritis.

Biomechanics: In a non-technical sense, it is the study of the way the body deals with its own weight – for example, the impact of walking or running on the weight-bearing joints. Using proper biomechanical techniques, you can greatly minimise the stress placed on the joints while moving, lifting, or even sitting.

Blahs: Generally feeling under-the-weather, off colour, and down-right yucky.

Borrelia burgdorferi: The bacteria that causes Lyme disease, transmitted to humans in bites from infected ticks.

Bursitis: A painful condition resulting from inflammation of the bursae, the fluid-filled pouches that keep certain joints moving smoothly. Shoulder joints are likely targets for bursitis.

Calcium pyrophosphate dihydrate crystals: Crystals that can accumulate in a joint and cause the symptoms of pseudogout.

Capsaicin: The hot part of chilli peppers. Capsaicin fights pain as it stimulates nerve cells to release large amounts of substance P, which sensitises the receptors that originate the pain signals. When cells run out of substance P, pain signals subside.

Carpal tunnel syndrome: A condition due to pressure on the median nerve as it runs through the *carpal tunnel,* a narrow opening between the ligaments and bones in the wrist. Symptoms include pain, weakness, tingling, burning, and muscle wasting (atrophy).

Cartilage: Connective tissue found in the joints and elsewhere in the body. Joint cartilage helps protect bone ends that would otherwise rub against each other and produce pain and other problems.

Chiropractic: A healing system based on the belief that disease arises when spinal vertebrae are out of alignment and press on nerves. Chiropractic healing techniques include spinal manipulation and possibly exercise, nutrition, massage, and other modalities.

Chondroitin sulphate: A supplement that, studies suggest, can relieve symptoms of osteoarthritis. Often used in conjunction with glucosamine, chondroitin sulphate helps pull water into the cartilage and fights the cartilage-eating enzymes that damage this precious tissue.

Chronic pain: Pain that lasts weeks or months, that accompanies long-term disease, or that keeps recurring. It may continue long after the apparent cause has disappeared, and can significantly reduce the quality of life.

Cognitive behavioural therapy (CBT): A form of psychotherapy that helps you discover how certain thinking patterns can exacerbate your problems, coaching you how to change your habitual reactions to these problems.

Complementary medicine: Non-standard, alternative healing approaches designed to work together with conventional, Western medicine.

Corticosteroids: A group of hormones naturally produced in the body that have wide ranging effects on metabolism, water balance, and organ function. Synthetic versions have powerful anti-inflammatory properties but also have some serious side effects.

COX-2 inhibitors: A relatively new form of NSAID with the same pain-relieving and anti-inflammatory benefits as other NSAIDs, but with less irritant effects on the stomach lining.

Deep tissue massage: The application of strong pressure to the muscles using fingers, hands, or elbows to relieve chronic tension in the muscles.

Dermatomyositis: A disease that produces muscle pain plus skin rashes and other problems.

Discoid lupus erythematosus: A form of lupus that may produce a rash and other skin problems, weakening of the immune system, and other symptoms, but that isn't as severe as systemic lupus erythematosus.

DMARDs: Disease-modifying antirheumatic drugs used for rheumatoid arthritis, psoriatic arthritis, and other forms of the disease. DMARDs appear to alter the behaviour of the immune system.

Fibromyalgia: A disease associated with inflammation of connective tissues, including the ligaments, tendons, and muscles. Symptoms include chronic achy pain, stiffness, disturbed sleep, depression, and fatigue.

Glucosamine: A supplement that studies suggest can relieve symptoms of osteoarthritis. Often used in conjunction with chondroitin sulphate, glucosamine is used in the body to manufacture proteoglycans, which draw water into the cartilage and keep it moist.

Gonococcal arthritis: The most common form of infectious arthritis; due to the *gonococci* bacterium that causes gonorrhoea.

Gout: A type of arthritis due to an accumulation of uric acid crystals in the joint, often the bunion joint of the large toe. Symptoms of gout include terrible pain, joint stiffness and swelling, and possibly fever, chills, and an elevated heart rate.

Herbalism: The use of the roots, bark, stems, flowers, or other parts of selected plants to relieve the symptoms of illness and/or strengthen the body.

Holistic medicine: An approach to healing and health based on treating a patient's mind, body, and spirit, rather than simply trying to counteract the disease or relieve symptoms.

Homoeopathy: An alternative-healing system developed in the 18th century, based on the belief that 'like cures like'. Thus, for example, patients suffering from nausea are treated with very small doses of a substance that can cause nausea when given in large amounts to healthy people.

Hydrotherapy: The use of water, both hot and cold or in the form of steam, ice, compresses, and so on to relieve symptoms and help the body heal itself.

Immunosuppressants: Drugs that dampen the immune system. These are used to treat rheumatoid arthritis, lupus, and other diseases in which the immune system is malfunctioning.

Infectious arthritis: Arthritis due to the invasion of bacteria, viruses, or fungi.

Joint: The place where two bones meet. Joints are either moveable or fixed. There are gliding joints such as the spinal vertebrae, hinge joints such as the elbows, saddle joints such as the wrist, and ball-and-socket joints such as the hip.

Juvenile rheumatoid arthritis (JRA): The most common form of arthritis to strike children, producing pain or swelling in the joints, fever, anaemia, and other symptoms.

Lyme disease: A disease due to the *Borrelia burgdorferi* bacteria, which is transmitted to humans through the bite of an infected tick. Lyme disease can produce a large bull's-eye-shaped rash at the bite site, swelling and pain in the joints, fever, fatigue, muscle aches, nausea, swollen lymph nodes, and other symptoms.

Mediterranean diet: The standard diet consumed in the Mediterranean areas of Greece, Italy, southern France, and parts of Spain, made up of plenty of fresh vegetables, fruit, whole-grain breads, pasta and cereal, nuts and legumes, plus good amounts of olive oil. This diet may help ease RA-related pain and swelling.

MSM (methyl-sulphonyl-methane): An anti-inflammatory supplement that's used to help treat arthritis.

Naturopathy: A healing art based on the belief that all diseases have natural causes and that the body has very strong, natural healing powers. Naturopathic physicians use diet, herbs, exercise, stress reduction, acupressure, and other modalities to help increase the body's healing prowess.

NSAIDs: Non-steroidal anti-inflammatory medications designed to reduce pain and inflammation, often prescribed for various forms of arthritis.

Occupational therapist (OT): A licensed professional who can help you cope with the day-to-day problems of living with arthritis (and other ailments) through finding easier ways for you to accomplish tasks, designing splints, recommending assistive devices, teaching you ways to protect your joints, and so on.

Omega-3 fatty acids: Sometimes called fish oils because their major source is certain types of fish, these substances can help reduce inflammation and other symptoms of rheumatoid arthritis, and possibly other forms of arthritis.

Omega-6 fatty acids: Found primarily in salad or cooking oils, these fatty acids can increase the inflammatory response. The exception is an omega-6 called gamma-linolenic acid (GLA), which helps calm inflammation. GLA is found in evening primrose oil, as well as blackcurrant-seed oil and borage-seed oil.

Orthopaedist – sometimes shortened to Orthopod: A medical doctor specialising in orthopaedics, who diagnoses and treats problems of the bones, joints, muscles, and related tissues.

Osteoarthritis (OA): A type of arthritis linked with the breakdown of cartilage, most often in the hips, knees, and other weight-bearing joints. Osteoarthritis is due to injury, obesity, metabolic errors, heredity, or other factors.

Osteotomy: A surgical procedure during which a piece of bone is removed to improve joint alignment. It is sometimes used to treat osteoarthritis or ankylosing spondylitis.

Paget's disease: A disease in which the body inappropriately breaks down and rebuilds bone, resulting in weaker bones, bone deformity, and other problems. Many people with Paget's disease are middle aged or older.

Pharmacogenomics: A rapidly evolving new branch of genetic science that studies the response of individuals to therapeutic drugs.

Physiotherapy: The use of massage, exercise, hydrotherapy, electrical stimulation, and other modalities to help relieve pain, increase range of motion, strengthen muscles, and stimulate healing.

Polarity therapy: An alternative-healing art based on the idea that the body contains energy systems that must remain in balance. Polarity therapists attempt to find and release energy blockages through touching specific points on the body, and sometimes using gentle massage.

Polymyalgia rheumatica (PMR): A rheumatic condition associated with severe, sudden stiffness in major joints, plus headaches, difficulty swallowing, coughing, and other symptoms.

Polymyositis: A disease that produces inflammation of the muscles and loss of strength. There is often, also, joint pain, weight loss, Raynaud's phenomenon, and other symptoms. Polymyositis is like dermatomyositis, without the skin problems.

Pseudogout: A form of arthritis similar to gout, but due to the accumulation of calcium pyrophosphate dihydrate (rather than uric acid) crystals in the affected joint.

Psoriatic arthropathy: Striking about five per cent of those who have the skin condition known as psoriasis, psoriatic arthritis causes inflammation, swelling, and sometimes joint deformity.

Raynaud's phenomenon: A disease in which arterial spasms cause pain, burning, tingling, numbness, and/or discolouration, primarily in the fingers and toes. Raynaud's disease is a more common and often milder form. Raynaud's phenomenon accompanies another ailment, such as lupus or scleroderma.

Reactive arthritis: A disease that may develop after an infection, reactive arthritis can produce mild-to-severe pain in the joints, inflammation of the eyelid, eyeball, and urethra, and other problems.

Reflexology: An alternative healing system based on the idea that specific areas of the feet and palms are linked to parts of the body. Manipulating the point on the foot corresponding to the lungs, for example, is believed to help relieve some of the symptoms of asthma.

Reiki: A Japanese healing art in which the practitioner channels energy into the patient through laying his hands lightly on or directly above the patient's body to help restore the body's flow and balance of energy.

Reiter's syndrome: An immune reaction to *Chlamydia,* very often causing arthritis in young men, and also develops following food poisoning such as Salmonella. Eight out of ten people affected with Reiter's syndrome have the HLA-B27 gene.

Rheumatoid arthritis (RA): The second most-common form of arthritis, rheumatoid arthritis is brought about when the immune system attacks the body. The result is joint pain and inflammation, generalised soreness and stiffness, fever, difficulty sleeping, and joint deterioration. The disease can also attack the lungs, blood vessels, and other parts of the body.

Rheumatoid factor (RF): An antibody found in some 80 per cent of those with rheumatoid arthritis. Its presence strongly suggests that one has rheumatoid arthritis, although it's possible to have RF and not develop the disease.

Scleroderma: An autoimmune disease in which the body produces and stores excess collagen, resulting in damage to the skin, joint pain and swelling, difficulty swallowing, digestive difficulties, injury to the blood vessels, and damaged organs.

Sjögren's syndrome: A disease that produces dryness of the eyes and mouth and certain other parts of the body. Depending on the extent of the dryness and which parts of the body are affected, problems can range from the manageable to the very serious. A fair number of those with Sjögren's syndrome also develop arthritis, but this arthritis is most often a separate entity.

Soft tissue rheumatism: An old term indicating inflammation or pain in the bursae, tendons, ligaments, and other tissues surrounding and/or supporting the joints. Carpal tunnel syndrome is an example of soft tissue rheumatism.

Swedish massage: The gentle kneading and stroking of muscles, connective tissue, and skin to relieve stress and soothe pained muscles.

Synovectomy: A surgery in which an overgrown, inflamed joint lining is removed; it's performed mainly for rheumatoid arthritis.

Synovial membrane: Part of the capsule surrounding certain joints, this membrane releases a lubricating fluid into the joint.

Systemic lupus erythematosus: An autoimmune disease that tends to attack women of childbearing age. Systemic lupus erythematosus (SLE) can cause a variety of symptoms, including joint pain and inflammation, fever, rash, hair loss, anaemia, weakness of the immune system, depression, and nervous system disorders.

Tendonitis: Inflammation of a tendon, associated with pain to the touch or upon movement. The upper arms, hands, fingers, and backs of the ankles are common targets of tendonitis.

TENS: Transcutaneous electrical nerve stimulation – the use of mild electrical currents to deliver small jolts to painful areas of the body. The electricity overrides pain signals.

Trigger finger: The locking of a finger in a bent position due to swelling and inflammation of a tendon.

Trigger-point therapy: Prolonged, deep tissue pressure applied to specific, tender and hard points on muscles to relieve tension and pain. The therapy may include injections of local anaesthetic into trigger points.

Tumour necrosis factor (TNF): When overproduced by the body, causes the severe inflammation and tissue damage often associated with autoimmune diseases like RA. A special subgroup of the BRMs, called the 'anti-TNF' drugs, can help to calm inflammation and protect tissue.

Urethritis: An inflammation of the *urethra*, which is the tube urine passes through to get from the bladder to the outside of the body.

Uric acid crystals: The offending agents in gout that accumulate in the joint, causing pain and other symptoms.

Vasodilators: Medications that relax blood vessels and help blood flow more freely.

Appendix B

Resources

• •

Organisations

Acupuncture/Acupressure

British Acupuncture Council: 63 Jeddo Road, London W12 9HQ; phone 0208-7350400; Web site www.acupuncture.org.uk.

British Medical Acupuncture Society: BMAS House, 3 Winnington Court, Northwich, Cheshire CW8 1AQ; phone 01606-786782; Web site www.medical-acupuncture.co.uk.

Alexander Technique

Society of Teachers of the Alexander Technique: 1st Floor, Linton House, 39–51 Highgate Road, London NW5 1RS; phone 0845-2307828; Web site www.stat.org.uk.

Alternative and Complementary Medicine

British Complementary Medicine Association: PO Box 5122, Bournemouth, Dorset BH8 0WG; phone 0845-3455977; Web site www.bcma.co.uk.

British Holistic Medical Association: 59 Lansdowne Place, Hove, East Sussex BN3 1FL; phone 01273-725951; Web site www.bhma.org.

Complementary Medical Association: Web site www.newcma.co.uk.

Institute for Complementary Medicine: PO Box 194, London SE16 7QZ; phone 020-72375165; Web site www.i-c-m.org.uk.

Aromatherapy

International Federation of Professional Aromatherapists: 82 Ashby Road, Hinckley, Leicestershire LE10 1SN; phone 01455-637987; Web site www.ifparoma.org.

Arthritis Information and Management

Arthritic Association: One Upperton Gardens, Eastbourne, East Sussex BN21 2AA; Freefone 0800-6523188; Web site www.arthriticassociation.org.uk.

Arthritis Care: 18 Stephenson Way, London NW1 2HD; Freefone: 0808-8004050; Web site www.arthritiscare.org.uk.

Arthritis Research Campaign: Copeman House, St Mary's Court, St Mary's Gate, Chesterfield, Derbyshire S41 7TD; phone 0870-8505000; Web site www.arc.org.uk.

BackCare – The charity for healthier backs: 16 Elmtree Road, Teddington, Middlesex TW11 8ST; phone 020-89775474; Web site www.backcare.org.uk.

British Sjogren's Syndrome Association: PO Box 10867, Birmingham B16 02W; phone 0121-4556549; Web site www.bssa.uk.net.

British Society for Rheumatology: Bride House, 18–20 Bride Lane, London EC4Y 8EE; phone 0207-8420900; Web site www.rheumatology.org.uk.

Children's Chronic Arthritis Association: Ground Floor, Amber Gate, City Wall Road, Worcester WR1 2AH; phone 01905-745595; Web site www.ccaa.org.uk.

Fibromyalgia Association UK: PO Box 206, Stourbridge, Shropshire DY9 8YL; phone 0870-2201232; Web site www.fibromyalgia-associationuk.org.

Horder Centre for Arthritis: St Johns Road, Crowborough, East Sussex TN6 1XP; phone 01892-665577; Web site www.hordercentre.co.uk.

Lupus UK: St James House, Eastern Road, Romford, Essex RM1 3NH; phone 01708-731252; Web site www.lupusuk.com.

Lyme Disease Action: Web site www.lymediseaseaction.org.uk.

Myositis Support Group: 146 Newtown Road, Woolston, Southampton, Hampshire SO19 9HR; phone 023-80449708; Web site www.myositis.org.uk.

National Ankylosing Spondylitis Society: PO Box 179, Mayfield, East Sussex TN20 6ZL; phone 01435-873527; Web site www.nass.co.uk.

National Association for the Relief of Paget's Disease: 323 Manchester Road, Walkden, Worsley, Manchester M28 3HH; phone 0161-7994646; Web site www.paget.org.uk.

Psoriatic Arthropathy Alliance: PO Box 111, St Albans, Hertfordshire AL2 3JQ; phone 0870-7703212; Web site www.paalliance.org.

Raynaud's and Scleroderma Association: 112 Crewe Road, Alsager, Cheshire ST7 2JA; phone 0800-9172494; Web site www.raynauds.org.uk.

Chiropractic

British Chiropractic Association: Blagrave House, 17 Blagrave Street, Reading, Berkshire RG1 1QB; phone 0118-9505950; Web site www.chiropractic-uk.co.uk.

Chiropractic Patients' Association: 8 Centre One, Lysander Way, Old Sarum Park, Salisbury, Wiltshire SP4 6BU; phone 01722-415027; Web site www.chiropatients.org.uk.

General Chiropractic Council: 344–354 Gray's Inn Road, London WC1X 8BP; phone 020-77135155; Web site www.gcc-uk.org.

McTimoney Chiropractic Association: 21 High Street, Eynsham, Oxon OX29 4HE; phone 01865-880974; Web site www.mctimoney-chiropractic.org.

Disability and Assistive Information

The Disability Information Services Web site, www.diss.org.uk, from the Queen Elizabeth Foundation, provides links to a number of organisations that can provide information on a range of topics, including benefits, mobility, self-help groups, disability rights, and assistive devices.

Feldenkrais Method

Feldenkrais Guild UK: phone 07000-785506; Web site www.feldenkrais.co.uk.

Help for Caregivers

Assisted Living Foundation: c/o 86 Hale Drive, Mill Hill, London NW7 3ED; phone 0208-9596474; Web site www.assistedliving.org.uk.

Carers Federation Ltd: 1 Beech Avenue, Sherwood Rise, Nottingham NG7 7LJ; phone 0115-9858485; Web site www.carersfederation.co.uk.

Carers UK: 20–25 Glasshouse Yard, London EC1A 4JT; phone 0207-4908818; Web site www.carersuk.org.

Crossroads Association: 10 Regent Place, Rugby, Warwickshire CV21 2PN; phone 0845-4500350; Web site www.crossroads.org.uk.

Princess Royal Trust for Carers: 142 Minories, London EC3N 1LB; phone 0207-4807788; Web site www.carers.org.

Herbalism

National Institute of Medical Herbalists: Elm House, 54 Mary Arches Street, Exeter EX4 3BA; phone 01392-426022; Web site www.nimh.org.uk.

Homeopathic Medicine

British Homeopathic Association: Hahnemann House, 29 Park Street West, Luton, Bedfordshire LU1 3BE; phone 0870-4443950; Web site www.trusthomeopathy.org.

Hypnotherapists

Association for Professional Hypnosis and Psychotherapy: 15 Clarence Road, Southend on Sea, Essex SS1 1AN; phone 01702-347691; Web site www.aphp.co.uk.

National Council for Hypnotherapy: PO Box 421, Charwelton, Daventry, Northamptonshire NN11 1AS; phone 0800-9520545; Web site www.hypnotherapists.org.uk.

Massage Therapists

General Council for Massage Therapy: Whiteway House, Blundells Lane, Rainhill, Prescot, Merseyside L35 6NB; phone 0151-4308199; Web site www.gcmt.org.uk.

Medical Societies

General Medical Council: Regent's Place, 350 Euston Road, London NW1 3JN; phone 0845-3573456; Web site www.gmc-uk.org.

Naturopathic Medicine

General Council and Register of Naturopaths: 2 Goswell Road, Street, Avon BA16 0JG; phone 08707-456984; Web site www.naturopathy.org.uk.

Nutritional Counselling

The term *nutritionist* is not protected by the Health Professionals' Council and anyone, regardless of qualifications and experience, can call themselves a nutritionist. Some nutritionists are registered dietitians or medical doctors. Some sound as if they are doctors, but have a PhD rather than a medical qualification.

The Nutrition Society is the main professional organisation for nutritionists in the UK. To register with them, a nutritionist needs to have a minimum of three years' relevant postgraduate work experience in nutrition and must hold a university degree in nutrition (a minimum of three years' full-time study) or a closely related subject such as nutrition or food science.

To find a registered nutritionist, visit the Nutrition Society Web site (www.nutritionsociety.org.uk/membership/register/) or send an A4 stamped envelope (60p for first class, 46p second class) to:

Nutrition Society: 10 Cambridge Court, 210 Shepherds Bush Road, London W6 7NJ; phone 020-76020228.

You can contact a registered dietitian via your local hospital or GP surgery. For details of registered dietitians working in private practice, e-mail the British Dietetic Association at info@bda.uk.com or send a stamped, addressed envelope to: **British Dietetic Association:** Private Practice, 5th Floor, Charles House, 148/9 Great Charles Street, Queensway, Birmingham B3 3HT; phone 0121-2008080.

A list of dietitians is also available at the Dietitians Unlimited Web site (www.dietitiansunlimited.co.uk).

British Association of Nutritional Therapists: 27 Old Gloucester Street, London WC1N 3XX; phone 08706-061284; Web site www.bant.org.uk.

BANT is a professional body that holds a register of nutritional therapists who are fully qualified in both the science of nutrition and its clinical practice.

British Society for Ecological Medicine – formerly the British Society for Allergy, Environmental and Nutritional Medicine: PO Box 7, Knighton, Leicestershire LD7 1WT; phone 0906-3020010; Web site www.bsaenm.org.

A professional body that provides support and contact for doctors who use the insights of allergy, environmental, and nutritional medicine to help patients get well and maintain wellbeing. Members are all medically qualified nutritional specialists.

Institute of Optimum Nutrition (ION): 13 Blades Court, Deodar Road, Putney, London SW15 2NU; phone 020-88779993 or 0870-9791122; Web site www.ion.ac.uk.

ION is an independent educational trust that runs training courses for nutritionists, as well as home-study courses for the general public. A register of therapists seeing clients is available on the Web site. Some members are also BANT registered.

Osteopathy

General Osteopathic Council: Osteopathy House, 176 Tower Bridge Road, London SE1 3LU; phone 0207-3576655; Web site www.osteopathy.org.uk.

Pain Management

British Pain Society: 21 Portland Place, London W1B 1PY; phone 0207-6318870; Web site www.britishpainsociety.org.

Pain Relief Foundation: Clinical Sciences Centre, University Hospital, Aintree, Lower Lane, Liverpool, Merseyside L9 7AL; phone 0151-5295820; Web site www.painrelieffoundation.org.uk.

Polarity Therapy

UK Polarity Therapy Association: Monomark House, 27 Old Gloucester Street, London WC1N 3XX; phone 0700-7052748; Web site www.ukpta.org.uk.

Psychotherapy

Association for Professional Hypnosis and Psychotherapy: 15 Clarence Road, Southend on Sea, Essex SS1 1AN; phone 01702-347691; Web site www.aphp.co.uk.

Reflexology

Association of Reflexologists: 27 Old Gloucester Street, London WC1N 3XX; phone 0870-5673320; Web site www.aor.org.uk.

Reiki

UK Reiki Federation: PO Box 1785, Andover, Hampshire SP11 0WB; phone 01264-773774; Web site www.reikifed.co.uk.

The Trager Approach

Trager UK: Web site www.trager.co.uk.

Information Sheets from Arthritis Care

Arthritis Care produces a range of publications to meet the needs of people with arthritis. Many booklets are downloadable from their Web site www.arthritiscare.org.uk and include:

A Day with Sam

Arthritis Care: What We Can Do for You

Arthritis Care: Making a Difference

The Balanced Approach

Benefits for Beginners

Chat – A Guide for Parents

Chat 2 Parents – Arthritis in Teenagers

Chat 2 Teachers

Fit for Life

Food for Thought

Information for People with Arthritis

Osteoarthritis – A Guide

Our Feelings, Our Emotions

Our Relationships, Our Sexuality

Reaching Independence

Rheumatoid Arthritis – A Guide

Surgery

Talk about Pain

Working Horizons

You can also obtain publications by contacting Arthritis Care at 18 Stephenson Way, London NW1 2HD. For a free copy of *Arthritis News* magazine, phone 0845-6006868.

Appendix C

Weight Loss and Management Guide

*E*ven if you're eating a balanced diet, getting plenty of omega-3s, and avoiding danger foods, you still need to take one more step – the one that puts you up on the bathroom scales. And if what you see on the dial doesn't look good, you know what you need to do!

One of the best things for those aching joints if you're overweight or obese is to lose weight. Cutting away the extra pounds takes a tremendous burden off your joints, especially those bearing your weight such as your hips and knees. Not only does it take the pressure off, but strong evidence suggests that dropping down to your ideal weight can even stave off at least one form of arthritis.

When researchers in the Framingham Study used X-rays to track the development of arthritis, they found that, in overweight women of normal height, every 11 pounds (5 kilograms) of weight loss reduces the risk of knee osteoarthritis (OA) by 50 per cent. Similar findings in another study agree that older and overweight women can significantly lower their risk of developing knee osteoarthritis just through reducing their weight.

Figuring Out Whether You're Too Heavy

Medical experts agree that slimness is better for health, especially where arthritis is concerned. But what's slim? Unfortunately, no one is good at knowing when enough is enough as, in general, women tend to think they're too heavy, and men usually assume they're doing okay – whatever their weight!

For years, people looked at height–weight charts to see if they should drop a few pounds, but these charts are only rough guidelines. Modern guidelines use the *body mass index (BMI)* as a more accurate way of defining the ideal weight for your height. Now you just look for one number, your BMI, to see how you're doing in the weight stakes.

The formula for determining BMI is simple: Divide your weight in kilograms by your height in metres squared. The formula follows:

BMI = Weight (Kg)/Height × Height (M2)

This calculation produces a number interpreted in Table C-1, which is based on World Health Organisation (1998) guidelines.

Table C-1	Interpreting BMI Measures
BMI	*Weight Band*
≤ 18.5	Underweight
18.5 – 24.9	Healthy range
25 – 29.9	Overweight
30 – 39.9	Obese
≥ 40	Extremely obese

So you ideally want your BMI to be no more than 25, and certainly less than 30.

Well, maybe working out your ideal weight is not that simple. Luckily, Table C-2 helps you skip the maths and gain a good idea of whether or not you're in the healthy weight range for your height.

Table C-2	Body Mass Index Chart	
Height	*Optimum Healthy Weight Range based on BMI range of 18.5 – 24.9*	
Metres/ Feet	*Kilograms*	*Stones*
1.47/4'10"	40.0 – 53.8	6st 4 – 8st 7
1.50/4'11"	41.6 – 56.0	6st 8 – 8st 11
1.52/5'	42.7 – 57.5	6st 10 – 9st 1
1.55/5'1"	44.5 – 59.8	7st – 9st 7
1.57/5'2"	45.6 – 61.4	7st 2 – 9st 9
1.60/5'3"	47.4 – 63.8	7st 6 – 10st
1.63/5'4"	49.2 – 66.2	7st 10 – 10st 6
1.65/5'5"	50.4 – 67.8	7st 13 – 10st 9

Height	Optimum Healthy Weight Range based on BMI range of 18.5 – 24.9	
Metres/ Feet	Kilograms	Stones
1.68/5'6"	52.2 – 70.3	8st 3 – 11st
1.70/5'7"	53.5 – 72.0	8st 6 – 11st 4
1.73/5'8"	55.4 – 74.5	8st 10 – 11st 10
1.75/5'9"	56.7 – 76.3	8st 13 – 11st 13
1.78/5'10"	58.6 – 78.9	9st 3 – 12st 6
1.80/5'11"	59.9 – 80.7	9st 6 – 12st 10
1.83/6'	62.0 – 83.4	9st 11 – 13st 1
1.85/6'1"	63.3 – 85.2	9st 13 – 13st 5
1.88/6'2"	65.4 – 88.0	10st 4 – 13st 12
1.90/6'3"	66.8 – 89.9	10st 7 –14st 2
1.93/6'4"	68.9 – 92.8	10st 11 – 14st 8

The BMI isn't an absolutely perfect guide to weight. The calculation only compares height to weight; it doesn't take into account that fact that some people appear 'fatter' and get higher BMIs because they have lots of muscle. For other people, the reverse is sometimes true because they don't have much muscle. Still, the BMI is a good starting point.

Losing Weight the Safe and Healthy Way

If you're overweight, the bad news is: No quick, simple, guaranteed way to lose weight exists. The gimmicks don't work, and the fad diets don't live up to their promises. Oh yes, you can lose weight on most fad diets, primarily because they all get you to restrict your intake one way or another. And many of them cause you to lose lots of water weight quickly. But most people just as quickly gain back all the water weight – and all the other weight as well. The overwhelming majority of people who lose pounds on fad diets gain them back – plus a few more. And to make matters worse, a fair number of fad diets are nutritionally unbalanced: Eating what these diets recommend for long periods of time can lead to trouble.

However, good news also exists: You *can* lose weight *without* sacrificing nutrition or health. We can't go into great detail on losing weight, because this isn't a diet book. Fortunately, many books present safe, sensible, and effective diets, including *Dieting For Dummies* by Jane Kirby (Wiley).

Most people already know how to lose weight. Notwithstanding the hype in the fad diet books, the basic principles for healthy people are simple: Eat a well-rounded diet emphasising fresh vegetables, whole-grains, and fruit; keep your fat content down to reasonable levels; enjoy sweets as occasional treats; and burn lots of calories through physical activity and exercise. In short, burn more calories than you take in.

Aiming for long-term benefits

Don't diet. *Dieting* is a bad word, because it means giving up favourite foods and eating a lot of stuff you don't like or starving yourself. Dieting is a short-term fix that's usually discarded as soon as possible.

Instead, eat for lifelong good health. Focus on the slow, steady, and permanent weight loss that comes when your diet and activity/exercise habits are in alignment.

Eating fruits and vegetables

Eat a variety of vegetables, fruits, and whole-grains to ensure that you get all the numerous nutrients in foods. No single food or food group gives you all you need, for there's no such thing as a magic food. Eat fewer meat, poultry, and dairy products, but when you do, eat many different kinds.

Limiting your intake of certain foods

Take it easy on cholesterol, saturated fat, sugar, and salt.

Eat sweets sparingly. Many people find that the more they cut back, the less they crave these foods. Don't look upon limiting your intake as depriving yourself: Just cut back a little bit at a time. Surprisingly, your desire for these foods falls off with your consumption.

Read the labels on tins and packages carefully. An amazing number of calories can squeeze into some foods you thought were fairly 'lite'.

Using psychological strategies

Put smaller portions on your plate – then you can clear your plate without stuffing yourself.

Avoid places and settings that normally trigger overeating. For example, if you always gobble down bowls of peanuts and olives when meeting your friends at a particular bar after work, try going somewhere else.

Don't shop when you're hungry, because the growl in your stomach tempts you to buy sweets and fattening foods.

Set a reasonable goal. Don't try to lose 30 pounds (14 kilograms) a month or squeeze into that teensy bikini next week. People who lose weight that fast usually put it back on almost as rapidly. If you stick to a good eating and exercise plan and only lose half a pound a week, you're doing well.

Don't be hard on yourself if you don't meet all your goals exactly on schedule. You're only human; you're allowed some leeway. And besides, you're eating for life; you're in it for the long haul. When you do something great, reward yourself with something other than food.

Understanding that losing weight is not just what you eat

Remember that what you do or do not eat is only half the equation. You must also burn up calories with physical activity and exercise.

Eat slowly. Your brain takes a while to catch up with what you're eating, so it's possible to eat more than you want or need to when you shovel it in. Take your time, and let your brain register the fact that you've eaten. You'll eat less that way.

'Pre-eat' a little bit of something before going to parties, the cinema, and other places where you can't get healthy food. If you eat a small portion of health-enhancing food before you go out, the temptation to overdo popcorn and chocolate after you're there is less. Instead, you can enjoy a little taste as a special treat.

Eyeballing those portions

Many diets suggest specific portion sizes, such as 100 grams (3½ ounces) of fish or 300 millilitres (about 10 fluid ounces) of milk. But because few of us carry little food scales around, we're often forced to estimate. Estimating by eye is difficult, as most people tend to underestimate the portion size of foods they enjoy eating and overestimate those they don't like (for example, 50 grams (just under 2 ounces) of ice cream looks like nothing, but 50g of Brussel sprouts looks far too much).

Table C-3 offers some tips for eyeballing food portion sizes. The tips are easy to remember, or if you like, you can cut the table out and carry it in your purse or wallet.

Table C-3	Visual Food Portion Guidelines
Quantity	*Visual Aid*
How big is a 3-ounce (85g) serving?	About the size of a deck of cards.
How much is 1 teaspoonful?	About the size of the tip of your thumb.
What's a normal serving of veggies, rice, pasta, or cereal?	Cooked, a mound about the same size as a small fist (or cricket ball).
How big is a small baked potato?	Roughly the size of a computer mouse.
What's a medium apple or orange?	One about the size of a cricket ball.
What's an ounce (28g) of cheese?	About the size of four dice.

Index

• C •

• N •

• R •

• S •

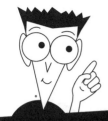

FOR DUMMIES

Do Anything. Just Add Dummies

UK editions

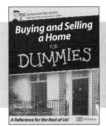

Buying and Selling a Home
0-7645-7027-7

Renting Out Your Property
0-7645-7016-1

DIY & Home Maintenance ALL-IN-ONE
0-7645-7054-4

PERSONAL FINANCE

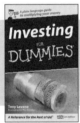 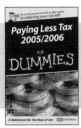 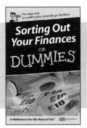

Investing
0-7645-7023-4

Paying Less Tax 2005/2006
0-7645-7053-6

Sorting Out Your Finances
0-7645-7039-0

BUSINESS

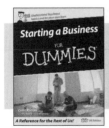 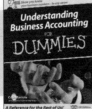 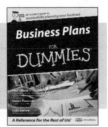

Starting a Business
0-7645-7018-8

Understanding Business Accounting
0-7645-7025-0

Business Plans
0-7645-7026-9

Other UK editions now available:

Answering Tough Interview Questions For Dummies
(0-470-01903-4)

Being The Best Man For Dummies
(0-470-02657-X)

British History For Dummies
(0-7645-7021-8)

Building Confidence For Dummies
(0-4700-1669-8)

Buying a Home On A Budget For Dummies
(0-7645-7035-8)

Cognitive Behavioural Therapy For Dummies
(0-470-01838-0)

Cleaning and Stain Removal For Dummies
(0-7645-7029-3)

CVs For Dummies
(0-7645-7017-X)

Detox For Dummies
(0-470-01908-5)

Diabetes For Dummies
(0-7645-7019-6)

Divorce For Dummies
(0-7645-7030-7)

eBay.co.uk For Dummies
(0-7645-7059-5)

European History For Dummies
(0-7645-7060-9)

Formula One Racing For Dummies
(0-7645-7015-3)

Gardening For Dummies
(0-470-01843-7)

Genealogy Online For Dummies
(0-7645-7061-7)

Golf For Dummies
(0-470-01811-9)

Irish History For Dummies
(0-7645-7040-4)

Kakuro For Dummies
(0-470-02822-X)

Marketing For Dummies
(0-7645-7056-0)

Neuro-Linguistic Programming For Dummies
(0-7645-7028-5)

Nutrition For Dummies
(0-7645-7058-7)

Pregnancy For Dummies
(0-7645-7042-0)

Retiring Wealthy For Dummies
(0-470-02632-4)

Rugby Union For Dummies
(0-7645-7020-X)

Small Business Employment Law For Dummies
(0-7645-7052-8)

Starting a Business on eBay.co.uk For Dummies
(0-470-02666-9)

Su Doku For Dummies
(0-4700-189-25)

Sudoku 2 For Dummies
(0-4700-2651-0)

Sudoku 3 For Dummies
(0-4700-2667-7)

The GL Diet For Dummies
(0-470-02753-3)

Wills, Probate and Inheritance Tax For Dummies
(0-7645-7055-2)

8185_p1

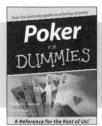
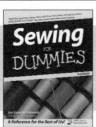
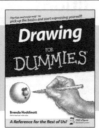
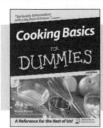
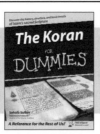
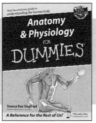
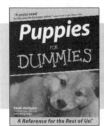
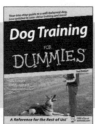
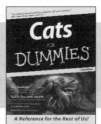